FROM SILENCE
TO VOICE

A VOLUME IN THE SERIES

The Culture and Politics of Health Care Work

Edited by Suzanne Gordon and Sioban Nelson

For a list of books in the series, visit our website at www.cornellpress.cornell.edu.

FROM SILENCE TO VOICE

What Nurses Know and Must Communicate to the Public

THIRD EDITION

Bernice Buresh

Suzanne Gordon

ILR Press

AN IMPRINT OF CORNELL UNIVERSITY PRESS

ITHACA AND LONDON

First published by Cornell University Press 2013
First printing, Cornell Paperbacks, 2013

Printed in the United States of America

Library of Congress Cataloging-in-Publication Data

Buresh, Bernice, 1941– author.
   From silence to voice : what nurses know and must communicate
to the public / Bernice Buresh and Suzanne Gordon. — Third edition.
      pages cm. — (The culture and politics of health care work)
   Includes bibliographical references and index.
   ISBN 978-0-8014-7873-4 (pbk. : alk. paper)
 1. Nursing. 2. Communication in nursing. 3. Mass media.
4. Public opinion. 5. Nursing—Social aspects. I. Gordon, Suzanne,
1945– author. II. Title. III. Series: Culture and politics of health
care work.
   RT42.B83   2013
   610.73—dc23   2012047182

Cornell University Press strives to use environmentally responsible
suppliers and materials to the fullest extent possible in the publishing
of its books. Such materials include vegetable-based, low-VOC inks
and acid-free papers that are recycled, totally chlorine-free, or partly
composed of nonwood fibers. For further information, visit our
website at www.cornellpress.cornell.edu.

Paperback printing   10 9 8 7 6 5 4 3 2 1

For our children

CONTENTS

Introduction   *1*

Part I   Silent No More

1   Ending the Silence   *13*

2   The Daisy Dilemma   *32*

3   From Virtue to the Voice of Agency   *67*

4   Presenting Yourself as a Nurse   *83*

5   Tell the World What You Do   *111*

6   Creating Anecdotes and Arguments   *129*

Part II   Communicating with the Media and the Public

7   How the News Media Work   *155*

8   Reaching Out to the Media   *174*

9   In Your Own Voice: Letters to the Editor, Op-Eds, and Blogs   *196*

10   Getting It Right   *225*

11   Appearing on Television and Radio   *243*

12   Opportunities and Challenges Ahead   *264*

Appendix: How We Came to Write This Book   *271*

Notes   *275*

Index   *287*

FROM SILENCE
TO VOICE

INTRODUCTION

We'd like to begin this new edition of *From Silence to Voice* with an exercise.

Imagine that you are at home and the phone rings. The caller from a research company tells you, "We're doing a survey about public attitudes toward nursing. Do you have time? It's really short. Only two questions."

Since it's about nurses you are eager to respond.

The pollster asks you question number one.

"Do you believe that the public trusts nurses as individuals and the nursing profession in general? Yes or no."

Question two. "Do you believe that most members of the public understand what nurses actually do? Yes or no."

If you're like virtually all the nurses we have talked to (and we have talked to thousands), you will have answered yes to the first question and no (unequivocally) to the second.

We have posed these questions to young and old nurses, to female and male nurses, to nurses of various races, nationalities, and ethnicities, and to nurses working in every area of the profession. We have presented these questions to groups of thirty, three hundred, and three thousand nurses at meetings and in hospitals and nursing schools in North America, the United Kingdom, Europe, Australia, New Zealand, Hong Kong, and Japan.

The response is always the same. When nurses are asked, "How many of you believe that the public trusts nurses?" virtually all the hands in the room go up. But when they are asked, "How many of you believe that most members of the public" ("and even many in the health care field," we sometimes add) "*understand* what nurses do?" few, if any, hands are raised.

The Trust Trap

Nursing organizations promote the fact that year after year nurses win top ranking in honesty and ethics surveys.[1] Nursing groups distribute these findings in news releases like one from the American Nurses Association headlined "Nurses Keep Top Spot for Honesty and Ethics in Poll Ranking Professions."[2]

It is wonderful that the public holds nurses in high esteem, but appreciation for nurses' honesty and ethics alone will not gain nurses the support that they need to do their work. Emphasizing trustworthiness and neglecting public understanding can lead to what we call a "trust trap." By winning the trustworthiness sweepstakes, nurses may be lulled into thinking they don't have to inform the public about what they actually do.

"People already trust us, don't they? So why do we have to talk about our work?" some nurses ask when we talk to them about moving from silence to voice.

The answer is that nurses need resources to do their work. Nursing is an organized institutional intervention, as Linda Aiken, a noted nurse researcher and authority on the consequences of nursing shortages, has pointed out. It depends on social and economic resources. To do their work, nurses need investments in education, research, equipment, technology, and most of all, appropriate staffing so that patients get the care they need. Today most members of the public do not fully understand the connection between nursing and quality patient care. As a result, nursing is under constant threat as hospitals and other health care institutions try to replace higher-paid, more educated professionals with cheaper lower-skilled staff.

Public ignorance of the importance of nursing work not only negatively affects nurses' practice and working conditions; it also influences societal beliefs about patient safety and care delivery. Consider the public discussion about medical errors and physician work hours. Ever since the Libby Zion case in New York City in 1984, there has been a robust debate about the hours worked by physicians in training. The preventable death of this young woman was linked to actions of residents who'd been literally up for days.[3]

It may have taken twenty years, but because of discussion and research about physician work hours, in 2003 the Accreditation Council of Graduate Medical Education mandated limiting residents' work to eighty hours a week with no more than twenty-four hours in a row along with more supervision by senior physicians.[4] Despite ongoing opposition from hospitals and many veteran physicians, the standard later was tweaked even more for first-year residents.

Still, the debate about resident hours continues. In an influential *New York Times Magazine* article, "The Phantom Menace of Sleep-Deprived Doctors," the writer and physician Darshak Sanghavi cited research that found no major improvement in patient safety after work-hour reforms were instituted. How could that be? Even researchers who had linked sleep-deprived residents with a high rate of medical errors were dumbfounded.[5]

What is dumbfounding is that anyone would imagine that changing one variable in a complex system like a hospital would have a revolutionary impact on patient safety. As Sanghavi explained, "Fixating on work hours has meant overlooking other issues, like lack of supervision or the failure to use more reliable computerized records. Worse still, the reforms may have created new, unexpected sources of mistakes."

He cited the work of the British psychologist James Reason, who asserted that medical systems are stacked like slices of Swiss cheese. There are holes in each system, but usually they don't overlap. "An exhausted intern writes the wrong dose of a drug, but an alert pharmacist or nurse catches the mistake," Sanghavi wrote. "Every now and then, however, all the holes align, leading to a patient's death or injury."[6]

Yet in his discussion of medical errors Sanghavi didn't take into account the working conditions of other hospital professionals. If he had been aware of nurses' escalating hours and, as researchers Alison M. Trinkoff and Jeanne Geiger-Brown have documented, their connection to medical errors and injuries, would he have written the same article?[7] If he had, would *Times* editors who had been aware of this problem have accepted his article without significant alterations? Or might they have insisted that the piece factor in, or at least mention, the workload and fatigue of nurses and other health care workers?

Because most health care writers and editors frame and anchor health care in a physician-centric manner—and because nurses have not altered that framework (except where emotional work is concerned)—discussions about the use of scarce health care resources have been shaped in a way that leaves nonphysician personnel out of the picture or assigned to a very narrow role within the system.

Whatever reservations people might have about physicians, the public clearly respects medicine as a profession and provides physicians with the lion's share of social resources—whether that be media attention, financial rewards, or control over their work, as well as control over the work of others in health care. This did not come about accidentally. It took many decades for medical doctors to consolidate their professional authority and convince the public that their medical services are indispensable.[8]

Nurses, as a group, do not enjoy this status. Rather than being defined by their own standards and practices, nurses are often described in comparison to physicians. A nurse who displays her intelligence and knowledge might receive the backhanded compliment "You're so smart, you could be a doctor." (Nurses who get PhDs in nursing are routinely asked why they don't just go to medical school.) Unlike individual physicians who, whether smart or not, benefit from the group's reputation for braininess, nurses, with their awards and rhetoric, tend to focus on the exceptional, or the exceptionally compassionate, to raise their status. While physicians solidify their profession by celebrating a legacy of medical knowledge and practice, nurses often try to elevate the modern nurse by denigrating the clinical competence of the "old nurse."[9] By embracing the traditional and highly gendered attributes of nursing while jettisoning nurses' cumulative knowledge and the realitics of patient care work, nurses may be communicating a muddled picture of what it is that nurses do and why health care's largest profession must be supported.

Frames and Anchors

In this third edition of *From Silence to Voice*, we use the twin concepts of framing and anchoring to analyze the ways that nurses and nursing groups describe nursing to the public.

Framing theory is derived from psychology and sociology. It is employed in media studies, and increasingly in analyses of political campaigns and voting patterns, to describe the mental filters we use to understand and respond to events. Framing is one of the ways our brains make sense of the world. According to the linguist George Lakoff, "People think in frames. . . . To be accepted, truth must fit people's frames. If the facts do not fit the frame, the frame stays and the facts bounce off."[10]

How nurses present themselves as professionals and how they explain their professional work has a bearing on how members of the public frame the practice of nursing. By the same token, how nurses are told they should act, behave, and present themselves to the world establishes a frame for them to understand their own work.

Framing effects play a role similar to *"anchoring effects."* Aptly named because it is hard to dislodge, an anchor is something—an idea, a price, a perception—that fixes a person's view of what that thing should be no matter what. As the cognitive psychologist Daniel Kahneman explains it, "an anchoring effect . . . occurs when people consider a particular value for an unknown quantity before estimating that quantity."[11] For example, you think something is worth ten dollars. That's your anchor. When someone tells you it's worth twenty dollars, you balk. This is why sellers try to establish an anchoring price as high as possible. The first figure that is named anchors the rest of the negotiation.

In what the great sociologist Erving Goffman calls "backstage" or "private spaces," nurses talk to one another about the realities of their work and the mastery of its technical, medical, pharmacological, and anatomical aspects. But when nurses engage in what Goffman calls "frontstage" presentations, they frame nursing in a discourse that casts kindness and compassion as almost innate attributes of the nurse, instead of as behaviors that depend on knowledge, judgment, and skill.[12] Because of complex history that we will explore further, nursing is often framed and thus anchored in a care narrative that suggests that nurses are valuable for their personal virtues alone—their trustworthiness, honesty, altruism, approachability, compassion, and, yes, niceness. This framework has led many nurses to present their work in particular ways and to view departures from this script as problematic. Reliance on this sentimentalized care narrative discourages the kind of critical thinking that would reveal its limitations as a vehicle for establishing the worth of nurses, supporting the practice of nursing, and helping the broad public understand why, as the Institute of Medicine has recently argued, nurses should have a greater role in shaping health care delivery.[13]

We are journalists, not nurses, but after decades of working with nurses and the media, we do not believe that promoting nursing on the basis of trust and care is sufficient. We are frequently asked what we think has changed in nurses' public communication since we wrote the first edition of *From Silence to Voice*. Certainly the scope of nursing education and practice has expanded, and that change is being communicated to the public through policy debates about primary care and other aspects of health care delivery. As we show in this book, there are many more nurse writers and communicators who are using their own voices and various media avenues to share many aspects of their practices with the public.

At the same time, in the United States at least, the defining of nursing for the public seems to have been outsourced to entities that have their own agendas. Johnson & Johnson's primacy as the go-to source for all manner of information on what it means to be a nurse comes to mind. Advertising circulars during Nurses Week supposedly aimed at "honoring" or "saluting" nurses solicit a kind of narrative from patients and colleagues that is heavy on compassion and weak on other factors. Even more remarkable is the growing number of chief nursing officers who are "partnering" with the DAISY Foundation to stage tearful Extraordinary Nurse Award ceremonies complete with marketing tie-ins to Cinnabon and Kleenex.

To a greater or lesser degree, these campaigns are communicating a feel-good message that may be more in the interest of the sponsors than of nurses. All claim to want to improve nurses' perceptions of themselves as nurses. Dealing with the working conditions or the lack of teamwork between health care professions and occupations—to name only a few critical issues in health care today—that so profoundly affect nurses' perceptions of their own value, however, is not their department.

These feel-good campaigns are missing the opportunity to connect with the important debates and discussions that are going on in health care. The national and international focus on patient safety, interprofessional education and practice, and evidence-based, quality care represents an opening that nurses can leverage to have a greater voice in their institutions and in the broader health care system. Physician advocates for patient safety such as Lucian Leape, Michael Leonard, and Michael Woods, among many others, are crisscrossing the globe and writing articles for major publications explaining why we need assertive nurses and why physicians should listen to them. When they talk with other MDs, these safety advocates explain that nurses have been ahead of the curve on safety practices. They encourage other physicians to stop barking out orders and to listen to nurses.

While these physicians are highlighting the potential of the assertive nurse as a leader in patient safety, the saccharinized care narrative avoids any references to nurses as the ones who, as the nursing theorist and educator Patricia Benner once put it, care enough to make sure that hospitals don't kill their patients. Sentimentalized awards encourage nurses to value themselves for such gestures as delivering a birthday cake or fruit plate to a patient, instead of for the professional acumen and caring that makes them an effective first line of defense against medical errors and injuries. The popularizing of a sugary care narrative threatens to deny nurses a leadership role in one of the most important movements in the history of health care delivery and to once again promote the illusion that nurses are followers, not leaders.

The truth is that promoting nurses' goodness is not going to redirect more health care resources toward nursing. Because the "virtue script,"[14] a descriptive term coined by Sioban Nelson and Suzanne Gordon, tends to dissociate and even trivialize the clinical knowledge and skill that it takes to be caring and compassionate with very sick individuals, it opens the door for nurse substitutes. It even undermines the necessity of nursing education by suggesting that clinical caring is not the product of instruction, learning, self-mastery, experience, expertise, and sometimes sheer grit, but instead "comes naturally," as a Johnson & Johnson nursing promotion puts it.

Nurses have told us that they fear that talking about their technical skills and medical knowledge somehow jeopardizes their reputation for caring and compassion. But parroting overly simplified slogans like "Doctors heal, nurses care," does little to define nursing and grants physicians credit for much of the work that gets reimbursed. Expressing horror—as nursing professors at one school did over a student nurse's anecdote describing how she prevented a vomiting patient from aspirating because it didn't highlight "holistic care"—reflects a perception within nursing that the public can't handle, or appreciate, the truth about nursing.

Reliance on a simplistic care narrative leads nurses to distort their own reality. Do many in nursing really feel that caring is exhibited only through talking, holding a patient's hand, giving a snack mix when someone is depressed, or rubbing a patient's back? Certainly in our assembly line–like health care system, niceness is very nice indeed. Shouldn't everyone be nice to sick people? But why isn't preventing someone from dying from an aspiration pneumonia conceptualized as an act of caring? Why isn't taking the time to wash your hands before you examine a patient an act of caring? Why isn't making sure that the proper OR equipment is available during surgery or that the team does debriefs and time-outs defined as an act of caring?

It is not only caring that is limited to a narrow register; so too is advocacy. Supporters of this care narrative argue that focusing on the conflicts and struggles that nurses engage in every day to advocate for their patients will inspire neither the public nor nurses themselves to have positive views of the profession. They seem to believe that a sugarcoated narrative is required for nurses to be appreciated (really almost to be loved) and to feel appreciated. In this narrative, nurses are rewarded for their heart work, not their brain work.

Holism Rather than Halfism

In this book we are arguing for communications that depict a holistic view of the profession by integrating the psychosocial/educational work of the nurse with the range of medical, technical, and even seemingly domestic activities involved in the hands-on care of patients.

The word *holistic* comes from the word *whole* (not *hole*). It is defined as "emphasizing the importance of the whole and the interdependence of its parts."[15] As you will see, as you move with us through an analysis of the images and words nurses often mobilize to describe their work and their profession, we usually get a "halfistic" picture of what it takes to be a nurse, to practice nursing, and to deal with the world in which nursing is practiced. That picture emphasizes the parts that doctors stereotypically don't do—caring, warmth, patient advocacy, compassion, and touch. (Although, as we will discover, with patient satisfaction assuming a larger role in reimbursement, hospital promotions are starting to laud physicians for their expertise *and* compassion.)

Echoing the kind of *Chicken Soup for the Nurse's Soul* construction of what nurses do, this halfistic narrative defines the role of the nurse as that of providing comfort, reassurance, prayer, spiritual succor, and even superstition. In this narrative we don't learn how hard it is to listen to a frightened and angry patient, how difficult it is to know when to give vital but anxiety-provoking information to a family, or how to challenge a physician or other coworker. Nor do we learn that nursing requires more than caring. It requires technical, medical, pharmacological, and other knowledge and expertise. The halfistic narrative downplays the extent to which nurses' professional judgment and experience lead to positive outcomes.

Nurses must expand halfistic accounts into genuinely holistic narratives that include dealing constructively with conflict, struggling, and fighting for what needs to be done. This is, of course, what nurses have done throughout their history and one of the reasons the public should trust nurses.

The truth is that nurses creatively employ many skills to confront the challenges that arise every day in their places of work. These skills are practiced and refined in accessing resources, maneuvering through the bureaucracy, negotiating with doctors and hospital administrators, and resolving conflicts in interactions with patients and colleagues.

Instead of defining patient advocacy as a kind of virtue, a more accurate account would see it as an act of daring. Most nurses will tell you that they are patient advocates. What does advocacy mean? As nurses in the book *When Chicken Soup Isn't Enough: Stories of Nurses Standing Up for Themselves, Their Patients, and Their Profession* depict it, it doesn't mean that nurses just want the best for their patients, wish them well, and hope no harm comes to them.[16] Advocacy demands action and risk. It comes from the word *advocate*, which in turn comes from the Latin *vocare*, "to voice." With the prefix *ad*, it means "to call out." Voice is a non-negotiable prerequisite of advocacy. You cannot, after all, call out in silence. And since advocacy usually requires risk, to be a patient advocate will sometimes involve taking some kind of risk and dealing with some kind of conflict. Advocacy is rarely sugar and spice and everything nice.

To get the resources and respect they need, nurses must advocate for themselves, not just for their patients. To do this, nurses must do more than "dare to care" as a Johnson and Johnson jingle puts it. They must dare to describe the breadth and complexity of nursing work. They must dare to explain the risks they incur every day as they advocate for patients. They must dare to assert that in order to do their heart work, they first need their brain to work. They must dare to deviate from the virtue script and help the public understand that nursing is more than smiles, good cheer, and friendship. Nurses and nursing organizations must go out and tell the public what nurses really do so that patients can actually get the benefit of their expert care.

Our mission in this book is to help nursing resemble medicine in one respect—in that its self-understanding does not repudiate the work of those engaged in the direct care of the sick but rather uses that work to construct a foundation on which to build an accurate representation of the profession as a whole.

It is designed to teach nurses how to do that. It is not about image marketing, social marketing, or any other kind of marketing. It is about helping nurses to construct messages that accurately inform the public about their work. Because nurses are busy, many of the communication techniques in this book are designed to integrate naturally into nurses' everyday lives and to complement nurses' work with patients and families.

A Note about Usage

We'd like to explain our choice of certain language in *From Silence to Voice*. Most of the time, for expediency, we use *we* in recounting situations involving one or the other or both of us. We refer to ourselves by name when it is necessary for clarity. As journalists, we have conducted interviews with many people for this book. Whenever a quotation appears without a note, it means that the material comes from one of our interviews with the source.

Although we talk a great deal about women's culture and its influence on nursing, we are not overlooking men who are nurses. Our purpose is to explore the legacy of women's socialization and gender stereotypes on nursing. Men in nursing are affected by these influences, just as women are.

Throughout this book, we use the word *patient* because it more accurately reflects the relationship nurses have with the people they care for than does the market-based term *consumer* or *customer*.

We are American journalists, not nurses. Like everyone else in journalism, and like much of the public, we started out knowing nothing about nursing. No doubt, without realizing it, we accepted many of the traditional stereotypes. Our views have been revolutionized. Nurses were our teachers. They have explained their work to us and expressed their insights about health and illness. We are profoundly in their debt. If we could be educated in this way, so can others.

Part I
Silent No More

CHAPTER 1

ENDING THE SILENCE

Envision how things would be if the voice and visibility of nursing were commensurate with the size and importance of the nursing profession.

Because nurses had educated patients, families, friends, relatives, neighbors, and community members about nursing work, patients would be fully cognizant that nurses are key to their survival and recovery.

When faced with medical treatments or procedures, patients would do more than inquire about the details of the procedures and their physician's qualifications to perform them. They would seek information about the qualifications of the nurses who would care for them during and after their treatments. They would want to know the nurse-to-patient ratio in their hospitals and the extent and type of nursing services available at outpatient centers, community clinics, and long-term care facilities. They would want to know how long their nurses had slept the night before and if their hospitals and health care institutions had lift equipment to help make them safe.

People would understand that many nurses, like physicians, have specialized expertise, even on a general medical floor. They would readily accept and often seek the services of nurse practitioners, mental health nurses, nurse midwives, nurse anesthetists, and hospice nurses. Similarly people would appreciate and support services provided by school nurses, public health nurses, and homecare nurses in their communities.

Because the public would understand the critical role of nursing in health care, hospitals could no longer rely on paring nursing staffs as their strategy for dealing with budget problems. Attempts to cut nursing staff, substitute aides for registered nurses (RNs), and stretch staff through floating and mandatory overtime would provoke public outcry. To the public, floating a nurse from an oncology to a pediatric unit would be in the same league as asking a medical oncologist to take over for a pediatrician.

Nursing salaries would more accurately reflect the expertise and responsibilities of nurses. This greater investment in nursing would mean that full-time jobs, with predictable schedules and decent benefits, would be readily available.

The visibility of nurses in the mass media would reflect the expanded participation of nursing in public discussions about health care. Nurses, not just physicians and policy PhDs, would be key participants in all health care forums whether they occurred in communities, before state and national legislatures, at economic conferences, or at international assemblies.

Physicians' views would no longer dominate the media. Nursing perspectives and expertise would be sought by journalists and radio and television interviewers and would be widely expressed on nursing websites, in blogs, in comments to news organizations, and in opinion pieces.

Everyone would know that nursing requires education and training, not just niceness. This understanding would translate into widespread public support for nursing education at the undergraduate, graduate, and postgraduate levels. Schools of nursing would be viewed as major contributors to the academic enterprise and would be fully integrated into higher education systems.

Just as people recognize that it takes someone with education and expertise to perform brain surgery, they would know that it takes someone with education and expertise to care for a patient who has just had brain surgery. Therefore they would oppose politicians and academic administrators who tried to eliminate or water down nursing programs or create less educated nurse substitutes.

A more complex and accurate image of a nurse would replace dated or distorted stereotypes. Respect for nursing would mean that young women and men who show an interest in nursing careers would be strongly encouraged, not grilled about why they aren't planning to go to medical school. With the challenges and rewards of nursing more fully appreciated, many talented women with other professional options would choose nursing. Nursing would be an increasingly attractive career choice for men.

The public would understand that medical interns and residents are not the only learners, and physicians are not the only teachers in medical centers. It would be known that hospitals are educational institutions for nurses and that nurses teach physicians as well as nurses in training. Institutional budgets would provide money, time, and extra staffing for continuing nursing education because everyone would know that veteran nurses, like physicians, need to keep up with the latest research and treatments. They would also understand that nurses do a lot of the teaching of doctors in training. In this new era of interprofessional education and practice, the concept of the teaching hospital would be transformed.

Medical research no longer would be perceived as the only scientific endeavor leading to health improvements. Health experts, journalists, policy makers, and the public would see nursing research as essential to health care and would support governmental and private funding for it.

Nursing shortages would not be tolerated because it would be crystal clear that human health and well-being depend not only on medically necessary care but also on *necessary nursing care.*

Nurses would receive the four *R*s that foster professional satisfaction:

- Recognition
- Respect
- Reward
- Resources

Does this vision seem like fantasy?

It's fantasy only if nurses are unwilling to make it reality. To be sure, a perfect world is not possible. But we are confident that nurses can significantly increase public understanding of and support for their work through effective public communication and sustained action. Without sustained action and communication, it's pretty much guaranteed that things will not improve.

Effective communication is essential because all areas of nursing—clinical practice, education, research, and policy—depend on public understanding of how and why nursing is indispensable to health care. Nursing is not practiced in a vacuum. It requires substantial resources, including physical space, equipment, staff, research, and higher education. If the public doesn't understand the significance of nurses' work and the context in which it takes place, it will be difficult to correct conditions that drive nurses out of the clinical setting and even out of the profession. Similarly, it will be hard to attract the best and the brightest young people into the profession and keep them in it.

If legislators, policy makers, and administrators are to allocate adequate financial resources to support nursing, they and the public must have a good idea of what nurses really do. If the work of contemporary nurses is unknown or misunderstood, then nurses cannot be appreciated or supported and cannot exert appropriate influence in health care. And if they can't do that, nurses will have difficulty delivering appropriate, high-quality care.

Missing in Action

The lack of accurate public information about nurses and their work allows insidious stereotypes to persist. Nurses tell us that many members of the public still believe that nurses are physician handmaids whose work is to carry out simple tasks under the direction of physicians. Others may idealize nurses as self-sacrificing angels of mercy. Even though surveys tell us that the public thinks highly of nurses' honesty and integrity, disturbing images of nurses as lewd sex objects or vituperative harridans also still circulate.

Being unseen and unknown in actual practice has been a perpetual problem for nursing. Studies of the visibility of nursing in the news media stemming from the 1990s found the largest segment of the health care profession to be virtually missing from coverage of health care.[1] Nurses were so rarely mentioned in health care coverage that they were essentially invisible even in those articles that dealt with hospital care.

In recent years news coverage of nursing has increased. For example, it is no longer astounding to see a news report based on *nursing* research. In general, we see more coverage of nurses in specialty practice. But we rarely see nursing covered as an integral part of health care and as a major source of expertise on health care and health issues.[2]

Health-related reporting by and large is defined as medical and focuses, often exclusively, on physicians. News stories concerning hospital care might refer to "doctors and nurses," but beyond that nurses are rarely named and quoted. Instead, nursing usually exists in the news as a separate category and stories are prompted by something going on within nursing, often something controversial. Nursing gets space in the mass media in connection with nursing shortages, staffing issues, dissention over the scope of nursing practice, and nurses' demands for better pay and working conditions. Nurses certainly aren't spared attention, or blame, for patient tragedies stemming from medication and surgical errors or from workplace system problems such as monitor-alarm fatigue or hospital-acquired infections.

So the public gets to see nursing in the mass media largely in connection with what we call "problem narratives." The public should be told about errors and nursing workforce issues to be sure, but nursing should be seen in broader contexts as well, as an essential part of health care. We should be exposed to "practice narratives," stories that integrate nursing into health care and enable us to see what nurses actually do.

Physicians also get caught up in patient tragedies and professional disputes. But that focus is only a small percentage of the media's coverage of medical practice and research. For decades, thanks to concentrated efforts by medical associations, the news and entertainment media have been telling stories about what physicians do. As a result, there is no information vacuum about physicians' work or a huge mystery about their contributions to health care. The work of nurses, however, has been and remains hidden. Hence, there is not a lot to balance or even challenge misinformation or stereotypes about nursing.

Although nursing, not medicine, is the largest health care profession and nurses, not physicians, are the largest group of clinical workers within hospitals, you would never know it from the coverage of health care and hospitals. For example, the *New York Times* carried an article about "a troubling picture of the care offered" at some for-profit long-term acute care hospitals that have proliferated in the United States in response to higher Medicare reimbursements.[3]

These hospitals are intended to deliver nursing care to very ill patients, not do medical diagnosis and treatment, a point the reporter, Alex Berenson, missed entirely, even though that is clear in the Medicare inspection report on which this story was based.[4] The story started with a description of the death of a horrendously neglected patient at Select Specialty Hospital of Kansas City, Kansas. The reporter seemed to attribute the death to the fact that "the sitter" whom "her physicians had ordered" had apparently not shown up, to "staff members [who] tied her down with wrist restraints," and to the fact that this hospital "has no doctors on its staff or its wards overnight."

Although the reporter said that these hospitals were not set up to do medical procedures and that "Medicare inspectors found that the hospital did not have enough nurses" on the night that the patient died, she did not give the details. In fact, the Medicare report said that the unit in question was supposed to have a minimum of six RNs. Two RNs were missing that night. Had this story been reported accurately, we would have seen how risky it is for patients when a nursing unit is short-staffed by a third.

There was a lot in this article about the high profits of corporations that run these step-down hospitals and their apparent reluctance to spend money on "staff." But we were never told what "staff" means in a facility that was supposed to care for (not "treat" as the story said) patients who need intensive nursing for an average of twenty-five days or more. The important players were "physicians." Everyone else was described as "staff" or "employees." "Nurses" came into the picture almost entirely in the assignment of blame for patient neglect.

There were so many misperceptions in this story about who does what, or who is supposed to do what in a hospital that it was almost laughable. But not funny at all was how the reporter and her editors allowed David Jarvis, a physician who spends a mere ten hours a week working as the national medical director for the Select Medical Corporation, to purposefully misconstrue the work of nurses in this excerpt from the article: "Dr. Jarvis defends Select and the industry, saying that long-term care hospitals play an important role by caring for patients who are not improving at traditional hospitals. Nurses and aides at traditional hospitals may grow frustrated with such patients, but Select's nurses and aides are used to them, he said. And after aggressive intensive care treatment, long-term patients need gentler care that will enable them to recover on their own. 'These people do better when we don't overdo it,' he said."

Another example of the effacement of nurses is a documentary film about the respected, but misleadingly named, organization Doctors Without Borders (Médicins Sans Frontières). The film, *Living in Emergency: Stories of Doctors Without Borders*, focuses on four physicians—three men and one woman. These physicians are veterans in providing medical care in dangerous and devastated war zones in such countries as Liberia and the Congo, and the film eloquently captures their commitment and the anguishing dilemmas they face daily.

The problem is that the majority of volunteers with Doctors Without Borders consists not of physicians but of nurses, statisticians, and other workers. Yet there is not a single depiction of a nurse or other specialist in the film. There are people shown in the surgery sequences who probably are nurses, but they are never identified as such. Of course the very name of the organization gives the impression that physicians either are the only people providing the health care in these circumstances or the only people who matter.

This film has serious implications. We know that health care, particularly in such circumstances, requires a team that functions with good team-member communication and relationships if it is to be safe and effective. But that is not what this documentary teaches. Rather, it reinforces stereotypes about physicians being the sole heroic deliverers of health care.

How is it that sophisticated journalists and producers miss the obvious—that nurses are central and essential in each of these cases? Perhaps they get this worldview from hospitals, the very institutions that would not exist without nurses.

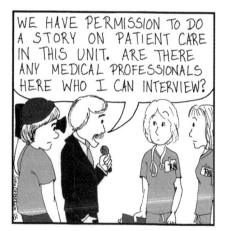

Sonia Oppenheim, www.familycomic.com

While we have not done a controlled study, we regularly look at North American hospital web pages, ads, and other marketing to see what members of the public might learn about nursing. The answer most of the time is little or nothing because nursing is either barely mentioned or ignored completely in hospitals' presentations of their clinical services and expertise. On their home pages some hospitals feature photos of smiling nurses who serve as attractive portal hostesses for the website but are missing elsewhere. The norm is that when nursing does appear, it is in a careers or employment section that tells you how and why you might apply for a job there.

This failure to integrate nursing into marketing materials does not mean that hospitals aren't sending messages about nursing. Quite the contrary: they are suggesting that nursing is not important to the services that they offer. In effect, it is hospitals themselves that issue blinders about nursing to various publics and especially to journalists.

Hospital web pages, advertisements, on-site posters and brochures, website videos, and other marketing devices are designed in large part to attract business. Health care centers strive to convince patients, potential patients, donors, businesses, government agencies, and others that there is something special about their services. Because they are competing for market share, they highlight what they consider to be their strengths. These often are medical specialties such as cardiac care, neurosurgery, women's health, and so on. For university-affiliated hospitals, the emphasis is likely to be on research and cutting-edge procedures and technology.

Even so, hospital websites carry a number of standard features. One is utilitarian information such as how to find a physician. Most post their clinical quality scores and highlight their awards. Essentially all the websites we've looked at offer health advice. This could be in the form of simple guides on blood pressure, diabetes, and exercise, for example, or more complex reports on such subjects as lung cancer, knee replacement surgery, or liver transplants. To a greater or lesser degree, hospital websites promote the work of physicians. We find that nursing is sometimes included or referred to when hospitals want to suggest that they are caring and compassionate in the delivery of services. Then again some hospitals talk about their compassionate care without ever mentioning nurses.

Almost always, when we've encountered information on nursing on hospital websites, it was segregated within a section on careers. Nursing information is there not to impress the public but to attract the attention of nurses for recruitment and retention purposes. In other words, medicine is marketed to the public, while nursing is marketed to nurses or potential nurses. Members of the public might happen on nursing sections and even learn something about nursing and the work of various nurses. Except in rare cases though, patients and the general public are not the intended audiences for information on nursing.

> **This failure to integrate nursing into marketing materials does not mean that hospitals aren't sending messages about nursing. Quite the contrary: they are suggesting that nursing is not important to the services that they offer.**

You might ask, is the same true of Magnet hospitals? When a hospital achieves Magnet Recognition from the American Nurses Credentialing Center (ANCC), it automatically gets bragging rights for the quality of its nursing. The ANCC asserts that Magnet Recognition correlates strongly with other quality awards, such as high best-hospital rankings by *U.S. News & World Report*. The ANCC's message is that excellence in nursing is not only an indicator of overall excellence but a catalyst too for attracting and developing excellence throughout the institution. If that is the case, you would think that hospitals would be eager to promote their Magnet status to the public. We found a lot of variation on that score. Some hospitals that we looked at featured the Magnet award on their home pages. What surprised us were the hospitals that didn't mention their Magnet Recognition at all, or buried it in the recesses of their websites.

Because web pages can offer so much information, many opportunities exist, even within the conventional hospital website framework, to end the silence by integrating nursing into standard website features.

End-the-Silence Opportunity 1: Show nurses in clinical action. Take the home page slide show. This is the first thing we encountered on virtually all the home pages that we visited. A series of photos scrolls across the screen. These slide shows generally have a theme. One sort centers on happy patients—either people who look as though they are patients or real patients who are identified by name. Often there is a link from them to written or video "patient stories." Another theme depicts medical personnel, predominantly physicians, in action often with high-tech devices and machines. When nurses make it into this sort of slide show, they are likely to be in the hostess pose, smiling at the camera.

End-the-Silence Opportunity 2: Construct patient narratives that include the work of specific nurses. In one way or another, sophisticated health care websites draw you into stories about real patients. The bare bones of the standard narrative is that patient X (who usually tells the story) had a problem that was identified by one or more physicians at the hospital. The patient was treated by a specialist or team of physicians who employed cutting-edge skill and technology, and the patient was fixed. There are no descriptions in these stories of how nurses helped the patient. Often there is no reference to nurses at all.

End-the-Silence Opportunity 3: Put Magnet or another nursing icon on the home page, and link it to stories for the public about nurses' innovations and research. When the hospital displays the Magnet Recognition icon, it is usually linked to a "for nurses" section that is not expected to be read by patients and the general public.

End-the-Silence Opportunity 4: Ask top administrators to mention the clinical work of nurses in their descriptions of their hospitals' services. Many of the websites we reviewed had a welcome video on the home page. In some of these, the CEO or president of the hospital welcomed patients and described the many excellent things that physicians do there. Some were better than others in mentioning nurses as a category instead of lumping them into "staff." Hospital leaders could do a much better job of highlighting nursing.

Later in this book we show how a few hospitals publicly promote nurses' work as a drawing card. Here let's take a look at some hospital websites that missed these opportunities.

Suppose, for example, you visit the website of the fabled Massachusetts General Hospital (MGH) in Boston. The home page (when we looked at it) tells you that MGH is "turning today's discoveries into tomorrow's care."[5] The ad copy continues: "At Mass General the world's leading clinicians and researchers work together to unravel the complexities of human disease and develop new and better treatments. Discover how our research improves patient care. Watch the video."

In the video, you learn from the president of the institution that MGH is a place where "firsts" happen. "First public demonstration of ether." "First use of X-rays." "First limb reattachment." A series of medical practitioners and scientists informs you that the institution is continuing its pioneering tradition— searching for cures for cancer, investigating a vaccine for HIV, testing a device that will restore mobility. MGH is unusual in that it is "a place where research and patient care are linked together. And what that does is it keeps scientific research focused on real patients."

How is the linkage effected? By bringing "engineers and biologists who have never seen a patient" to the bedside so that they can observe how their work helps patients. Throughout the three-minute video, we do not hear a single mention of nurses or nursing. In this presentation, nurses have nothing to do with the clinical care that the presentation trumpets. Neither are nurses referred to in any of the information displayed on the home page (although a training program to improve residents' empathy with patients is).

MGH, "the oldest and largest hospital in New England," gets around to mentioning its Magnet Recognition in the hospital's "Overview" and on an "Awards" page. But to find out anything at all about nurses at this institution you need time and determination to excavate your way through mazes, subsections and sub-sub-sections, until, voilà! you find the nursing department. (It is so difficult, we almost couldn't do it a second time.)

There we learn that the "essence of nursing practice at Massachusetts General Hospital is caring. Our every action is guided by knowledge, enabled by skill, and motivated by compassion."[6]

Beyond this portal exists a surprising multidimensional, multilayered, multimedia world of nursing. You could spend a lot of time here learning about nursing education, certification, professional development, clinical research, clinical management of various conditions, patient care standards, staff collaboration, ethics—you name it. For example, under the "Excellence Everyday Portal" you will find nursing descriptions and instructions on preventing and dealing with falls, pain, pressure ulcers, restraints, and other matters.

In another section, we found a fascinating video, "Two Hundred Years Later: A Spotlight on Quality and Safety," commemorating MGH's bicentennial in 2011. It was a recording of a Nurses Week lecture at the hospital by Susan M. Grant, chief nursing officer (CNO) of Emory University Health Care, on medical errors and the development of systems and standards to reduce them.[7]

One of Grant's slides showed a story headlined "Doctor's Orders Killed Cancer Patient" from the March 23, 1995, issue of the *Boston Globe*. Grant explained that she was the nurse manager on the unit of the Dana Farber Cancer Institute where two patients were given four times the amount of chemotherapy drugs that they should have received. The story referred to one of the patients, Betsey Lehman, who happened to be the *Globe*'s health writer, and who had repeatedly protested that there was something wrong with her chemotherapy. Lehman died from the overdose. The case was covered extensively by the *Globe* and became a national issue. Grant, who became the chief nurse at Dana Farber, explained that this tragedy led to ongoing data collection and analysis to improve patient safety.

Dana Farber, like MGH, is a Boston institution famous for its cutting-edge research and treatments to the detriment, at the time, of patient care. Grant blamed the overdoses on inadequate systems of care that existed rather than on individual nurses and pharmacists, most of whom, she asserted, did their jobs correctly. She explained that patient safety assessments since the late 1990s have produced quantifiable nursing-sensitive performance measures that are key to patient outcomes. She told the nurses at MGH that "this is a golden moment for nurses to lead" because hospital reimbursement is increasingly connected to patient-centered outcome measures that are "directly influenced by nursing care."

This point is being reiterated in health care centers throughout the United States but usually only by nurses for nurses. If nurses are crucial to both patients and pay, why, one may ask, are they absent in MGH's home page pitch? Why do "geeks," engineers, and biologists get mentioned, but not nurses? Why do hospital presidents go to Nurses' Day events to tell nurses how important they are and then fail to mention nurses in their overtures to the public? Why is nursing, when it is discussed at all, treated in such a separate and unequal way from medicine?

We were impressed with the video on the importance of nursing to patient outcomes, so we moseyed over to the website of Emory Health Care, where Grant is CNO, to see what it might have to say about nursing. The only nurse thing we found on the home page was an "Ask A Nurse" link to a questionnaire that you could submit online to receive a call from a nurse to determine what kind of services you might need.[8]

> In our surfing, we made a point of looking at Magnet hospitals with the idea that nursing would be more visible on their web pages. It wasn't.

In the numerous pages describing Emory's forte as an academic medical and research center, there were no mentions of nursing.[9] We were told that "Emory is Georgia's 'medical safety net'—the place where other hospitals send their patients with the most serious and complex health issues." The doctors and specialists at Emory were cited as the reason for this. There was no hint that patients "with the most serious and complex health issues" desperately need nurses to monitor and care for them.

The closest we got to the "*N-word*" was in Grant's title, following a quotation by her: "'Patient- and Family-Centered Care is doing things with patients and their family members instead of doing things to and for patients and their families.' *Susan Grant, Emory Healthcare's Chief Nursing Officer.*"

In our surfing, we made a point of looking at Magnet hospitals with the idea that nursing would be more visible on their web pages. It wasn't.

According to the ANCC, Vanderbilt University Medical Center achieved Magnet recognition April 2012. The hospital promoted it by featuring the Magnet icon in its home page slide show. The headline above the icon said, "Thank you Vanderbilt Nurses for all you do."

This hospital convention of publicly thanking its nurses puzzles us. On the one hand it implies that it values nurses. On the other, this statement addresses nurses as though they are outsiders instead of part of the clinical team, and the "for all you do" could mean almost anything. The hospital has an opportunity with Magnet to "own" nursing by saying something like "Our nurses have been recognized for the clinical excellence they bring to Vanderbilt."[10]

You can link to Vanderbilt Nursing from a "For Employees" section on the home page. Once again, this is a section about nurses for nurses. Under "Spotlight and Events" we found a page called "Our Nurses' Stories" and this statement: "VUMC is very proud of our nursing staff. The individuals featured below have been nominated by management or co-workers to appear on our home page" (meaning the nursing home page, not the main hospital home page). "They each have unique stories to share that include overcoming obstacles, professional challenges, and the perks of practicing at Vanderbilt University Medical Center."

The nurses whose headshots appear were identified in what we call kindergarten style—a first name and a last-name initial, as in Pam A., RN. When we clicked on individual nurses, however, we found his or her full name in the nomination for recognition written by a colleague. Then the kindergarten labeling returned ("Pam A.'s Story,") followed by photos and personal narratives in which nurses described how they got into nursing, their feelings about it, the obstacles they overcame, and the help that they were given. The nurses also talked about their families and other interests. The nominations and first-person narratives rarely gave much information about the nurse's actual work, but when they did, we found it enlightening. One such nomination gave a glimpse of how a mental health nurse had coordinated services to ensure safe administration of medications to mental health patients.

The public should know that nurses do these things. Why not feature nurses describing their work on the public web pages?

Stanford Hospital and Clinics received renewed Magnet Recognition in April 2012, but as of June, that news hadn't made it to its home page. Inasmuch as Magnet was tucked away as the last item on an "Awards" page, and inasmuch as a link from the icon took you to the ANCC website instead of to nursing at Stanford, it appeared that Stanford didn't see Magnet Recognition as significant enough for public promotion.

Nursing was referred to in the announcement of Stanford's ranking as one of the top twenty hospitals by *U.S. News & World Report*: " 'This distinction reflects the outstanding efforts of our doctors, nurses, clinicians, researchers, educators, support staff and managers,' said Amir Dan Rubin, President and CEO of Stanford Hospital & Clinics."[11]

But nurses were pretty much passed over in a series of text and video patient stories. These narratives followed the form we've come to expect: a patient with a particular health problem is treated expertly and successfully by a physician specialist. On this website, patient stories were accompanied by educational material on the particular health issue. It seemed to us that there were opportunities in these patient narratives to name individual nurses and describe what they did. We read seven narratives and found only one instance of a nurse being named. In one of the stories, "interdisciplinary collaboration" was described as something that happens "among surgeons, radiologists, medical oncologists, radiation oncologists, pathologists, researchers and support programs."

Nursing was also missing from Stanford's extensive lists of clinical services but found, as usual, under "For Health Professionals." There, in issues of *Stanford Nurses*, a quarterly publication, we found material that would help patients and the public understand nursing if it were presented to them. Much of the content was educational material for nurses. But the topics were stimulating, like one article on the history of Stanford's patient airlift program. This piece could be rewritten to show the work of flight nurses. We think it would make a nice feature on the public part of the hospital website.[12]

When we speak with nurses, they express concern about letting the public in on the difficulties of delivering care. The result is that individual nurses get blamed for things that go wrong because of inadequate systems. This problem was described in the following excerpt from a *Stanford Nurse* article on unit-level pain management: "Since each individual experiences pain differently, pain control is complex and addressing uncontrolled pain can be very challenging for nurses. Nurses are frequently caught between a chronic pain patient and a doctor who will not order any more pain medication, which can lead to patients believing that nurses are not adequately controlling their pain."[13] We thought this statement confirms that silence about the realities of patient care serves neither nurses nor patients.

Our surfing was guided by state-by-state listings of Magnet hospitals on the ANCC's website. We picked the Banner Good Samaritan Medical Center in Phoenix at random, clicked on the link from the ANCC, and were taken not to that specific hospital but to the home page of Banner Health, a nonprofit system with facilities in Arizona and six other states.

In general, we found that Banner did a better job than most of integrating nurses and nursing into its descriptions and illustrations of clinical services. But it had a peculiar practice of decredentialing its nurses. For example, Banner devotes a lot of web space to its Simulation Medical Center ("a one-of-a-kind learning opportunity for health care professionals"). It has a link to a video that is clearly directed to a public audience ("A Nurse Talks about How the Center Helped Her"). The people in the video look like nurses and the accompanying text refers to them as nurses and gives their first and last names. But, except for one person (Samantha Hasso, RN, PICU), their credentials are missing. The leading person in the video is Carol Cheney, director of Simulation and Innovation. Is she a nurse? We're not told.

This missing-credential habit carries over into Banner's first issue of its *Simulation Newsletter*.[14]

It leads off with a "Note from Karen." Karen's full name is at end of the article, Karen Josey, but her credentials are missing. She thanks others for their work, so we assume she is in charge of something. There is also an article by Carol Cheney, the director who is in the simulation video. We still are not given her clinical credentials. But the physicians are referred to as Dr. Chu and

Dr. Smith. We wondered why nurses who are writing articles and appearing in videos aren't making their clinical credentials part of their identification.

We zipped over to the "For Nurses" section of the website and found a page titled "Nursing Research at Banner Health."[15] Here we were told that "Banner Health is constantly looking at new ways to improve patient care. Learn more about our nurses and their research projects." We were eager to learn more about Banner's nurses and their research, but this page turned out to be largely a tease. It contained headshots of nurses and their full names, but no credentials. Research titles appeared, as in "Melanie Glaze, peritoneal dialysis patients." We would liked to have known more about Nurse Glaze's research, but the link took us only to the home page of the facility where she works. A few projects had links to posters, but the information on these was presented in research-study style and was incomprehensible in terms of learning how the research in question benefitted patients.

Asymmetrical naming practices communicate as much to the people within health care systems as they do to the public. Decredentialing nurses or referring to them by only their first names promotes nursing anonymity in the workplace and trains those in the organization to overlook the contributions of nurses. Taken to the public sphere, these conventions instruct the public (and journalists) about how to regard nurses. This is why we think it is important for hospital promotions to desegregate nursing and to treat nurses with parity.

New York University's Langone Medical Center, a Magnet institution, tells us a lot about education and training on its website—but only about the education and training of physicians in connection with NYU's school of medicine. NYU also has a renowned nursing school, but you would not find that out on this website.[16] Nor would you learn that nursing research is conducted at Langone. The website's extensive "Research" section deals only with medical and biochemical research. In that section, we found that Langone hosted "Doctor Radio" that featured "experts from NYULMC [NYU Langone Medical Center] who drew on knowledge in their areas of expertise to answer questions that take research from the lab bench to the patient's bedside."[17] We didn't see any evidence that nurses are involved in this process. Nor did nursing appear in Langone's welcome-to-the-medical-center text that touted the institution as "a world-class, patient-centered, integrated, academic medical center."[18]

In fact, we couldn't find a reference to Magnet Recognition in the "About Us" section of the website, but the institution's rankings in three categories by *US News & World Report* were prominently displayed. The Magnet icon was tucked into the website's "Department of Nursing," again a cloistered section designed for nurses. There nurses could learn about the achievements of other nurses whose full names actually appeared along with their credentials.

In an Office of Communications subsection, intriguingly labeled "Advertising & Branding," we pored over "advertising campaigns that distinguish us within an increasingly competitive healthcare market." We had already presumed that Langone doesn't consider nursing to be a big selling point. That was confirmed in expensive Langone Medical Center ads that appeared on the radio, on billboards, on buses, in bus shelters, online, and in print publications such as the *New York Times*, the *Wall Street Journal*, the *New Yorker*, *New York* magazine, the *Economist*, and *Crain's New York Business* between 2009 and 2011. This "Any Given Moment," ad campaign, Langone stated, "captures some of the most powerful, intimate and uniquely human experiences to emerge from the Medical Center and highlights its core clinical care and research strengths."[19]

The template for most of the ads is a photograph, usually of a physician, at the center of the page. A very large single word appears above or in the image, then a smaller word in parentheses in the following manner: "Brain (trust)," "Speedy (recovery)," "Heart (beats)." A short narrative appears under the photo.

We saw one of these ads in the *New Yorker* in 2010. It read, "Intensive (support)." The photograph was of a man in scrubs next to a patient's bed. We thought he might have been a nurse. We were wrong. "Sometimes it's what happens in the hours immediately after surgery that makes the difference," the caption read. "The Critical Care Unit at NYU Langone Medical Center Tisch Hospital is staffed 24/7 by physicians board-certified in critical care medicine, ensuring the intensive support you deserve at the moment you need it most."

We always find it strange when critical care is defined as physician care, given that the critical care unit was developed to provide intensive nursing. According to the historians Julie Fairman and Joan Lynaugh, in the 1950s and 1960s "in erratically staffed but expanding hospitals, nurses found themselves responsible for desperately ill and dying patients whose medical and nursing needs exceeded the nurses' availability, knowledge, and authority. Left on their own to cope with these difficult and frustrating situations, some physicians and nurses were powerfully motivated to find a better way." This dilemma led nurses to found intensive care units. As one early intensive care nurse said, because of "the problems that came from a patient being desperately ill and needing one nurse. . . . Finding a way to respond to that situation multiplied by thousands of times forced us to change the hospital."[20] Nurses also found a way to develop their knowledge and skill in this area by creating the American Association of Critical-Care Nurses.

Langone's ads focus on physicians' work in other areas. One titled "Brain (trust)," highlights the work of neurosurgeons. According to the ad, "No case is too complex for John Golfinos, Chief of the Department of Neurosurgery and the team of world-renowned neurosurgeons." Another ad, "Whole (hearted)," shows a white-coated physician holding a baby in his arms and states, "No heart is too small for Dr. Ralph Ma, who leads the accomplished team that treats pediatric and adult congenital disease."

The ads that feature physicians show their entire bodies and identify them by name. In contrast, the "You (come first)" ad in the series shows what we presume to be a nurse's hand holding that of a patient who is in a bed. We don't know if the nurse in question is a man or a woman since the image of the nurse is cut off. The ad copy reads, "Our nurses anticipate patient needs, making call buttons virtually obsolete."[21] And there is a "Magnetic (energy)" ad, with the Magnet icon in the lower corner, picturing a nurse dangling what appears to be an inflated latex glove to amuse a young pediatric patient. It reads, "World-class nursing care comes from unmatched skill, dedication and a human touch." The nurse is anonymous.

When nurses describe their work, they almost always mention at some point that they work as members of a team. They acknowledge what the most authoritative reports on health care assert—that patient safety depends on teamwork. Would that other team members and team "owners" acknowledged this as well. The NYU critical care ad copy, for example, would have been far more accurate if it had said, "Sometimes it's what happens in the hours immediately after surgery that makes the difference. The Critical Care Unit at NYU Langone Medical Center Tisch Hospital is staffed 24/7 by critical-care-certified physicians and nurses, ensuring the intensive support you deserve at the moment you need it most."

Patients are in hospitals because they need nursing care as much as, or even more than, medical treatment. Yet much of the marketing and development material we read from hospitals sets up two categories of personnel: MDs and "staff." While all the "staff" people are essential to the team, there is a good argument for making nurses distinct—they make up the one group that is indispensable to the hospital. Health care can be delivered by physicians, therapists, and others in various settings, but these practitioners cannot provide hospital care without nurses. This reality is reflected in the fact that nurses are the largest personnel group in hospitals and represent 50 percent of a hospital's labor budget. Ignoring this leads to the slanted media coverage that we described earlier.

> **Patients are in hospitals because they need nursing care as much as, or even more than, medical treatment.**

Your Turn

Examine the website of the place where you work. Who and what are highlighted on the home page? This is what visitors see first. Any sign of nurses there? How many clicks does it take to find nurses? What impression do you get of nurses and nursing? How would you redesign the website to show the work of nurses?

Media Friendliness versus Accuracy

Contrary to what many nurses think, omissions and distortions don't come about because journalists and television writers, or even hospital communications staff, are hostile to nurses. We've heard complaints that the media are not "nurse friendly" and that they pick on nurses. Even the television show *Nurse Jackie*—a show we believe actually depicts nursing in a favorable light—is cited as proof positive that the media are unfriendly to nursing and deliberately broadcast stories about killer nurses, incompetent nurses, poorly trained nurses, and, for entertainment purposes, "naughty" nurses.

Nursing groups say they want "positive" coverage. But how are *friendly* and *positive* defined? There is little clarity on this score. Do these words mean that nurses would like to be treated with kid gloves by the media, perhaps even cast as an extra-special angelic group? We think that stereotyping nurses as extra human will not lead to a fair shake from the media.

In fact, the media are not particularly unfriendly toward nursing. A lot of journalists, like members of the broader public, feel very friendly toward nurses. The problem is they aren't interested in reporting on nurses because they don't know much about what nurses do and they are not helped by the kind of hospital promotional material discussed above. That may well have been why the *New York Times* reporter, or her editors, while preparing the story on the shortcomings of for-profit acute care hospitals, didn't ask, "Hey, aren't patients in those hospitals because they need nursing care?" Just raising that question would imply some grasp of nursing practice.

A longing for a kinder, gentler press should be jettisoned in favor of a quest for attentive and accurate coverage. An accurate picture of nursing will emerge only when nurses and their organizations tell journalists not who nurses are and how virtuous they can be but what they do and why it is so important. The public needs to know that nursing care is *consequential*—as much so as medical treatment. Accurate reporting on nursing—warts and all—would be an indication that nursing is being taken seriously.

Ending the Silence

Today every profession must speak for itself and justify its existence. No one can do this for nurses. If nursing is to acquire public *significance* commensurate with its role in health care, many more individual nurses and nursing organizations must be actively reaching out to influential and broad publics. To move toward the ideal that we described in the beginning of this chapter

- Individual nurses must make public communication and education about nursing an integral part of his or her nursing work.
- Nurses must communicate in ways that highlight nurses' knowledge rather than their virtues.
- Nurses must insist that their hospitals and other workplaces promote nursing to the public.

Public Communication

Some basic concepts are helpful in exploring how to communicate with the public effectively. The phrase *public communication* contains two words, both of which we define broadly.

The *public* is not a singular mass. There are many "publics," or audiences, that nurses need to communicate with. These publics include patients and family members, doctors and other nurses, managers and administrators, a nurse's own family and friends, members of community and religious organizations and social groups, marketing and public relations professionals in hospitals, professional organizations and colleges and universities, regulators and legislators, and journalists and other media professionals. Putting it simply, a public or audience is anyone a nurse is in contact with or can reach via the media.

Similarly *communication* is multidimensional. There is more than one way to communicate. Verbal communication can be oral or written, and some forms of communication are nonverbal. The fact is that we all communicate in various ways with many publics everyday. A great deal is being communicated about *nursing* whenever a nurse introduces her- or himself to a patient, whenever a nurse calls a doctor, whenever a nurse talks to a patient about his or her treatment, whenever a nurse makes a complaint to managers or administrators, whenever a nurse tells stories about nursing, and even whenever a nurse remains mute. Similarly, what a nurse wears to work and the body language that a nurse employs speak volumes.

The question is, do these communications convey what nurses want them to? Do they contribute to a strong professional identity, or are they, at times, at cross-purposes to that goal?

Three Tiers of Communication

In subsequent chapters we organize communication into three tiers and discuss the opportunities in each for educating the public about nursing. These are

1. Public communication through professional self-presentation.
2. Public communication through anecdotal descriptions of nursing work.
3. Public communication through various media.

The essential thing to remember as we continue is that while communication skills are important, *willingness* to communicate about nursing is crucial.

CHAPTER 2

THE DAISY DILEMMA

One of the fundamental questions that animates this book and that has driven our work for almost three decades is: Why does the public so misunderstand nursing?

The answer to this question is what we have come to think of as the Daisy Dilemma: nurses who have long fought for greater professional and social respect promote themselves, and allow others to promote them, in ways that undercut their claims to seriousness and crediblity.

Nurses universally say that they need more resources, university education as entry into practice, higher salaries for educators, better staffing in health care institutions, broader awareness of the multiple areas in which nurses work and the myriad roles they perform, more money for research, improvements in wages and working conditions, better workplace equipment to protect both patients and staff, and greater efforts to increase support both from within health care systems and from the larger society. Yet messages that that emerge from the profession explaining what nurses really do and why investments in nursing are crucial are few and far between. Many of the messages that originate with nurses, or that are put forth on their behalf, focus more on who nurses are or how they feel about their work rather than on what they do and how it relates to crucial health care concerns like patient outcomes, safety, suffering, or costs. Nurses, in other words, are frequently applauded for their virtues instead of for their knowledge, skill, and actions.

There is a big cultural and commercial investment in the "goodness" of nurses. This trait gets expressed in cute and sentimental words and images that, in the words of social marketing expert Christina Young, "SweetiePieize" nurses. These messages conceal and sometimes even denigrate nurses' clinical knowledge and skilled practice. Problematical messages about nursing are widely apparent in hospitals and other health care facilities, in nursing school activities, in promotions from nursing organizations, in nursing award programs and celebrations, and in recruitment campaigns. In this chapter we analyze several ways that nurses communicate their work through words and images and how they have partnered with companies and marketers to promote traditional gendered images of the profession.

Nurses' Juvenalia Problem

Humans have a gift for simultaneously holding opposing views and acting in contradictory ways. This is exhibited when nurses who yearn to be taken seriously associate themselves with childishness. Sometimes this tendency is found in surprising places. Let us give you a few examples.

In the fall of 2011, one of us spoke at a North American school of nursing. As we exited the elevator on the floor where the administrative offices, the library, and some classrooms were located, we noticed that numerous little butterflies and hearts dangled from strings attached to the ceiling. What was all this, we asked? We learned that one of the nursing professors had asked students to draw and cut out these hearts and butterflies to soften the concrete cinder-block look of the institution.

None of the other schools in the university housed in similar concrete cinder block buildings had cutesy decorations adorning their halls. It's hard to imagine that students of the law, medicine, the social sciences, or the humanities would produce kingergartenish hearts and butterflies to pretty up their educational environment, much less be asked to do so by a professor. Nursing has struggled to gain academic acceptance on a par with other disciplines. What do these decorations communicate to others in the university about nursing?

In another example, first-year students at another North American university school of nursing were asked to make a trace of their hands on a piece of paper and then, on each of the fingers and thumbs, write an attribute they believed to be that of a nurse. According to students, the professors seemed to be soliciting attributes like caring and empathy rather than clinical expertise or scientific knowledge. One student told us, "I felt absolutely stupid. It made us (nursing students) feel inferior. The assignment was like something you'd give a kid in the first grade—you know, what we wanted to be like when we grew up."

When nursing organizations use juvenile images in their logos and campaigns, they contradict the professional acumen and status that the organizations promote. For example, the American Association of Heart Failure Nurses is made up of nurses who deal with complex cardiac problems. The association

> When nursing organizations use juvenile images in their logos and campaigns, they contradict the professional acumen and status that the organizations promote.

offers instructional workshops at its conferences aimed at applying the latest research to such clinical challenges as managing complex cardiac problems and medication regimens. The group's logo, however, is a series of childish cut-out doll characters strung on a ribbon.

This isn't a North American phenomenon only. When the New Zealand Nurses Organization, a labor union representing nurses in that country, launched a safe-staffing campaign, it put extensive effort into developing seven components of safe staffing. To illustrate these components, it chose images of cut-out dolls in seven different colors.

Cute, lovable, and juvenile illustrations are so common within nursing culture that it is easy to overlook how they trivialize nursing. Nurses may not notice this effect, but it speaks loud and clear to influential publics that need to be taking nursing seriously.

Certainly not every nurse buys into this. But enough nurse-angel pins, scrubs imprinted with hearts and teddy bears, coffee cups bearing cute child-nurse images and stuffed animals representing nurses show up in the nursing workplace to keep the juvenalia market alive.

Mercifully they seem to be decreasing in number, but every once in a while we encounter a Precious Moments figurine depicting a nurse either as a small child or as a baby with tiny wings, nurse's cap, and stethoscope. This is an interesting image in that it represents the practitioner as being as helpless as a very young child.

The juvenile theme is not only produced *for* nurses. It's sometimes produced *by* nurses. At one hospital we spoke at for Nurses Week, staff nurses had taken pictures of their colleagues with their arms around one another smiling at the camera. These photos were displayed on circular paper balloons attached to green poster paper and adorned with ribbons drawn with magic markers. The collage was exhibited on two large panels positioned at the entrance to the hospital's main cafeteria. It looked more like an elementary school art project than a depiction of professional practice.

A juvenile theme is often echoed in the trinkets and food treats that hospitals give to nurses at Nurses Week events. In one Magnet hospital that we spoke at during Nurses Week, staff nurses were rewarded with Halloween-type candy in cellophane pouches tied with adorable pink ribbons. These candy trinkets were displayed

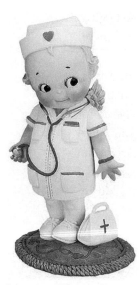

Baby nurse-angel figurine

outside the auditorium where we observed a number of professional-looking personnel casting dismissive glances at the exhibition. One website devoted to selling Nurses Week trinkets exhibits balloons festooned with cutesy flowers and a Nurse Antenna ball—an adorable yellow ball with a smiley face topped with a white nurse's cap.[1]

Images and activities that depict the nurse as childlike raise a serious question: Who needs care more, the patient or the nurse? A homemade "nurse survival kit" sold at a conference that we attended included a "bandage, to mend hurt feelings; a crayon, to color every day cheerful and bright; and a cotton ball, to help soften disappointments"—not for the patient but for the nurse. Undoubtedly, given the difficult and stressful work they do, nurses need decent working conditions and need to take care of themselves and each other. That is not the issue. The issue is what these childish symbols and messages communicate, intentionally or not, to the public. Patients' lives depend on the maturity and clinical mastery of nurses. Nurses make this claim rhetorically but often contradict it iconographically.

The Nurses Week Problem

During Nurses Week hospitals and other health care institutions honor nurses and invite others to do so. While there are many professional and educational activities held during Nurses Week, the annual observation timed to observe the May 12 birthday of Florence Nightingale also seems to call forth a veritable orgy of sentimentalized images. This is ironic inasmuch as the mother of modern nursing famously declared in her recruitment notices that "sentimental women need not apply."

In the next chapter we explore the origins of such images and how they came to be embedded in nursing culture. Here we are concerned with what they communicate to various audiences—including non-nurses.

National, international, and specialty nursing organizations choose a theme each year for Nurses Week and promote it with paraphernalia like banners, posters, mugs, and tote bags. These are often sold to hospitals and health care institutions. Hospitals display these items in lobbies, corridors, and individual units and sell them or give them as gifts. Some health care institutions create their own celebratory messages and items.

From year to year Nurses Week clichés and icons get recycled into slightly new designs. For example, in 2002, the American Nurses Association (ANA) used an image of a gauzey angel in pastel colors to illustrate its theme "Nurses Saving Lives, Touching Lives." In 2006, the organization's image was that of a green heart being offered in an outstretched hand, to accompany a much stronger theme, "Strength, Commitment Compassion." In 2011, the ANA's Nurses Week theme was "Nurses Trusted to Care" Illustrated with the clichéd image of two clasped hands, thus reinforcing the mistaken idea that nurses complain about, that nursing is mere hand-holding.

As nursing descriptors, hearts and clasped hands send a feel-good message but they don't begin to capture what is so important about nursing. Yet these icons are so ubiquitous in nursing promotions that they have come to represent nursing itself.

When patients, families, and other members of the public thank nurses, they often feed back these themes and images in cards, poems, and trinkets, and then some. A particularly patronizing Nurses Day card we bought in 2011 came with the printed message "You're such a kind and caring and thoughtful nurse, they ought to put R.R.R.N. after your name. For Real, Real, Real Nice."

In some Nurses Week messages, nurses are encouraged to be self-sacrificing for a greater or spiritual good. If you look up poems for Nurses Week on the web, you might encounter one that starts, "A Nurse is more, Why?" and then answers the question like this:

> Nurse's desire for service is pure.
> Not for themselves, it has to be for others . . .
> Above and beyond, their duty comes first.
> Their patient's needs paramount, before even hunger and thirst.[2]

In his idealization of nursing as self-sacrifice, it's clear this author is unaware of studies documenting that tired, hungry nurses are actually dangerous to patients.

Nurses Week Supplements

The public participates in another Nurses Week staple, the annual advertising supplements that newspapers put out. These are quasi-public vehicles in that patients, as well as nurses and other health care professionals, are solicited via hospital posters and newspaper and website announcements to nominate "their favorite nurse." Some newspaper supplements publish a number of these letters along with photos of the respective nurses.

Presumably members of the public read these widely distributed supplements. But their real purpose is to serve as recruitment and retention vehicles for hospitals and as cash cows for newspaper companies. In the case of the

Boston Globe, hospitals, health care chains, and nursing schools pay from sixty-five hundred to thirty thousand dollars per ad to position themselves in the nursing market. One of the things we've noticed about these supplements is that patients sometimes do a better job of linking the various aspects of nurses' knowledgable care than do those who write the headlines or the hospitals' ad copy. Consider the following letter submitted by a student at Weston High School in Massachusetts about Nurse Kathy Becker:

> As a high school nurse, Kathy Becker deals with absolutely everything, from minor headaches to broken bones and seizures. I have been lucky and honored to get to know her well due to my severe allergies. When I have an allergic reaction, she ably assesses the situation, making sure that I am comfortable with the decisions made. Furthermore, she respects my opinion, even though I am only 18 and have no medical training. She stays calm throughout the process, even as she dials 911 and watches me self-inject my EpiPen. She makes sure to keep my mind off of the reaction by telling me about her weekend or asking about my last soccer game. When another student comes in for Advil or a Band-Aid, she firmly but politely tells them to come back later. She keeps a smile on as she records my blood pressure, oxygen level, and time of injection. She knows when to throw in a joke, and when to be serious. When the paramedics arrive, she gives them a rundown of my medical history in a timely manner. The next day, she is sure to check in with me and let my teachers know what happened. Ms. Becker's compassion and expertise have allowed me to stay calm and positive during situations that might otherwise be terrifying. Words cannot describe how truly thankful I am to have worked with such a terrific nurse and person during my high school years.
>
> *—Nominated by Kate Freedberg* [3]

This sophisticated view of a nurse's work is headlined "A Calm Presence," which represents the nurse as being in a static mode rather than the active one that the student described.

It isn't easy to be comprehensive or to capture nuance in a few words. But labels and themes need not reduce nurses' work to simplistic sentiment, as in the headline "He Dispenses Hugs, Humor" for a story about Nurse Gordon "Ed" Newbert of Massachusetts General Hospital. Newbert was nominated by a patient who wrote that Newbert had hugged her and that he has a sense of humor. But the context she put it in is anything but simple.

"I cannot say enough good things about how he has treated me," the patient wrote, saying that Newbert had been her nurse since she started chemotherapy for pancreatic cancer almost a year previously. "Every week, he will ask all the questions about my physical health but will also want to know about my mental health: Was I able to go out? Have I seen friends? What activities have I done? . . . The week my mother died, he was the first person to give me a big hug and express his condolences." The patient, unlike the headline writer, grasped the professional context of Newbert's caring and went on to cite his medical knowledge. "When I started treatment I could not understand why things took so long," she wrote. "He carefully explained the timeframes required for the medications and the clinical trial infusion. No one else had taken the time to give me the details."[4]

A striking feature of the supplements is how they set up a contemporary view of professional nursing in a lead article, then devote the rest of the publication to dismantling it. For example, the *Boston Globe*'s 2011 "Salute to Nurses" supplement led off with an article titled "The New Nursing Landscape: Nurses Extend Influence throughout Medical Community." The article talked about "the sweeping changes that have transformed the nursing profession over the past decade." It asserted that shared hospital governance gives today's nurses more control over staffing, scheduling, policies, and procedures. It cited research on the perils of understaffed hospitals and stated that nurses have "fabulous ideas" for reducing the cost and improving the quality and safety of patient care. "Nurses today are better educated, more respected, and more tech-savvy than ever," it declared.[5]

However, the banner headline that ran across the top of the front page captured what the supplement was really about: "Stories That Warm the Heart: Nurses Who Were There When It Mattered Most." That take on nursing prevailed in the rest of the publication. Once again Educated, Respected, and Savvy Nurse was transformed into Real, Real, Real Nice Nurse in such headlines as "Amy's Friends," "A Big Heart," "Blood Sisters," "Nurturing Patient and Family," "Labor, Delivery, and Love," "HIV, Hugs, and Healing," "A Friend to Our Mother," "A Gentle Messenger," "A Gentle Teacher," "A Cheerful Presence," "Holding the Smallest Hands," and "A Port in the Storm."

The *Boston Globe*'s 2012 "Salute to Nurses" repeated the pattern. Its front-page article, "Nursing through the Decades" asserted that nursing involves science as well as art. It discussed the Institute of Medicine's report *The Future of Nursing* that calls for nurses' contributions to be more fully used in our health care system. However, the banner across the top of the front page read, "The Drama of the Simple Gesture: Stories of Nurses Whose Actions Speak the Language of Compassion." In this positioning, the simple gesture trumps the science.[6]

There are so many messages that counterpose nursing science and nursing compassion that it's not surprising that patients and others who nominate nurses for salutes or awards pick up on them. In some of these stories, knowledge is cast as almost a threat to compassion and kindness. As one patient said of a critical care nurse, she "had it all: an unbelieveable clinical and didactic base tempered with everything that is good and right with nursing."[7] It's hard to imagine a patient saying that of a physician. A physician would be lauded for being both knowledgable and caring. In the case of the nurse, "everything that is good and right with nursing" functions to "temper" her clinical and didactic skills as though they might be dangerously strong.

Nurses Week supplements seem to specialize in this kind of disconnect. The *Virginia-Pilot*'s 2012 supplement contained an interesting story about neonatal nurse–researcher Ashlynn Baker, who cares for premature infants *and* does data collection and analysis to develop better protocols for treating newborn infants. The headline on the article boils this down to "Child's Play: Ashlynn Baker Makes Pediatric Nursing Look Easy."[8]

From the four posed photographs on the front page of the *Virginian-Pilot* supplement, you would not learn that nurses do anything of significance, much less complex care and research. One of the photos shows a nurse smiling at a patient; another has five nurses smiling into the camera; the third shows two nurses hovering over a child patient, one of them stroking the child's hair; and the last presents a nurse smiling at an older patient, her hand resting on the patient's forearm.

The *Portsmouth (Ohio) Daily Times* Nurses Week supplement didn't bother with subtlety in conveying its idea of what is important about nurses. Its cover featured a full-page photo of a nurse with an enormous red heart superimposed on her chest.[9]

Contradictory messages are so prevalent that one has to wonder if nursing executives and nursing academicians have become contortionists. When they talk among themselves, and certainly at our workshops, they emphasize the key roles that nurses play in clinical outcomes, patient safety, and newer specialities like infomatics, which deals with communicating, managing, and interpreting information. But that take on nursing rarely goes beyond special reports on nursing and often gets undermined elsewhere.

For example, the lead article in the *Boston Globe*'s 2012 supplement asserted that nurses can play a significant role in shaping health care redesign. It quoted Jackie Somerville, chief nursing officer at Boston's Brigham and Women's Hospital, as saying, "The system, and most importantly our patients and their families, need the voice of the nursing community at the table now more than ever. It is critical that every nurse articulates his or her practice, their unique contributions and the skill set that makes them equal partners in the conversation about the future of health care."[10] That may be, but you won't find these "equal partners" articulating their practice or anything else on the Brigham and Women's website. You will be led to believe from the hospital's presentation that health care's science, technology, expertise, and knowledge belong to physicians.

Even more puzzling is the extent to which nursing leaders turn a blind eye to, support, or even actively participate in obscuring or undermining the nursing functions they say are so essential. There is no better example of this than the uncritical adoption of the DAISY awards program by chief nursing officers of health care facilities, by some deans of nursing schools, and by professional nursing organizations. For us the DAISY Award is emblematic of a broader phenomenon that we have come to think of as the Daisy Dilemma: the institutionalizing of an image of nurses that directly contradicts what nurses say they want the public to recognize about their profession.

The DAISY Foundation

The DAISY Foundation was formed in 1999 in memory of J. Patrick Barnes, who died at age thirty-three of complications of the autoimmune disease idiopathic thrombocytopenia purpura (ITP). Right after he passed away, Patrick's family—his father, J. Mark Barnes; his stepmother, Bonnie Barnes; his widow, Tena Barnes; and other relatives—got together to create a nonprofit foundation that would focus on ITP. The acronym DAISY was derived from the last part of the foundation's official name—Foundation for the Elimination of Diseases Attacking the Immune System.

In its application for tax exempt status with the United States Internal Revenue Service, the foundation stated that it would offer "financial, emotional and educational assistance to families who have a member afflicted with an immune system disease." It also planned "to provide support for research to find cures for immune system diseases."[11] However, the family, according to Bonnie Barnes, "very quickly learned that we didn't have the resources or wherewithal to really make a dent in medical research on ITP."[12]

The DAISY Foundation website describes how the family came to focus on nurses: "As we brainstormed what to do in Pat's memory, the one really positive thing we could hold onto from the experience of his eight-week hospitalization was the skillful and amazingly compassionate care he received from his nurses—even when he was totally sedated. When Pat died, we felt compelled to express our profound gratitude to nurses for the work they do for patients and their families every day. This is the primary mission of The DAISY Foundation."[13]

The foundation's mission is stated somewhat differently in the description of its purpose that it filed with the State of Washington and elsewhere:

to "provide a recognition program to support health care organizations' nurse retention and recruitment efforts."[14]

The most visible part of its mission is the DAISY Award for Extraordinary Nurses, created to honor "the super-human work nurses do in direct care of patients and families every day." The foundation has two other programs: a recognition award for instructors in nursing schools, and a small-grants program for nursing research projects that deal with the care of patients with cancer or autoimmune diseases. The nurses' award, however, remains the foundation's centerpiece and its most marketable activity. It has morphed from an expression of gratitude to nurses into a kind of nurse recruitment and retention franchise that is supported financially by corporations that sell products or services to the health care industry and to nurses and that is endorsed by national and international nursing organizations. In 2011, the foundation celebrated its one thousandth health care facility to "commit to the DAISY Award." In October 2012, that number had risen to 1,333 facilities in the United States and six other countries.[15]

DAISY award ceremonies are highly noticeable, standardized events that take place in hospitals and other health care facilities. They are scripted and feature certain commercial products, namely, Cinnabons and Kleenex tissues. Award winners receive a certificate, a small daisy flower pin, and a hand-carved statue named *A Healer's Art*. Most award winners are pictured with their names and institutions on the foundation website along with the text of the nomination that was the basis for their award.

The DAISY home page when we looked at it in 2011 and 2012 was almost a textbook example of how to deprofessionalize professional practice. Snapshots from nurses' awards ceremonies, bracketed by daisies, scrolled across the top of the home page. In one a nurse received a huge bouquet of daisies. Another

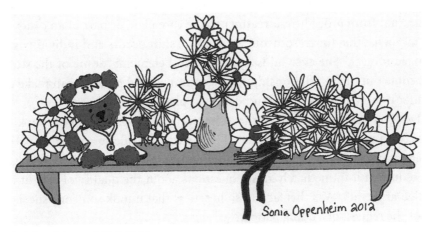

Sonia Oppenheim, www.familycomic.com

featured a nurse with a small child with a daisy headband next to dog wearing a collar of daisies. Another picture showed a glass display case filled with daisies and a teddy bear dressed in a nurse's uniform and cap.[16]

The elements on the home page reflected the image of nursing that the foundation promotes. The Barneses insist that health care facilities signing on to the program "create their own criteria (for the awards) according to their own mission and values and culture of the hospital and nursing practice." The stories that appeared on the website, however, guided anyone nominating a nurse to a preferred constellation of characteristics. The first cue was the header introducing the award winners—"DAISY Was Created to Say Thank You to Nurses Like You." To find out which kind of nurses DAISY values the viewer was told to "read their stories by clicking on their name. Get your Kleenex Ready!"[17]

The theme of the stories is niceness and self-sacrifice. Just as they have been for centuries, women/nurses (and now men/nurses) are recognized for coming in to see a patient on a day off, for spending money on a present for a patient, for organizing a hospital romance, or for getting someone a birthday cake. Like public school teachers who are asked to make up for the deficiencies of the system by working longer hours and spending their own money on supplies, DAISY reinforces the traditional vision of nursing as sacrifice by rewarding nurses who contribute their unpaid labor to the hospital.

In her column in *Nursing Economics*, Kathy Douglas, president of the nonprofit Institute for Staffing Excellence and Innovation, and CNO of API Healthcare, Hartford, Wisconsin (a corporate sponsor of the DAISY Foundation), wrote that the recipient of a DAISY award is expected to "demonstrate great clinical skills and leadership skills, but also a strong sense of compassion for patients and their families." Yet in her article she goes out of her way to downplay the role of clinical skills in "remarkable and life-changing interactions" between a nurse and a patient or a patient's family. She says these occur, "not from procedures, treatments, the care plan, or part of an order set, but moments that touch someone so deeply a shift occurs and individuals are changed forever." She even adds a supernatural element: "Some of the stories that come out of the relationships between nurses and patients can make one wonder if there is not some grand design at play."[18]

Douglas writes that one of her favorite stories is about a "simple act of kindness" by "a nurse who was nominated for getting an elderly and dying patient a plate of fruit" that the patient had been requesting for days. It's an odd story to cite in that it immediately raises questions about the quality of care at that particular facility. Was this facility so heartless that it took someone special to honor the request of a dying patient?

Another story that Douglas cites is about a patient "who claimed his nurse 'saved his life.'" Speaking of the nurse, Douglas writes, "She did not do this by virtue of her clinical excellence. Rather, when he refused to get out of bed after heart surgery to begin his rehab, she came to his room on her day off and would not leave until he got up and took his first steps. Her not very gentle push made him work through his depression and turned his desire to die into a strong will to live." In fact this story could be a perfect example of nurses' clinical knowledge. What brought the nurse back to the hospital was her knowledge of the clinical dangers this patient faced if he did not get up and move. Instead of making the connection between clinical knowledge and the nurse's action, Douglas severed it.

The anecdote is interesting in another regard. When Sean Clarke, a renowned nursing workforce researcher, read this story, his first questions were "Where is the team in this hospital? Where is the plan of care? Why does this patient have to depend on a nurse coming in on her day off to be ambulated? This says very serious things about the standard of care in this hospital."

Sioban Nelson, dean of the faculty of nursing at the University of Toronto and a historian of nursing, had a similar reaction after reading Douglas's article and perusing the foundation website. She posed these question about the DAISY awards: "Why is simple kindness defined as an extraordinary measure? Did these actions really need to have been done by a nurse? So many of these actions could have been equally effective if undertaken by a volunteer. Why do these awards not find that the knowledge and skill that nurses have merit recognition?"

There is no question that many of the stories are touching. They are intended to be. Some do reflect nurses' clinical knowledge and skill. But anyone who looks at the DAISY Foundation website, with its admonition to "get your Kleenex ready!" is being prepared to frame the actions of nurses as virtuous not as knowledgable.

This is obvious in a story about a critical care nurse who works in a trauma/surgical ICU in Illinois. She was nominated by the mother of a boy who had a craniotomy following the discovery of a brain tumor. The mother wrote that when her son was comfortably resting, the nurse came in to check on her. "I sensed she knew all of the things that were going through my mind," the mother said. The two talked about the fall season and compared the snack mixes that they make in fall. Later the surgeon came in with "news that we would rather not hear." At some point, a jar of the nurse's fall snack mix arrived in the room. The mother wrote, "I was so touched that [the nurse] was thinking of us and called in during the middle of her night. I tasted the mix and it was delicious, but I have kept the jar as a reminder of one nurse's special touch. We had great care during our stay, but this kind gesture truly came at a much needed moment."[19]

The DAISY stories often describe actions that a kind person could take. This is different from what the nursing theorist and educator Patricia Benner has called the "skill of involvement"—social and emotional skills that require effort to master and even more to exhibit in the stressful environment of the modern hospital.

DAISY's definition of nursing excellence is the same as the one often promoted during Nurses Week. Except with DAISY it's promoted year round. Mark and Bonnie Barnes have set up the program so that DAISY facilities commit to eight to twelve award ceremonies a year, depending on the size of the staff. Bonnie Barnes says that because "we knew how busy nurses are" the program needed to be "turnkey," meaning that "we would do most of the work," such as supplying the script and the award materials. For chief nursing officers, as one explained to us, the awards program is an inexpensive way to recognize nurses on their staff. Initially the Barneses paid for the award materials. Now facilities that "commit to" the program are charged on average $100 per award, according to the Barneses.

Committees at the facilities seek nominations from patients, family members, and colleagues. The type of story sought, according to Bonnie Barnes, is "all about patient care—not clinical ladder involvement, not academic or certification achievement, or other things that are so important—just great nursing care." She described this as "specific things that a nurse has done to care for a patient whether it is a life-saving clinical act that made a huge difference or some of the smaller things that make a huge difference in the patient experience or the family's experience." An element of the stories, she said, is "the emotion that is caught up in that care delivery."

Some of the stories that are posted on the DAISY website indeed reflect very small things that are suffused with the kind of sentimentality that Nightingale deplored. Although we believe that there is no such thing as a "small thing," when it comes to the care of the sick and vulnerable, DAISY seems to go out of its way to minimize the clinical significance of nurses' actions. For example in 2012, a postanesthesia nurse won an Extraordinary Nurse award for ordering a birthday cake for a patient. "Both the patient and his wife were so grateful for this gesture and attention to detail," the nomination noted.[20]

Bonnie Barnes told us that when the nominations are read at the award ceremony, "usually they are very emotional, particularly because the patient or family has told this story when they were in pain, or joyful over the birth of a baby. There's just a lot of emotional content around great nursing care, at least that's our experience, clinical as well as supportive."

The highly orchestrated ceremony takes place in the unit of the awardee and is often sprung as a surprise to her or him. The stage is set with a seven-foot-long green vinyl congratulatory banner—"a very coveted thing to have in the nursing unit," according to Bonnie—imprinted with the DAISY logo and also the logo of Cinnabon, the DAISY foundation's "premier sponsor." Nursing colleagues decorate the banner with congratulatory messages and, not surprisingly, with daisies. Boxes of Cinnabons (or a reasonable cinnamon bun facimile if the locale lacks a Cinnabon franchise) are on a table.

The ceremony starts with a story about Patrick that describes what happened during the eight weeks that he was hospitalized. If Mark Barnes is present, he tells the story. Otherwise it is read by someone else, preferably by the chief nursing officer or by another hospital executive. The foundation strongly encourages leaders of the facilities to participate.

A key element in the story is the role of Cinnabons. As Mark tells it, "The reason for Cinnabons being served is that when Pat was in the hospital he wasn't eating anything at all. We tried everything to get him to eat. He had no appetite. I brought a Cinnabon in for myself one morning and he asked for a bite of it. Then he ate the whole thing. That night he said, 'Please bring me one in the morning and make sure you bring enough for all my nurses.' So that has been Pat's gift to his nurses."

There is another reason, he told us, for serving Cinnabons, and that is "to celebrate teamwork . . . so that everybody in the unit can share in the kind of feel-good moment with that particular nurse."

The emotional tone set by Patrick's story continues with the reading of the winning nomination. Often the patient, family member, or colleague who wrote the story is present to read it. "And that can be," Bonnie says, "of course, a tremendous reunion for the nurse (and the patient and family) and again emotionally packed." The ceremony so reliably produces tears that the Barneses sought and won sponsorship from the Kimberly-Clark corporation, which provides small packets of Kleenex bearing congratulatory stickers. Hence the special mention of Kleenex (rather than tissues) on the foundation's homepage.

The equation of nursing and feminine emotionality is reinforced in the presentation of the three DAISY gifts to the awardee. One is the daisy pin. Another is a certificate "presented in a beautiful portfolio" that reads, "The DAISY Award for Extraordinary Nurses: In deep appreciation of all you do, who you are, and the incredibly meaningful difference you make in the lives of so many people." It is signed by an executive of the facility and by Mark Barnes. The certificate carries the DAISY logo and that of the American Organization of Nurse Executives (AONE). It notes that the award is "in collaboration with AONE, the voice of nursing leadership."

The third gift is a hand-carved sculpture from Zimbabwe representing a large and a small figure with entwined arms. According to the Barneses, the foundation employs fourteen artisans full-time in that impoverished country to create these sculptures in a classic Shona design called *Mother and Child*. Although mothering and the provision of professional health care are entirely distinct, the Barneses renamed the design *A Healer's Touch*. "When we saw it (the Shona sculpture) we thought it was just a perfect representation of the relationship between nurses and patients, going both ways," Bonnie told us. If that is so, then the sculpture suggests that the patient is at times the mother figure and the nurse the child, implying that it can be the nurse who needs care from the patient. This hardly portrays nurses in a serious professional light. In fact, a reversal of roles between the nurse and the patient, or even a confusion about the needs of the nurse and those of the patient, can constitute a professional boundary violation, according to the National Council of State Boards of Nursing.[21]

Furthermore, this view of nursing as a maternal activity also disempowers the patient by casting the patient as a baby. Dominick Frosch of the Palo Alto Medical Foundation Research Institute and principal investigator for studies on patient involvement in clinical decision making, told us that the mother-baby image "reflects a very antiquated view of the relationship between patients and doctors, nurses and other members of the healthcare team." It harkens back to the kind of thinking prevalent in the 1950s and '60s, when the sociologist Talcott Parsons elaborated his conception of the "sick role." "This view," Frosch explained to us, "held that patients were excused from normal social and professional obligations because they are ill. To be excused from these obligations, however, they must submit to the directives of the physician—or other healthcare professional. This no longer reflects modern thinking." He said that modern health care thinking and today's patient advocates encourage patients to play a greater role in decision making and to take more responsibility for their care.

Cinnabons assume a pivotal role at the end of the award ceremonies. The Barneses are convinced from nurses responses—"I was just doing my job"—that nurses don't grasp the "meaningful difference" that an act of theirs has made in the life of a patient. Nurses thus are urged to use the smell of Cinnabons in a mall or airport as a cue for them to "stop for a moment and remind themselves that they are special people that are making a difference in the lives of others."

This positioning is quite extraordinary given the connection junk food has to one of the most serious health crises in history—the obesity epidemic. Hospitals have long been criticized for the kind of food they serve patients and staff. Today, with over 30 percent of the American public obese, it seems mind-boggling to place Cinnabons center stage in hospital award ceremonies and link the product to nurses' self esteem. The public might well wonder why a profession that claims to have a leadership role in health promotion and disease prevention would even consider such a thing. According to Science in the Public Interest, a single classic Cinnabon has 880 calories, more saturated fat than many popular bacon cheeseburgers, and 830 mg of sodium (the total recommended daily intake of sodium is less than 2400 mg).[22] Why would the AONE, the American and Canadian Associations of Critical-Care Nurses, the American Association of Colleges of Nursing, the Emergency Nurses Association, the National League for Nursing, Sigma Theta Tau International, and Advancing Men in Nursing, all of which are listed as "supportive associations" on the DAISY website, condone an association between their profession and this product?

The issue goes beyond what this symbolizes to patients and the public. Nurses' job stress and shift work put them especially at risk for obesity, according to researchers at the University of Maryland School of Nursing who found that 55 percent of nurses in a survey group were overweight or obese,[23] a condition linked to diabetes and heart disease among other illnesses. The authors of the study specifically recommended that healthful food be more widely available in the workplace and that nurses have sufficient time to consume it.

Bringing Cinnabons into health care facilities, associating them with a "feel good moment," and urging attention to their smell is more likely to lead nurses to food cravings than to self esteem. The physician David A. Kessler, a former U.S. Food and Drug Administration (FDA) commissioner, defines craving as "cue-induced wanting" in his book, *The End of Overeating: Taking Control of the Insatiable America Appetite*. He says that humans are already wired to enjoy and seek foods with high amounts of sugar, fat, and salt even in the absence of hunger. But there is a difference between liking a food and *pursuing* it. Cues associated with pleasure can strengthen our focus on a particular food and our pursuit of it. "Along with taste and other sensory characteristics, the location where the food has previously been available and the events associated with past consumption can be reinforcers," Kessler writes. "In time, these cues become as important in food-seeking behavior as the food itself."[24]

Food corporations are well aware of the factors that get people hooked on their products. They put them into effect by increasing the amounts of sugar, fat, and salt in their foods, increasing portion sizes, making the foods readily available, and associating them with certain places and with pleasurable events. It's a real marketing coup for Cinnabon to be able to move from the mall to the hospital and to become the food mascot for nurse recognition ceremonies.

For his book, Kessler interviewed Jerilyn Brusseau, the woman who created the Cinnabon and who worked assiduously to enhance its appeal. Ironically, she told him that she'd "probably think differently" about creating the product today. "I'm very concerned that kids are growing up eating too many things like Cinnabons every day of their lives," she said.[25]

Carla Wolper, a professor in the Eating Disorders Research Unit of Columbia University College of Physicians and Surgeons, and a dietician who works with the "super-obese," told us that she saw the Cinnabon sponsorship as another example of how the food industry uses charitable giving to expand its market, in this case to some three million nurses in the United States alone. "You would think that nurses would be intelligent enough to pick another symbol," she said.

Some nurses also have second thoughts about the product. When one nurse learned that each classic Cinnabon has almost 900 calories—almost half the daily caloric requirement of the average adult—she told us, "Why don't they just give us a gun so we can put it to our heads and shoot ourselves?"

The Barneses are aware of criticism about the Cinnabons. Bonnie finesses it by suggesting that nurses can just use cinnamon, "a very healthful spice," as a sensory trigger to appreciate "how special you are because you are a nurse." The concern about Cinnabons is mitigated, they say, when people understand their role in the context of Patrick's story. The fact that a dying patient ate Cinnabons when he could eat nothing else is, of course, entirely different from promoting Cinnabons to nurses as does the DAISY homepage. During Nurses Week, the first thing that came up on its link to Cinnabon was an offer of free Cinnabons for nurses.

Some observers see the DAISY award as trivializing the practice of nursing by emphasizing the "little things" that nurses do to the neglect of the big things. That is the view of Isabel Marcus, a legal scholar who teaches at the State University of New York at Buffalo, who had a double mastectomy after she was diagnosed with breast cancer. Each week for four months Marcus received chemotherapy from nurses in a Buffalo hospital. What impressed her was the nurses' knowledge.

"Every time I go for chemo, I talk with the nurses at great length about patients' responses to the chemo process," she told us. "They are a fount of useful, insightful, and thoughtful information, which, I suspect, if they are not asked to give, they may feel unwilling to put forth. They explain the physiological processes affected by my chemo so beautifully and intelligently."

When we asked Marcus if she would consider nominating one of these nurses for a DAISY award she was aghast. "Never!" she replied. "It seems so silly and superficial. I wrote letters to the head of the oncology department to tell this physician what an extraordinary unit the oncology nursing department was and how nurses shared their knowledge, expertise, and experience with me. I told her they were always willing to talk about concerns I had. They didn't just provide cut-and-dried answers to my questions but engaged in discussion with me and often used examples from their experience. It was nice that the nurses were kind and supportive, but remembering my name and asking me how I was feeling was only the first step in creating the context in which they could provide much needed information from their years of experience. Most had been on that unit for at least ten or twelve years."

Cynthia Enloe, research professor of politics and women's studies at Clark University in Worcester, Massachusetts, told us, "The DAISY awards look like a very organized process of trivialization. Nursing is a profession that has been historically feminized. Part of that 'feminization' involves asking nurses to work very hard but to not take their expertise seriously. One should be content to be seen as good, virtuous, and dutiful, but not as serious in the sense of having expertise that one has put into nursing practice. This Cinnabon ceremony just plows that process even deeper and makes nurses complicit in the process. Nurses have been socialized to feel that through this trivialization, they are actually being rewarded and acknowledged. But they are being acknowledged only in the safest and narrowest patriarchal zone of the trivialized caretaker." Enloe, who has a forthcoming book about who and what are taken seriously in our society, poses a relevant question: "Would you ever consider giving these kinds of awards to a surgeon?"

In contrast, the Barneses receive positive feedback from nurses in response to the DAISY awards. Mark says that nurses tell him, "Thank you for reminding me why I became a nurse." This kind of assent may be expresed in what the sociologist Erving Goffman would call the "public space" of the award ceremony.[26] In "backstage and private spaces," it turns out, not every nurse is so uniformly grateful to DAISY. "I told the manager that I really didn't like all these flowers, and teddy bears, and statues of mothers and babies," a male nurse told us at a recent conference. Although Advancing Men in Nursing is an organizational supporter of the DAISY awards, this nurse does not concur with its endorsement. "I mean, what kind of message does this send to men in nursing?" he asked. "I was told by my manager to stop being such a hard-ass."

Another nurse said she dislikes the DAISY paraphernalia and has raised the issue in her hospital. She said her comments were not well received by managers and she was essentially told to keep them to herself. One nurse bemoaned the fact that two nurses at her hospital who received the award for leaving work to buy a present for a patient, had actually left their colleagues to shoulder heavy patient loads while they went shopping.

One staff nurse whose hospital has signed on to DAISY explained, "When you focus on what they're giving out, it's awful. But most of us don't consider the content. We just think, 'Oh, that's nice, another attempt to recognize nurses. Great.' So this becomes another example of how we let others define how we talk about ourselves and don't think enough about the implications."

A hospital CNO told us she finds it difficult to counter the DAISY sentiments and images even though she finds them demeaning. "But what can you do to object to this?" she asked. "It makes it seem as though you are against recognizing nurses. So I kind of ignore the DAISY stuff, hope no one will notice, and just try to focus on nursing excellence."

The Barneses worked in advertising and marketing prior to running the DAISY program. Although they present themselves as having been naive about nursing, they have become sophisticated about selling the DAISY awards to employers as a low-cost tool for improving organizations' ability to recruit and retain nurses. A review of studies on the impact of recognition programs on employee performance that was done gratis for the foundation in 2009 butresses their claim that the DAISY awards can help employers with their staffing issues. The review was coauthored by Cindy Lefton, a nurse and PhD who is with Psychological Associates in St. Louis, "a firm of behavioral scientists who apply behavioral science principles to the work place to improve staff performance." Lefton's report explains that "meaningful recognition has been linked to such positive outcomes as job satisfaction, organizational and career commitment, cohesion and collaboration, and perceived organizational support. A lack of meaningful recognition has been linked to negative outcomes such as absenteeism and turnover, stress and burnout, and decreased quality of patient care."[27] The DAISY foundation borrowed the term "meaningful recognition" from the AACN's (American Association of Critical-Care Nurses) list of six "Standards for Establishing and Sustaining Healthy Work Environments."[28] The foundation emphasizes the "meaningful" part of its recognition program presumably to differentiate it from employee-of-the-month type programs associated with fast-food franchises and supermarkets.

Although studies have found that other factors such as competitive wages contribute to lower turnover and job satisfaction, Lefton's literature review focuses only on the outcomes of recognition programs. At one point it warns that "recognition can become an entitlement instead of an extra gesture of appreciation," and that "communication regarding why the recognition was given should be clear to all." It cites a 1994 study on public posting recognition programs entitled "How about a Lollipop? A Peer Recognition Program." It found that employers could save from $600 to $105,000 a year on personnel costs by adopting such a program. We don't know what the savings would be in

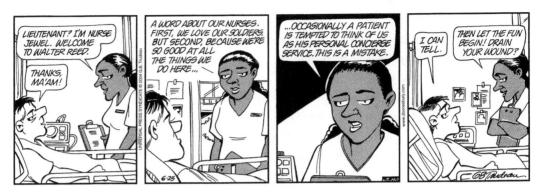

today's dollars. The study did note that "return on investment will be easier to achieve with cheaper recognition programs."

One of the questions raised by nurses' recognition programs is whose interests do they serve? In its presentations, the DAISY Foundation has described its awards program as "meeting strategic needs of hospitals." Kathy Douglas, in her *Nursing Economics* article, states: "The DAISY Award is focusing attention on the specific behaviors administrators want to encourage to bring the organization's vision and values to life." To that end, Cindy Lefton headed a study to identify the themes or behaviors that were prevalent in the stories about the DAISY award winners with the idea that they might be used to model behavior in the workplace. When we went to press, the content analysis was being prepared for publication under the title "Impact of the DAISY Award on Nurses' Perceptions of Their Work Environment."

To enhance the perception of nursing work, Kathy Douglas, who has defined the role of the DAISY awards in her writing, directed a documentary film on nursing entitled, "Nurses: If Florence Could See Us Now." The film, completed just as this book was going to press, was produced by On Nursing Excellence (ONE), a nonprofit organization that Douglas founded in 2009 to "expand the effectiveness, efficiency, well being, and recognition of the healthcare workforce."[29] In an interview about the film, Douglas was quoted as saying, "It's really important that everyone—from policymakers to the public—understands who nurses are and what we do. It's essential that they comprehend this as we form our future in healthcare." Douglas said she had three goals for the film: "to help people understand what it means to be a nurse; to bring out the realities of nursing and how it touches people's lives; and to show nurses how beautiful and powerful they are."[30]

More than one hundred nurses from nine states were interviewed for the feature-length documentary. According to Douglas, "There was no scripting or prepping. We showed up with a camera and had candid conversations. It's authentic and real." Douglas said in her description of the work that it was not easy to identify nurses to interview for the film. But she thanked the Barneses for making it easier by providing a select group of candidates to choose from—DAISY award winners.[31]

As a U.S. tax-exempt 501(C)3 organization, ONE, like the DAISY Foundation, functions as a charity in that corporations and individuals that fund them get a tax break for their contributions. The film, according to ONE's website, was financed by contributions from a long list of health care industry consultants, vendors, insurers, medical centers, and nursing organizations (some of which also support DAISY Foundation activities). ONE also solicited small donations via Indiegogo, a website that people use to raise money for their projects. The film premiered October 11, 2012, during the American Nurses Credentialing Center (ANCC) National Magnet Conference in Los Angeles.

API Healthcare, a DAISY Foundation sponsor that bills itself as the largest health care vendor of workforce management solutions, was a leading supporter of the film. Douglas is chief nursing officer at API. Although the film's promotional representative at API encouraged us to write about the it, our requests to view the actual documentary were not fulfilled. We were able to view online promotions for the film including a poster and the trailer.

The poster for the film shows an attractive smiling nurse hugging a toddler who wears a purple headband decorated with an enormous flower. The trailer for the film opens with a soft female voice saying: "It is hard to find a person whose life has not been touched by a nurse." With soothing music playing in the background, we are told that nurses are there "at our birth . . . through wellness, illness, recovery, and loss." Then a nurse describes a spiritual function of nurses: "It's being able to bear witness to that couple who's had a baby and it's not the perfect baby or the baby dies. Or a young woman who's just finished her college degree and got her first job and she feels a lump in her breast, she's 29 or 30 and you tell her she's got cancer."

The trailer asks: "How much do we know about these people (nurses) who beome a vital part of some of the most difficult and intimate moments in the human experience? Who are nurses? What do they really do?" Most people have a difficult time describing what nurses do, it says. Therefore, "it seems easier to describe the way they make people feel. They might use words like compassionate, caring, and supportive."

We then learn that, "Nursing is critical because we don't put barriers on how we engage. You can do this work and you can engage at a visceral soul-to-soul level in a therapeutic way." A man with a stethoscope on his neck refers to a woman who "changed my path in my life." It is not clear if he is a nurse describing a patient or a patient describing a nurse. His words are accompanied by an image of someone placing what looks like Buddhist prayer beads on another person's wrist.

The trailer does acknowledge that the feelings nursing engender are based "on science, critical thinking, clinical judgment, communication, research, education, leadership, and innovation." The trailer then undercuts the concept of nursing as knowledge by concluding with a question, "Is nursing a job, a profession, a calling?"[32]

If the trailer is a true preview, it seems that *Nurses* is a film that is firmly anchored in the tradition of nursing's comfortable and ostensibly comforting virtue script. For nurses, it may be compelling to see themselves projected on the screen doing soul work instead of some of the work they actually do. But along with raising the question of professional boundaries, the trailer's depiction of nursing distorts reality in terms of the demands made on nurses in stressful workplaces.

A serious question is how do these recognition activities that idealize nurses affect nurses' workplaces? Do they lead to a deeper understanding of nursing so that those in charge can supply the resources that nurses need to give quality care? Or do they function to simultaneously make up for and reinforce nurses' invisiblity within their larger institutions? Genuine recognition, for nurses' real—rather than idealized—work, still eludes nursing within the majority of institutions in which nurses work. Like Nurses Week itself, idealized recognition produces a kind of placebo effect, convincing nurses that something is really being done to acknowledge their work, when they may, in fact, be receiving a sugar pill.

The DAISY awards and the film *Nurses* appear to be a springboard to a number of workplace and staffing consultanting services including Douglas's ONE spinoff, the Institute for Staffing Excellence and Innovation, which describes itself as "your non-profit resource for healthcare staffing."[33] Over the past twenty-five years, nurses have had ample experience with workplace engineers, not all of it to their or to their patients' benefit. Will the DAISY awards and the *Nurses* film convince health care consultants to recommend more resources for nurses' "soul-to-soul" work, or will this new rendition of the virtue script simply justify business as usual?

As for the DAISY Foundation, it has mushroomed from a modest mom-and-pop project into an assertive revenue-raising operation with increasing clout with nurses, health care facilities, and the corporate world. Its national sponsors, in addition to Cinnabon, listed on the foundation home page, include API Healthcare; Cherokee, a health care worker's apparel company; GetWellNetwork, a patient care consulting company; Hill-Rom, a medical equipment and device company; Kimberly-Clark, a maker of health care products as well as consumer paper products; NIH Federal Credit Union, which bills itself as "the nation's largest credit union serving the biomedical industry"; and Wells Fargo, a bank.[34]

The Barneses say they visit some fifty to a hundred health care facilities each year where they do presentations, meet with DAISY award committees and nurses who have won DAISY awards, and consult with nurse executives on staffing concerns. Bonnie Barnes said that when they travel, "we usually have at least one sponsor with us so that they can experience the DAISY award. We want them to see nurses as we see nurses, not as users of their products but as partners in celebrating their work." She said the couple particularly enjoys having the salespeople from Kimberly-Clark and GetWell Networks accompany them.

Presumably sponsors also use these ceremonies to make contacts with executives at the facilities and to refine their sales approaches. When we asked the Barneses what the companies get from their contributions to the DAISY Foundation, Bonnie put the benefits firmly into an idealistic DAISY context. "Of course they get something out of it," she said. "They know the award is a beloved program in so many facilties and they feel that being associated with us is good for their brand." But, she added, "they also get something else. Many of the salespeople at Kimberly-Clark will tell us at the end of a sales presentation, they feel so good, it reminds them of why they're in the business they're in. It's not just about selling a drape for an operating room. It reminds them that there's a patient on that operating table."

Your Turn

Suppose a foundation, corporation, or family offers to set up a program at your facility to honor nurses for "all the good things that they do." What criteria do you establish for "the good things?"

Johnson & Johnson

In recent years, corporations have been targeting their charitable support toward activities that are in sync with their business goals. In business, charitable contributions are more and more seen as social investments that are expected to bring quantifiable returns to the corporation. Johnson & Johnson—a holding company of some 250 subsidiaries in sixty countries that produces pharmaceuticals, medical devices, and consumer products—has formed this sort of association with nursing through its Campaign for Nursing's Future. Launched in 2002, the campaign outlined an ambitious strategy to improve public understanding of nursing and attract and recruit more people into the profession. Since its launch with TV advertisements in the 2002 Winter Olympics, the campaign, by its tenth anniversary in 2012, had expanded into a multi-activity, multimedia blitz, all of which can be accessed through a nursing website, Discovernursing.com, that is unequaled in scope.

Among the campaign's offerings are free brochures, posters, bumper stickers, car magnets, "Be-a-Nurse" T-shirts, and other promotional items; nurse recruitment television commercials; video profiles of working nurses packaged in a "Day in the Life" series on YouTube; "You Can Be a Nurse" coloring books for children and "Nursing Gang," videos for middle schoolers; a Facebook fan page for the monthly newsletter *Nursing Notes*, with spaces on the page's wall for comments, Twitter messages; nursing games and apps; "Maintaining the Magic of Nursing" conferences for nursing students; regional fund-raising galas to raise money for "undergraduate student scholarships, nurse educator fellowships, and capacity expansion grants for nursing programs"; and, to celebrate the project's tenth anniversary, a "Portrait of Thanks Project," a photo mosaic of ten thousand photos of nurses—all smiling—because "your smile will help nursing students get a picture perfect start."[35]

Through these and other efforts, Johnson & Johnson, or J&J, has created a network of involvement with almost every stakeholder in nursing—professional organizations, nursing administrators, nursing educators and researchers, and nursing media. Among the nursing organizations and schools of nursing that have allied themselves closely with the campaign are the American Nurses Association, the American Association of Critical-Care Nurses, the American Hospital Association and its close affiliate the American Organization of Nurse Executives, the American Association of Colleges of Nursing, Sigma Theta Tau International, Vanderbilt University, the National League for Nursing, the American Student Nurses Association, the American Academy of Nursing, and *Nursing Spectrum*.

The stated goal of the J&J campaign is to end a worrisome nursing shortage. Using a practice that is common in the pharmaceutical industry, the company funded research on the efficacy of its own product—in this case the Campaign for Nursing's Future and its success in heightening awareness of J&J among those who might be a position to send business its way.

In their research on the campaign, Peter Buerhaus of Vanderbilt University and his colleagues surveyed nurses and asked them how they reacted to campaign images. Most were delighted that their public profile was being raised and reacted positively to the image of the nurse who makes a difference every day. Some nurses reported that they have a more positive feeling about nursing as a result of the campaign. One of the other questions the J&J-sponsored research posed was whether nurses were aware of the identity of the corporate sponsor of the Campaign for Nursing's Future. Close to one-third of RNs surveyed accurately identified J&J by name, while two-thirds of CNOs did so. Of the CNOs who identified J&J's sponsorship, 91 percent had a "positive attitude toward private companies that sponsor these initiatives."[36]

The company used these research findings to claim that its campaign (and thus J&J) has been instrumental in "making headway" toward ending the nursing shortage. In two progress reports, J&J takes credit for increasing public interest in the profession, increasing nursing school enrollments, and encouraging "more people than ever before to go back to school to enter nursing," as well as for creating a "growing optimism among the nursing profession."[37] The company claims, "Nursing school enrollment numbers are up; more nurses than ever are becoming nurse educators; and we're spreading the word in larger numbers than ever about the nursing profession."[38]

J&J is indeed spreading the word about nursing. The question is what message is it spreading?

The Campaign for Nursing's Future intentionally uses emotional and feel-good images to market nursing. An article about the strategy of Andrea Higham, J&J's director of corporate equity and nursing campaign, listed the following steps:

- "Attempt to make an emotional connection with your audience first. Decisions are ultimately made when *emotions* are changed, not just *thinking*.
- Once the emotional connection is forged, add only a few more factual selling points, such as the knowledge and skills required for the career and the variety of career paths available.
- Emphasize the opportunities and job stability, not the workforce shortage.
- Use images that assist students in identifying and visualizing themselves in the shoes of a nurse.
- Use "content-lite" materials for initial encounters as information overload can be an intimidating deterrent to learning more.[39]

Although the approach is supposedly "content-lite," its messages are content heavy in terms of their implications for nursing. Because the campaign wants its audiences to make a positive emotional connection with nursing (and J&J, by association), its messages simplify the complexity of nurses' work and sugarcoat the realities of the delivery of patient care in the contemporary nursing workplace. The campaign also portrays nurses as modern-day angels of mercy, angels who are perhaps a bit smarter than average, but who remain on the job because of their "natural" altruistic inclinations. For example, in one TV spot, a patient is lying in a hospital bed attached to myriad tubes and lines. The patient looks very sick indeed. A nurse walks up the bedside. What does she do? She puts a pair of headphones over his ears.

In a 2007 spot, a group of nurses take care of several patients. As in many of the ads, nurses are shown in action, skillfully employing all manner of high-tech equipment. The final image is of a nurse hugging a patient. One voice-over states that nurses save lives, make lives easier, and make a difference. Another voice sings lines from an alternate script—"You're the one who's born to care. Seems you've always been right there . . . making smiles appear again. You're a nurse; you make a difference."

In another spot about emergency room nurses, a nurse races to a man who's brought in on a stretcher, and manipulates high-tech equipment in his care. As the team is cutting away his clothing, a set of keys, a dime, and a four-leaf clover pendant fall from the patient's pocket onto the stretcher. The nurse's voice explains, "I'm a nurse, I believe in the power of science and medicine." The nurse approaches the bedside of the intubated patient and says, "But I'm also a human and I believe in stacking the deck" as she presses the four-leaf clover into his hand.

In their "Patient's Perspectives" videos, available on DVD and on YouTube, various patients talk about their experiences with nurses. The nurses are credited with having knowledge and skills. The dominant discourse is, however, one of comfort and support. To the patients who speak here, the nurses are "friends" who will always be a part of their lives, as though nurses' primary work is to bond with patients and forge lasting relationships rather than save lives and prevent complications.

A video directed toward middle school children titled "The Nursing Gang," repeats these themes. The video's introduction features a cartoon character and the words "Making a Difference Everyday, and Never Stop Caring.[40] Then you see Kiki ER Nurse, Danny Pediatric Nurse, Ashleigh Visiting Nurse, and DeVaugh OR Nurse. DeVaughn spies on a child in a waiting room. He sees "someone looking really down" and goes into nursing action. "I want to let them understand that I want to lend a helping hand/We sit and talk for just a while, and soon I see a smile/ Yeah, yeah, making a difference every day/ With everything we do and say."

The other nurses work with a child whose arm is bandaged and with an old woman at home. The jingle tells us, "Walking in someone else's shoes, you can feel their hurt, you can feel their blues." As the nurses play ball or hug their patients, DeVaughn tells us that "showing you care is what I've found to really turn a life around." The jingle goes on with "Just trying to help a friend, keeping an open heart, that's the way to start." The video continues with its refrain, "Making a difference every day, with everything you do and say." When the cartoon characters and their patients dance together, the following flashes across the screen to describe nurses: "They're cool, They're smart. They're the best of friends."

Johnson & Johnson and its campaign advocates say they are trying to transform the public image of nursing. The words and images analyzed above, however, repeat every societal stereotype about nursing and then add some. In its major public offerings, nursing is depicted as not brain work but heart work. Nurses' psychosocial work, which is enormously complex cognitive work, is reduced to hugs and smiles—to providing a helping hand, or being the best of friends—as if patients need nursing care because they all have a friendship disorder.

Unlike medicine's promotional advertising—and DAISY's—where real physicians and nurses are identified by their last names and titles, none of the nurses featured in the J&J campaign are identified with their last names. In the "Profiles in Nursing" on the home page of the campaign's website, nurses are labeled kindergarten style, with a first name and last initial—Paula D. or Andre P. This naming practice, as we will discuss in chapter 4, places nurses lower on the health care hierarchy than physicians and gives the profiles of real nurses a juvenile tone.

The campaign's main themes have changed very little over time. Additions to the campaign include well-designed bios of working nurses in which nurses talk about the satisfaction of their own work and their own well-rounded lives. The recipe also includes a nice dose of high-action nursing heroism. Underlying the positive aspects of the campaign is a subscript that is expressed in the repeating jingle, "The care you give comes naturally; you dare to care, dare to cry, dare to heal, dare to try." The campaign's underlying theme is a sophisticated version of nursing's nineteenth-century-virtue script, disguised in twenty-first-century production values.

Nursing Shortage

In both their research and campaign materials, J&J ignores the main drivers of the nursing shortage. While the shortage is exacerbated by poor public understanding of nursing, research strongly indicates that the shortage is fundamentally a product of the kinds of conditions under which nurses work today. Whether in hospitals, home care, schools, rehabilitation facilities, nursing homes, community clinics, or psychiatric institutions, nurses work in settings that increasingly fragment nursing care duties in order to wrest them from higher-paid, more highly educated personnel so that they can be performed by cheaper, less educated staff. Nursing hours have been extended alarmingly so that, as studies document, nurses are routinely working thirteen-plus-hour days, which produces more medical errors and injuries and more health problems for nurses who do not get enough rest.[41] As patient acuity has increased because of reductions in length of stay, nurses are also caring for more, and sicker, patients. Many nurses shoulder unbearable workloads and suffer from more stress-related illnesses than other professionals. As patients have got progressively heavier, most hospitals continue to refuse to purchase the kind of lift equipment that has proved to be cost effective and could make nursing work safer for nurses and their patients; hospitals have also resisted legislation to require it. As a result, nurses—largely women—suffer from more back, neck, and shoulder injuries than those of men who work in construction, baggage handling, and even shipping. Indeed, studies estimate that the average hospital loses between 6 to 11 percent of RNs every year because of musculoskeletal injuries. This higher percentage often represents the number of extra nurses it would take to end nursing shortages. Similar conditions apply in every setting in which nurses work—including schools, nursing homes, home care, community clinics and rehabilitation facilities, and even in primary care and other facilities that employ advanced practice nurses.

Having spoken with thousands of nurses over the past twenty-five years, we know that most nurses actually love nursing. They feel very positive toward their profession. What they don't like are the conditions under which they are forced to practice in the contemporary market-driven nursing workplace—where an obsession with speed-up, through-put, and cost cutting has assembly-lined care and made it difficult for nurses to feel that they are putting their hard-won knowledge and skills into practice. It's the classic case of loving your work and hating your job. That is why many nurses discourage younger people—even their own children—from going into nursing.

In a fascinating study on why people enter the nursing profession, professors of business and management and of nursing surveyed nurses in the first year of a university baccalaureate nursing program. They discovered that the group they surveyed was almost evenly divided between what they called "traditionals" and "instrumentals." Traditionals went into nursing because they wanted to be in a profession that "provided the opportunity to make a difference by helping others."[42] These people "prefer nursing because it provides tangible evidence of positive outcomes."[43] The other half, the instrumentals, were interested in another set of tangible rewards—economic stability, job security, and mobility.[44] All those who chose nursing said it was "important for them to see tangible and timely connections between their activities at work and positive outcomes for patients."[45] This sense of efficacy was equally important to both groups, as was having some independence on the job.

Since health care reengineering began in the mid-1990s, a majority of nurses surveyed over the past decade or more have repeatedly stated that "tangible and timely connections between their activities at work and positive outcomes for patients" has been compromised. A profession that has long been plagued by subordinate status is now not only subordinate to medicine and hospital administration but also to health care consultants who are trying to micromanage and even script nurse-patient encounters. In spite of reports of nursing shortages, employers are cutting nursing jobs and replacing nurses with lower-skilled, lower-paid workers, which is why one nurse responded to an article that Peter Buerhaus and his colleagues did in *Health Affairs* discussing employment opportunities for nurses, with the following letter to the editor.

> I have experienced some new caveats to our current situation that I believe may be of interest. I graduated May 2008 with my BSN in Northern California and did everything by the book (hundreds of apps, spoke with managers, thank you notes, ACLS, BLS, professional resume, LTC, SNF, etc.) and was unable to locate employment. When an offer was made, my children and I relocated to a rural town four hours away. Sadly, after four months of orientation, I was told I "failed orientation" and they needed an experienced RN. My children and I moved again. Recently I applied to a Versant New Grad Residency. I made it through their first round of interviews but was told that I was no longer a "New Grad" due to my previous four months of experience!
>
> So, not only am I not experienced enough to work as a staff nurse, but I am no longer considered a New Grad! So, where do I fit in? I feel that if I cannot get into a New Grad program I will have the same unstructured learning demands and unrealistic expectations placed on me similar to my first failed hospital experience. It also appears that the longer it takes for me to find employment, the more reservations the employers have towards me.
>
> I have researched my situation. It appears my peers from nursing school are experiencing similar situations. www.allnurses.com, an all-nurses Web site, further elaborates that my situation is happening all over the U.S.A. to new nursing graduates.[46]

On the Allnurses.com website, one new nurse explained why so many choose to leave the hospital or even the profession: "So finally, I'm a new grad day shift RN working on a cardiac progressive care unit. It's been almost 6 months and

I'm beginning to really dread going to work. I didn't want to do med-surg because I wanted a challenge and now I'm beginning to regret it. At work, I'm so overwhelmed and I have so much to do that I never take breaks and I eat really late lunches. And even then I get interrupted during lunch. . . . I switched from my previous career to pursue nursing and now I'm beginning to wonder if I had made the right choice."[47]

In its progress reports, J&J suggests that its campaign is having a positive effect on remedying the nursing shortage. The implication is that attracting new recruits to the profession and retaining nurses in their jobs is attributable to J&J's efforts. While it is true that more people seem to be interested in nursing, and that people who would have left the profession are choosing to stay rather than retire, this has a lot to do with the state of the U.S. economy. As prominent researchers on and advocates of the campaign wrote in a 2009 study published in the journal *Health Affairs*, hospitals have always increased RN FTE employment during bust periods.[48] The article documents that current surges in RN employment, like those in the past, are recession related and that interest in nursing might not last should the recession end. Once the current economic crisis is over, will nurses decide they want to stay on the job? If the campaign is having such a positive effect, why do so many new nursing school graduates continue to leave the workforce after just one year?

Over the past decade, J&J has put at least seventy million dollars into nursing. What is a pittance to an international conglomerate (in 2011 alone J&J made over $13 billion) seems like a huge amount of money to a profession that has been so long neglected. Many nurses thus feel grateful for this financial and public relations attention and tend to ignore the reasons why J&J has embraced a profession that survey respondents rate number one in honesty and integrity. Without exception, every message that the Campaign for Nursing's Future puts out is branded with the J&J corporate name and logo. Without exception, when J&J salutes nurses for their goodness, it also salutes itself. Without exception, when J&J improves the public image of nursing, it does the same for itself. J&J's association with nursing may thus have a lot more to do with profits and corporate reputation than altruism.

In fact, the Campaign for Nursing's Future fits the model known as "cause-related marketing", a philanthropic strategy that has grown in scope and sophistication over the past twenty years. It is widely used, according to Samantha King, the author of *Pink Ribbons, Inc.: Breast Cancer and the Politics of Philanthropy*, "because it is understood to

> **Without exception, every message that the Campaign for Nursing's Future puts out is branded with the J&J corporate name and logo.**

accomplish efficiently the integration of a corporation's philanthropic activities with its drive for profit." King writes: "Unlike traditional charity promotions in which a brand or company simply donated money to a cause or sponsored a range of unrelated charities without a coherent strategy, cause-related marketing seeks to ensure that the brand and the cause share the same 'territory' in a 'living, altruistic partnership for mutual benefit.' Thus, since the mid-1990's, cause-related marketing has evolved from what were mostly short-term commitments from corporations to their chosen causes . . . to major, long-term commitments to an issue through an alliance that links the company brand name with the issue in the consumer's mind."[49]

As an article in the *Journal of Marketing* explains, "One of the most basic objectives firms strive to realize by participating in CRMPs (Cause Related Marketing Programs) is to increase the sales of their product." Other objectives include gaining national visibility, thwarting negative publicity, generating incremental sales, promoting repeat purchases, broadening customer base, and increasing and reinforcing brand recognition."[50]

Curt Weeden, as a J&J vice president, was instrumental in 1990 in starting the Wharton (School of Business) Fellows Program for Nurse Executives. "The business purposes were extremely well defined" before launching that program, Weeden told us. Weeden, an expert on corporate philanthropy no longer with J&J, emphasizes in his presentations and writing that there has to be a strong business reason for corporate giving. In his ten-step model for "corporate social investing," the number two step is "Identify a significant business reason for every corporate social investment and obtain as much business value from social investments as is allowable and practical."

Although we generally think of physicians as the chief decision makers when it comes to the purchase of drugs and medical products, nurses make many such recommendations and decisions. J&J's connection to nursing, Weeden explained, came out of what was then J&J's division of hospital services, which marketed "just-in-time" products directly to hospitals. The company's executives realized that the person often making the point-of-sale decision about hospital products was a senior nurse on the unit or at department level rather than a top administrator. When it comes to making a decision about purchasing products that are similar in price, J&J believes it has an edge with the many nurse executives who received J&J-funded fellowships to attend the Wharton program.

J&J's large consumer products division—which sells everything from Band-Aides to Tylenol—also benefits from the company's investment in nursing. In the corporation's analysis of its marketing, said Weeden, "the people who were most responsive to the J&J name were females. All the advertising centered around mothers and babies." Weedon noted that the majority of nurses are women. Thus when J&J expanded its social investment with nursing to its name-enhancing Campaign for Nursing's Future, it also expanded its potential consumer base from CNOs to virtually all of nursing.

From Texaco's sponsorship of the Metropolitan Opera's Saturday afternoon live radio broadcasts, to Kimberly-Clark's support of the American Heart Association, to Exxon Mobile's underwriting of Masterpiece Theatre on PBS, the recipe is tried and true. Bernice Buresh, an opera fan who has been listening to the Metropolitan Opera broadcasts since she was a child, went out of her way to buy gasoline at Texaco stations out of gratitude for Texaco's sixty-three years of sponsorship that made these live broadcasts possible.

J&J could not have found a better vehicle than nursing to help in another aim of cause-related marketing, "thwarting negative publicity." The company that once gained public trust because of its speedy acknowledgment and recall of tainted Tylenol tablets has in recent years been plagued by recurring scandals. Among these are J&J's overseas marketing of its flawed metal-on-metal ASR Hip Resurfacing System even though the FDA refused to approve the use of the device in the United States.[51] Another is the company's agreement to pay seventy million dollars in fines after pleading guilty to bribing European doctors to use its products.

In her recent book, *Blood Feud: The Man Who Blew the Whistle on One of the Deadliest Prescription Drugs Ever*, the investigative journalist Kathleen Sharp details how J&J's biotech division promoted the drug epoietin alfa—brand name Procrit, street name epo—which treats anemia resulting from chronic kidney failure, chemotherapy, HIV, or other problems. J&J's subsidiary company Amgen put so much pressure on its pharmaceutical representatives to sell the drug in unsafe doses and for off-label uses that two of those representatives actually blew the whistle on company dealings. According to Sharp, Amgen bribed physicians and pharmacists to purchase the drug. Later it was discovered that the drug caused blood clots and heart attacks and acted almost as a "tumor fertilizer" for those with cancer and was responsible for numerous patient deaths.[52]

In 2011 *USA Today* published this capsule summary on J&J: "The company has been found liable or reached settlements totaling $751 million in taxpayer health care fraud claims; paid $70 million to settle foreign bribery charges; been sued by consumers who say J&J's hip replacement devices failed inside their bodies; and seen the shut-down of a major plant that produces Tylenol and other best-selling pain relievers because it failed to meet federal safety standards."[53] In 2012, the company replaced its chairman of the board.

All this has led to criticism of how J&J now does business. "There are so many mistakes being made now, it is shocking," said Elliot Schreiber, a marketing professor at Drexel University's LeBow College of Business, who is an expert in brands and corporate reputations. Curt Weeden told us that in the past, "We were careful about what motivated people and made sure that the name of J&J resonated with dependable products. . . . The question now is whether J&J is putting more intent into the end effect [profits] and less into the product." Weeden doubted that the halo effect of J&J's partnership with nursing would survive if its products continue to be defective. "You can buy some of that halo effect in a broad campaign," he said, but with product problems "the halo goes away. You can't substitute it for product quality."

Even if Johnson & Johnson had maintained its reputation for product quality, such an unprecedented alliance with an entire health care profession is questionable in the contemporary health care world. Critics like physicians Jerome Kassirer and Marcia Angell, former editors of the *New England Journal of Medicine*, have disparaged medicine's cozy relationship with the pharmaceutical industry. Medicine's reputation for trustworthiness has taken a hit because of revelations of physicians' financial arrangements with the industry. Doctors cannot claim to be serving their patients if they are prescribing medication, conducting research, teaching other physicians about particular pharmaceuticals, and making treatment decisions if these activities favor corporations with which they have a financial relationship. Public and professional debate has prompted calls for tougher regulations to curb these practices.

Nursing appears to be ignoring this broader critique of how professions should relate to private, corporate interests and is allowing one of the largest for-profit corporations in the world to trade off its reputation for trustworthiness and patient advocacy.

This critique has significantly affected medicine and has caused a number of key medical leaders to not only question medicine's close contacts with the pharmaceutical industry but actually resign influential posts in protest. One of those leaders is Kassirer, the *New England Journal of Medicine* former editor and now distinguished professor at Tufts Medical School. In 1999 Kassirer was fired from his post as NEJM editor because the Massachusetts Medical Society, which publishes the journal, wanted to use the NEJM's stellar reputation, via its name and logo, to market other publications that were not, in fact, under the NEJM's control. When Kassirer refused to go along with the marketing deal, he was fired. Since leaving the NEJM, Kassirer has written a book about the dubious relationship between physicians and the pharmaceutical and other industries, titled *On the Take: How Medicine's Complicity with Big Business Can Endanger Your Health*. In it, Kassirer asks a critical question: "Where does the line exist between advancing the cause of science and the betterment of patient care on the one hand and the pecuniary interests of physicians collaborating with industry to produce these advances on the other?" His book answers this question quite clearly as he warns that "whether intentionally or not, too many physicians have become marketing whores, mere tools of industry's promotional efforts."[54]

"Making alliances with industry is a shady practice," Kassirer said when we discussed the J&J Campaign for Nursing's Future with him. "When the American Medical Association wanted to align itself with Sunbeam in the 1990s, there was a great outcry about how the connection with Sunbeam would taint the AMA and the AMA dropped it. The AMA was going to directly profit from this alliance, which," Kassirer acknowledged, "is slightly different than this case." Nonetheless, he continued, "there is still a serious problem with aligning a profession with a commercial company. The profession endangers its own reputation by connecting itself with a company that hasn't always been upstanding. It's a shady practice whether or not the company has done something wrong, and it's one that should be shunned. . . . If nursing prides itself on public trust it ought to get a divorce from J&J."

We wonder whether nursing's alliance with J&J will diminish public trust for the profession. How can nurses claim to be acting as patient advocates when major nursing organizations and schools of nursing are allowing themselves to be branded with the name of a company whose products are hurting—even killing—some patients? How can it enhance the image of nursing if the public suspects that nurses are recommending preferential purchases of products from a company that has seriously compromised patient safety?

When we have discussed campaigns like Johnson & Johnson's Campaign for Nursing's Future and the DAISY awards, many nurses explain that they are grateful for outside attention and financing—any outside attention and financing—and try to bracket or ignore any objectionable strings that are attached to these so-called gifts.

With the 2010 publication of the Institute of Medicine/Robert Wood Johnson Iniative report *The Future of Nursing: Leading Change, Advancing Health*, nurse leaders all over the United States expressed delight that finally health care decision makers were taking nursing seriously. One of the report's recommendations is that "nurses should be full partners with physicians and other health care professionals, in redesigning health care in the United States."[55] It is hard to imagine how nurses can claim an equal, leadership role with physicians to lead change and advance health if they are promoting Cinnabons and allowing profit-making corporations to sculpt their image.

We urge nurses to think critically about these images and messages. To advance this critical thinking, in the next chapter, we consider why so many postmodern nurses (women who have, after all, grown up in a culture that has rejected the sugar-and-spice-and-everything-nice definition of the feminine) still cling to and even promote traditional, trivializing images of nurses' work. We then discuss how nurses can speak in a different voice—a voice of agency—to explain their work to their patients, their institutions, and the broad public so that they can help lobby for the the resources on which necessary nursing care depends.

CHAPTER 3

FROM VIRTUE TO THE VOICE OF AGENCY

Several years ago, Marion Phipps, a clinical nurse specialist in Boston, wrote a narrative for a writing class Suzanne Gordon taught for nurses. Over several pages, Phipps described how she had helped a patient to die in peace and with dignity and how she worked with his family so that they could cope with his dying process.

In the final paragraph, however, Nurse Phipps got stage fright. Instead of summing up her accomplishments, she undercut her actions by arguing that it was the family that did everything worthwhile.

Gordon pointed out that by retreating into the background at the end, Phipps erased the point of her story, which was to show the important work *nurses* do. Why did she drag the nurse from the center of the action to the periphery? Gordon asked Phipps. "My role as a clinical nurse specialist," Phipps explained, "is to support the primary nurse, and to do that, I tend to pull back. I feel very good about my work, but I don't talk much about it. I see my work as supporting others. I'm a sort of a behind-the-scenes person. There are many people in the hospital like this. We're the ones who hold the place together but we don't stay very much in the forefront."

An oncology nurse we'll call Ruth Jones similarly placed herself in the background in her description of her work with a cancer patient. Nurse Jones had cared for a young woman with breast cancer for several years. During this time, the woman not only had to grapple with cancer and chemotherapy but also contend with beatings from her abusive husband. As her nurse, Jones administered, monitored, and managed the many side effects of the young woman's chemotherapy and also helped the patient to bring an end to the abuse.

When Nurse Jones told us about her work with this patient, she added that the patient had filed for divorce. "Terrific," we said. "You helped her get away

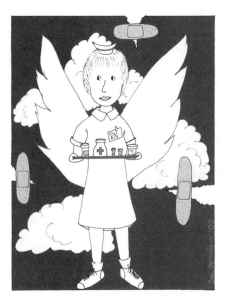

Sonia Oppenheim, www.familycomic.com

from a person who was harming her." Rather than acknowledge her accomplishment, Jones demurred. "Oh no, I didn't really do that much," she protested. "The patient's doctor helped a lot." When we suggested that the doctor's contribution sounded minimal, she agreed. But then she attributed the pivotal role to others—the social worker, the patient, the patient's family. After a full ten minutes of discussion, this nurse finally owned up to her essential work. Then she described in detail exactly what she did and how she did it.

Why would nurses diminish their agency?

Why would nurses believe that backstage players should not be allowed to come to center stage and take a bow?

Why would nurses resist taking credit for their accomplishments even when the credit is given to them?

Why would nurses allow their profession to be defined in ways that trivialize their skills and knowledge and settle for "rewards" that do not maximize the resources they need to do their work?

To answer these questions, it is useful to look at the religious and secular influences that shaped nursing and are still influential today.

The Virtue Script

For centuries in the Western world, nursing as an organized institutional intervention was delivered through Christian religious institutions. Most nurses were monks or nuns. They belonged to and obeyed the rules of Christian religious orders and adapted to what feminist scholar Isabel Marcus has called a strict "moral script."[1]

This "virtue script" framed nursing in particular ways, according to nursing historian Sioban Nelson and Suzanne Gordon.[2] While religious nurses had great technical and even, for their day, medical mastery, their work was cloaked in a veil of deference, submission, obedience, self-abnegation, and anonymity. Religious nurses were taught to view themselves as God's agents, to attribute their own skills and accomplishment to the divine.

Most important for the purposes of this discussion, they were taught to be self-effacing. Religious nurses were devoted to the performance of good deeds through which souls were saved—their own as well as their patients'. To talk about a good deed, to hint at one's own accomplishments, was to be guilty of the sin of pride, which turned the good deed into a sinful one. When nursing was professionalized and feminized in the nineteenth century (men were no longer allowed to register as nurses), reformers did not rebel against this religious-virtue script. Instead they used the religious template to help women navigate the treacherous passage from the domestic to public sphere, from unpaid work within the family to paid work outside the home.

"Respectable" women who entered this first large profession for women were moving into dangerous moral territory. In an era that prized blushing innocence and one in which women were not allowed out of the house unchaperoned, nurses were taking care of strangers' bodies—many of which were male. They were learning and seeing things that no respectable woman should ever encounter. In this context, nursing could be practiced by women only if it were desexualized. The calling to do God's work provided the proper context. The cloak of God's agency allowed nurses to develop their agency, but not to claim it as their own. Nurses were discouraged from ever talking about their work because if they did so a good deed would be turned into a bad one through the exhibition of the sin of pride.

Nurses were taught to "say little and do much," a phrase that Sioban Nelson used for the title of her history of nineteenth-century hospital formation. As one mother superior in San Antonio admonished a teaching and nursing nun, "Remain hidden, Alphonse. I cannot recommend this as much as I would like to, and beg you to give this spirit to our sisters. It is better that people take us for imbeciles, in no matter what, than to consider us clever and intelligent, agreeable to popular or worldly opinion."[3]

Another force that encouraged nurses to deny their agency was the entrance of physicians into positions of power in hospitals. When medicine (perhaps the quintessential patriarchal profession) and nursing met on the "contested terrain" of the hospital in the nineteenth century, medical men were not at all eager to allow a cadre of educated women (either as nurses or as physicians) to have authority or autonomy within the hospital. Many favored the idea of a better-trained nurse, but only if that nurse was conceptualized as the physician's servant, or handmaid. To function in the hospital, nurses thus had to negotiate a deal with medicine, one that gave doctors a dominant role over nursing as well as medical practice. Just as nurses had, for centuries, deferred to the divine, they now would learn to defer to the doctor and view themselves as fulfilling his medical mission.

If the modern doctor's authority stemmed from education and special knowledge, and if doctors would cast their profession as unique in that regard, then what could nurses claim as their own province that would not provoke competition with physicians? The answer was already in the culture—women's moral superiority and so-called natural caregiving abilities. As Susan M. Reverby has noted, nursing's very mission was "based on womanly duty requiring service to others."[4]

Patriarchal culture places women's work under the control of men and conceptualizes it as an extension of male agency. Women have been, and in some countries still are, seen as being men's possessions. In patriarchal culture, when the man leaves the home, he temporarily assigns his agency to his wife, but he reclaims it when he returns. Exciting, dynamic work is reserved for men. In such a culture, caregiving is defined not as an opportunity for self-assertion or self-fulfillment but as self-sacrifice. Nineteenth-century nursing thus established a template that endures to this day: Nursing is self-sacrificing, altruistic, devotional, poorly paid, anonymous, silent work. The idea that women are "naturally" caring and that caring is instinctual or hormonal or is guided by divine intervention or "design"[5] also lives on and conceals both the complexity of caregiving and the agency of the caregiver. "Women's work" is said to rely on instinct rather than knowledge, intelligence, or judgment. The complex caregiving that is described by such feminist scholars as Sara Ruddick, Laurel Thatcher Ulrich, and Patricia Benner is missing from the patriarchal conceptualization of "women's work."[6] Most important, the traditional definitions of *women's work* deny women belief in their own agency. The female caregiver (and this extends to the male nurse as well) isn't an actor, she is the container for the genetic engine that drives her actions.

It is remarkable today, given nursing's educational and scientific advances, its claims to professionalism, and its incorporation of increasing numbers of men, that the virtue script remains so powerful.

The first commandment of the virtue script is that nurses must remain silent about their work, meaning they must not claim credit for their mastery and accomplishments. We saw examples of this in the two anecdotes at the beginning of this chapter. One way to avoid the danger of "pride" is to give the credit to someone else.

A Singular Strength: For Nurse Lake, Caring Is Instinctual

—Headline on article honoring nurse practitioner Nancy Lake in "Salute to Nurses" advertising supplement, *Boston Globe*, May 2005

The response of one nurse caller to a radio talk show where one of us discussed the need for our society to recognize the work of nurses is an example of this dynamic. "I don't need credit for my work," the nurse said. "Working with patients is reward enough." She continued with heated remarks that diverted attention from nurses to physicians. She told the audience that physicians are hardworking, highly educated, and intelligent. Her statements diminished nursing, reinforced the stereotypical notion that the nurse exists to support the physician, and, in a larger sense, legitimized the traditional allocation of resources to medicine.

Human beings need to be recognized for their accomplishments. If nurses feel that they can't claim recognition for their real contributions, then the need might mutate into a plea or demand for recognition, or even for love, based on something other than accomplishment, something like personal goodness, moral superiority, or even the ability to cloak the need for recognition in inoffensive or juvenile imagery.

When members of the public (journalists, politicians, policymakers, and regulators, as well as patients) walk into hospitals and other health care settings, they see the cloaking of adult agency exhibited in scrubs printed with teddy bears, hearts and flowers, and smiley faces; stuffed animals and toys; all manner of angel paraphernalia—pins, artwork, key chains; and now daisies and sculptures of mothers and babies.

Members of the public see nurses with pens decorated with hearts writing on notepads emblazoned with endearing slogans, like that on a notebook we saw in 2005 at St. Mary's (Magnet) Hospital in Madison, Wisconsin: "With love we wrap you in our quilt of caring." In 2012 on its website, St. Mary's depicted the role of the nurse in similarly virtuous terms. It featured a smiling middle-aged nurse in scrubs with a big headline: "Would you go above and beyond just to put a smile on someone's face? A St. Mary's nurse would."[7]

When hospitals do make nursing visible in their promotional materials, nurses are photographed smiling at the camera or at the "patient" (who is usually the picture of health) rather than concentrating intently on the work that they are doing. In these posed pictures, nurses even smile at the complex machines they use to monitor patients. Doctors, on the other hand, are usually depicted with serious expressions. These pictures invariably suggest that physicians are the ones with the knowledge while nurses are there to pat the patient on the head or provide reassurance and comfort. The fact that providing reassurance and comfort to the sick is actually complex cognitive work is absent in this dichotomized iconography.

Some nurses recoil at the idea of explicitly explaining their work to patients and families in a way that highlights the *nurse's*, rather than someone else's, clinical knowledge and judgment. Just a few months ago, we were talking to a group of working nurses about our observation that few hospital websites include nursing in their depiction of the mission of the institution. An ER nurse in one of the hospitals we cited—Massachusetts General—insisted that she wasn't at all concerned about the invisibility of nursing on the MGH home page. All she cared about was the fact that patients recognized the value of nursing work.

Nurses like the one who called in to the radio show or the other who sloughed off website visibility construct recognition as personal. Because there is confusion in nursing about the professional versus the personal, we want to be clear about where we stand. We come down solidly on the side of *professional* visibility and voice, which is not to say that the nurse as a person is effaced. Quite the contrary. The individual nurse who talks about her or his work is present front and center, but the qualities of the nurse that should get public attention are those that pertain to the nurse's work, such as clinical judgment and skill and knowledgeable caring.

Confusion on this point is hardly surprising since so many institutional efforts to recognize nurses focus on who they are, rather than what they know and do. Indeed, when many of the DAISY stories, and nurse leaders' interpretations of them, actually dismiss nurses' clinical knowledge and emphasize the personal (or the divine), any suggestion that individual nurses should act to attract public attention is bound to stir up unease about possibly violating the age-old taboo against exhibiting the sin of pride.

We encountered an extreme example of elevating the personal over the professional in a Nurses Day composition that a student nurse sent to her friends and family and that was then sent to us.

> Being a nurse isn't about grades. It's about being who we are. No book can teach you how to cry with a patient. No class can teach you how to tell a family that their parents have died or are dying. No professor can teach you how to find dignity in giving someone a bed bath. A nurse isn't about the pills, the IVs, and the charting. It's about being able to love people when they are at their weakest moments and being able to forgive them for all their wrongs and make a difference in their lives today. No one can make you a nurse. . . . You just are.

Lest anyone think this is merely an individual view of nursing, its sentiments were applauded by almost every member of a graduate-level nursing class at a major nursing school where Bernice Buresh distributed it, and also by more than half the working nurses at a large workshop she conducted at a midwestern hospital. The latter group wrote testimonials about it, among them, "This is absolutely true!"

Your Turn

Write a paragraph describing what "being a nurse" is really about.

Is it? It's not surprising that a student nurse might, in a roundabout way, reveal a lack of confidence in her clinical skills. But this composition says learning and clinical activities aren't important and that nursing professors and scholars don't have much to offer. What is important is the natural moral superiority of the nurse.

Consider the irony. Some of the same nurses who expressed their concern about nurses becoming self-aggrandizing if they talked about their work found the hubris in a student nurse's claim that she could "forgive" patients "for all their wrongs" acceptable.

> *You're always there when someone needs you,*
> *You work your magic quietly,*
> *You're not in it for the glory,*
> *The care you give comes naturally,*
> *You take my hand,*
> *Touch my life,*
> *When I need you.*

CAUTION

As we saw in the previous chapter, the idealized nurse works well for companies that would like to be associated with the "goodness" that such a nurse emanates. The staple jingle, quoted above, that accompanies Johnson & Johnson's nurse recruitment ads expresses the virtue script writ large.

This promotion undercuts the skilled caring that nurses do and the knowledge that nurses have. How does a nurse know what question to ask a patient, what tone of voice to use, or when to hold the patient's hand? These actions stem from attentiveness, knowledge about the patient and his or her condition, clinical judgment, experience, and well-developed caring skills. But this promotional material argues that such caring is not knowledgeable work; it's "magic." According to J&J, caring isn't learned and practiced, it just comes naturally. So, one might ask, why should we support nursing education if nursing comes naturally?

Another way that these ads negate the idea that nursing requires other resources is in their assertion that you as the nurse are always going to be there no matter what. Are you always going to be there when someone needs you if you don't get paid, if the nursing agency you work for goes bankrupt, or if you are stretched so thin by a shortage of staff that you can't tend to all your patients? A literally minded member of the public might wonder, why should I worry about nurse staffing since you're always going to be there "when I need you"?

The J&J jingle presents an idealized version of the kind of care nurses might like to give and patients might like to receive. These virtue script messages are also appealing because they reflect our yearning for a mother who will care for us when we are sick. This is what resonates from the mother-and-child sculptures that the DAISY Foundation gives as awards.

Boston Medical Center

Exceptional Care

Without Exception

A place where nurses walk on water

—headline in *Hospitals 2004*, advertising supplement to the *Boston Globe*

The virtue script exploits this yearning by casting nurses, if not as mothers, then as trusted friends or "like family" to patients. Quite a few patients in the Nurses Week supplements that we have studied interpret a nurse's recognition of them as a real person, with specific needs, as friendship or as being treated "like family."

That theme is picked up in hospitals' promotions like one by the Newton-Wellesley Hospital in Massachusetts in the 2012 *Boston Globe* Nurses Week supplement. It depicts a nurse's hand laid on top of a patient's hand and reads, "Newton-Wellesley nurses are second to none. Your dedication and compassion ensure that our patients are treated as beloved family members. We thank you for your kindness, commitment and clinical excellence."[8]

Do most people really believe that hospitals treat patients "as beloved family members?" Probably not. In these promotions it's the feeling that counts, not the facts. Health care facilities will do a lot to foster that feeling even if it means promoting nurses from the angelic to the messianic in the above ad by the Boston Medical Center.

The virtue script in hospital advertising, nursing awards, and Nurses Week supplements is picked up by the news media, which might headline stories about nurses' accomplishments with such descriptions as "Angel in Our Midst," or "St. Joseph's Angel of Mercy" or might well illustrate articles with pictures of nurses in caps and with angel's wings. This process is an example of a negative feedback loop. The concept of the "feedback loop" is critical to communication theory. It was developed by Claude Elwood Shannon and Warren Weaver in 1949 and describes the process through which people provide feedback to one another as they communicate.[9] Feedback loops can be positive or negative.

In this case, nurses inherit what they perceive to be safe-communication framing then rebroadcast the framing of nursing work as altruistic and self-sacrificing to the public. Small publics, like the Barnes family, or some hospitals in their advertising, recirculate virtuous-nurse images and messages to a more general audience. Patients look at a website like DAISY's and are guided to tell stories about nurses that bring tears to the eyes and a Kleenex out of the box. Hospital administrators, and even physicians who attend awards ceremonies, absorb the messages delivered at Nurses Week or by Johnson & Johnson's nursing promotions. They may choose to believe that, for nurses, virtue really is its own reward and that nurses will be content to work for the gratitude in a patient's eyes or for certificates of appreciation. The cycle continues ever on-ward, feeding back and reinforcing messages and images that contradict nurses' claims to a serious role in health care leadership, system redesign, and health promotion.

We believe this negative feedback loop can be broken if nurses deliver different messages and educate various publics that depict their work—J&J, DAISY, newspapers that put out Nurses Week supplements, and others—about what nurses really do and why they should have a leadership role and far more voice in health care generally and within the institutions for which they work. We believe they can do this by replacing the virtue script with what we call a "voice of agency" that accurately describes nurses' complex and critical work.

Moving to a Voice of Agency

When we've talked about replacing the virtue script with a reality script some nurses have expressed the fear that "this is all we have and now you're trying to take it away from us."

Quite the contrary. The appropriate use of voice is not a threat to either nurses or nursing. *Silence* is the threat to nursing. Nursing recognition that leads to respect, reward, and resources hinges on individual nurses' employing a voice of agency that accurately represents the experience of illness as well as the experience of those who care for the sick and vulnerable.

What do we mean by *voice of agency*? The word *agency* stems from the Latin verb *agere*, meaning "to act" or "to do." Agency is the capacity for acting or the condition of acting or exerting power. An agent is a person who is instru-mental, "through whom power is exerted." *Agent* can denote someone who is acting on behalf of someone else, such as an agent for a movie star. But we are concurring with the view of Nobel Prize–winning economist Amartya Sen, who describes *agent* in "its older—and 'grander'—sense as someone who acts and brings about change, and whose achievements can be judged in terms of her own values and objectives, whether or not we assess them in terms of some external criteria as well."[10]

In writing about the social, economic, educational, and employment inequities that women suffer in a number of countries, Sen applauds the increasing emphasis on "the ac-tive role of women's *agency*," as contrasted with the state of women's "*well-being*." Well-being,

> An agent is a person who is instrumental, "through whom power is exerted."

The voice of agency is the voice that says, "I helped the patient to walk after surgery so that she wouldn't get blood clots in her legs." "I taught the patient how to take his medications so that they would be effective and produce fewer side effects." "I listened to the patient's fears about the surgery and I was able to give her some information that reassured her."

The voice of agency is the voice that conveys the message "I'm here. I am doing something important."

according to Sen, offers "a very restricted view of the personhood of women," whereas "the agency role is . . . central to recognizing people as responsible persons [who] can choose to act one way rather than another." This shift of emphasis is especially significant in developing countries, Sen writes, where women, "no longer the passive recipients of welfare-enhancing help[,] . . . are increasingly seen, by men as well as women, as active agents of change: the dynamic promoters of social transformations that can alter the lives of *both* women and men," as well as the entire society.[11]

For nurses, developing a sense of agency depends on *recognizing* the importance of nursing work *and* their own importance in carrying out this work.

To speak with a voice of agency is to admit the incontrovertible fact that the seventy-nine-year-old patient did not teach himself how to take his diabetes medication; that the sixty-one-year-old stroke patient did not read her own EKG; and that the man with dementia did not assess his own skin, discover the beginning of a decubitus ulcer, and act to prevent further skin breakdown. Most patients do not monitor and evaluate their own conditions themselves. When they are most vulnerable, they do not have the ability to prevent catastrophes or educate themselves about their conditions, treatments, and medication regimens; moreover, they do not have the responsibility to do so. Nor can patients always effectively negotiate the complexities of the system and advocate for themselves. This is what nurses do for them through their professional agency.

All the classic definitions of nursing incorporate the idea of agency in the sense that they emphasize the importance of the nurse's making her or his own observations and acting on them. In nursing theory, mastery is seen as developing from the nurse's own informed experiences. It is present not just because one is a "good" woman or man. Mastery is active, not passive, and thus leads to agency.

Without using the term "*agency*," Florence Nightingale saw that quality as essential to nursing and derided the trivialization of qualifications needed for the profession. In *Notes on Nursing* she wrote:

It seems a commonly received idea among men and even some women themselves that it requires nothing but a disappointment in love, the want of an object, a general disgust, or incapacity for other things to turn a woman into a good nurse. This reminds one of the parish where a stupid old man was set to be schoolmaster because he was "past keeping the pigs." . . .

The everyday management of a large ward, let alone of a hospital—the knowing what are the laws of life and death for men, and what the laws of health for wards—(and wards are healthy or unhealthy, mainly according to the knowledge or ignorance of the nurse)—are not these matters of sufficient importance and difficulty to require learning by experience and careful inquiry, just as much as any other art? They do not come by inspiration to the lady disappointed in love, nor to the poor workhouse drudge hard up for a livelihood.[12]

Patricia Benner's more recent analysis of nursing practice in *From Novice to Expert* is grounded in the daily reality of agency. One can't possibility move from novice to expert without being an agent. Even such seemingly passive nursing work as "being with the patient" and "maximizing the patient's participation in his or her recovery" requires skill, knowledge, and action, according to Benner's analysis.[13]

While leading nurse theorists seem to emphasize agency as the heart of nursing work, many nurses have been taught to deny the agency involved in their work. "We were taught in nursing school that nurses are 'facilitators,'" a nurse interjected when the concept of agency was brought up at one of our workshops. "We facilitate healing and we help people to get better, but we don't do it for them."

To *facilitate* is to make something easier. The word connotes agency, but agency in a different form. Interestingly, the nurses at the workshop saw the act of facilitating as counterposed to agency and were wary about embracing agency lest it take them beyond the acceptable bounds of nursing.

These boundaries can be very harmful to nurses in the current health care environment. In recent years, even the U.S. Centers for Medicare and Medicaid Services (CMS) has inadvertently helped to encourage hospitals to see nurses as virtue workers. With the CMS using patient satisfaction scores as a factor in determining reimbursement, consultants have created a mini-industry advising hospitals on how to increase their patient satisfaction scores. Consultants like Disney and the Studder Group, among many others, charge hospitals millions of dollars to teach staff—particularly nursing staff—how to smile and act solicitously to patients who will then be surveyed following their hospital stays.

Nurses in various parts of the country have told us that smiling has even become de rigueur for continued employment. At one hospital in Rochester,

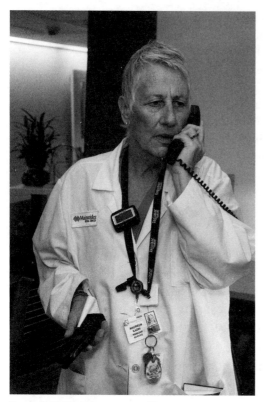

Maureen Kadri, RN, night nurse-manager: What a real nurse looks like when she's troubleshooting. (Photo by Earl Dotter.)

New York, nurses were instructed to smile at patients or visitors in the hospital regardless of the clinical situation they were dealing with. Nurses were instructed to smile before they answered a phone or called a patient, to ensure that they "had a smile in their voice." This hospital installed mirrors near phones at the nurses' stations so nurses could check that they were smiling. In a New Jersey hospital, a nurse was suspended for two days because she was caught talking on the phone without smiling.

In this misconstruction of caring as commercial friendliness, we see a direct connection between what society expects of nurses and some of the messages that nurses communicate about themselves. It's not clear how long this hospital trend will continue in the form of scripting nurses like hotel concierges with the intention of getting patients to feed back certain positive phrases on patient satisfaction surveys. Nurses complain that hospitals' patient satisfaction surveys focus too much on hotel-like amenities and not enough on actual clinical care. To get patients to grasp what really matters, nurses will have to take advantage of opportunities to educate patients about what is involved in clinical care. This means being willing to communicate what nurses know and what they do—not who they are. In the next few chapters we describe how to do that.

Nurses can no longer afford to observe the traditional physician-nurse Maginot Line expressed in the mantra "Physicians cure and nurse care." They cannot do so because physicians are now breeching this line. Physicians have strong impetus to do so if they want to remain at the top of the health care hierarchy, particularly when studies and reports recommend that advanced practice nurses provide more primary care. The same hospital consultants who are advising nurses to smile are also telling physicians that patients are not satisfied with quick drop-ins to hospital rooms and brusque demeanors.

With hospital reimbursements linked to patients' perceptions of care, it was only a matter of time before marketing companies would expand the image of physicians as being not just competent medically but caring as well. An example of this is a full-page ad that Beth Israel Hospital in New York ran in the *New York Times* in 2012.[14]

The top half of the page shows a large photograph of Martin S. Karpeh Jr., M.D., chairman of surgery. We know who he is because his name is on his badge (along with his title) and embroidered on his white coat. He stands center stage, focused and alert as he listens to another physician who is off to the side. Karpeh's demeanor is full of intelligence and competence. It reflects the caption at the bottom of the photo: "Expert medical care." The image is so compelling, we think, who wouldn't be willing to put his or her life in Dr. Karpeh's hands?

But there is more. The second half of the page illustrates, as the caption puts it, "medical experts who care." The photo under this caption shows two men in scrubs and OR caps expertly helping an infirm patient (wearing a hospital smock, ID wristband, and hairnet) to ease off of an examining table. The photo doesn't reveal the credentials of the men, but we are meant to understand that they are physicians. Two doctors helping one patient to stand—how reminiscent of TV docs in hospital series hovering over patients in their rooms, monitoring them, and nursing them, all in the absence of nurses.

The essence is summed up in two sentences: "At Beth Israel Medical Center, we understand there is so much more to medicine, than medicine alone. With state-of-the-art medical technologies and a vast array of proven therapeutic resources, we're committed to total patient care. Beth Israel, Where Health and Healing Come Together."

A later full-page Beth Israel ad suggests that docs have appropriated even those mystical qualities that have long been associated with nursing. The top half of the page pictures a female physician studiously looking at the back of a clothed male patient, perhaps assessing his posture. The caption is "Medical Know-How." A different photo at the bottom of the page shows her hands positioning his head. The caption reads, "Magical Somehow."[15]

So now physicians have it all. They provide "expert medical care," they are "experts who care," and their work evokes the "magical." Introducing magic into their work doesn't diminish their expertise because they, unlike nurses, have never counterposed caring with curing even though they may not have always exhibited the former.

Nurses must communicate more accurately about their work to get the kind of resources they and their patients so desperately need. Today more than ever nurses need the four *R*s for RNs—recognition, respect, reward, and resources—that are the non-negotiables of quality patient care. The four *R*s are essential in this professional framework if our societies are going to have necessary nursing care. The four *R*s are sequential. The various publics with whom nurses work and upon whose support nursing depends must first *recognize* what nurses do. People must perceive what goes on in nursing in order to *respect* the work and *reward* it by providing the *resources* that allow nurses to do their work, refine their practice, maintain their health and thus protect the health of their patients. By *reward* we do not mean token acknowledgment in the form of Nurses Week trinkets and DAISY Cinnabons. We do mean, in addition to appropriate pay levels, institutional supports that provide nurses with appropriate caseloads, time with patients, authority and autonomy in their workplaces, and continuing education.

To succeed, we believe, nurses must employ the voice of agency in their descriptions of their work. An example of how to use agency to transform a *half-istic* description into a *holistic* account follows.

Here is the original excerpt from a Johnson & Johnson public service advertisement in which a nurse describes his work:

- *Being a nurse is all about holding someone's hand . . . or getting the wrinkles out of the back of a sheet that's causing someone to be uncomfortable . . .*
- *And sometimes just rubbing someone's back is the answer to all their prayers.*

What do you think about this description of nursing? How could it be improved? Suzanne Gordon did this makeover:

- *Being a nurse is about saving patients' lives.*
- *Being a nurse is about making sure a patient doesn't develop a fatal complication before, during, or after surgery.*
- *It's about paying attention to the "small" but significant details such as smoothing out the wrinkles on a sheet so a patient doesn't develop an excruciating and costly bedsore.*
- *Sometimes by sitting and talking to someone, I find out the most important things—like whether patients understand how to take their medications, whether they have support at home, and whether they are frightened and anxious.*

Which script do you think more accurately captures the essence of nursing? Which script is more convincing? Which script makes it clear that not just anyone can do the work of nurses?

We conclude this chapter with an excellent example of how nurses can use the voice of agency. It is a reprint of an op-ed column by oncology nurse Theresa Brown that was published in the *New York Times*.

Hospitals Aren't Hotels

Op-Ed

BY THERESA BROWN, PITTSBURGH

March 14, 2012 (*New York Times*)

"You should never do this procedure without pain medicine," the senior surgeon told a resident. "This is one of the most painful things we do."

She wasn't scolding, just firm, and she was telling the truth. The patient needed pleurodesis, a treatment that involves abrading the lining of the lungs in an attempt to stop fluid from collecting there. A tube inserted between the two layers of protective lung tissue drains the liquid, and then an irritant is slowly injected back into the tube. The tissue becomes inflamed and sticks together, the idea being that fluid cannot accumulate where there's no space.

I have watched patients go through pleurodesis, and even with pain medication, they suffer. We injure them in this controlled, short-term way to prevent long-term recurrence of a much more serious problem: fluid around the lungs makes it very hard to breathe.

A lot of what we do in medicine, and especially in modern hospital care, adheres to this same formulation. We hurt people because it's the only way we know to make them better. This is the nature of our work, which is why the growing focus on measuring "patient satisfaction" as a way to judge the quality of a hospital's care is worrisomely off the mark.

For several years now, hospitals around the country have been independently collecting data in different categories of patient satisfaction. More recently, the Centers for Medicare and Medicaid Services developed the Hospital Consumer Assessment of Healthcare Providers and Systems Survey and announced that by October 2012, Medicare reimbursements and bonuses were going to be linked in part to scores on the survey.[16]

The survey evaluates behaviors that are integral to high-quality care: How good was the communication in the hospital? Were patients educated about all new medications? On discharge, were the instructions the patient received clear?

These are important questions. But implied in the proposal is a troubling misapprehension of how unpleasant a lot of actual health care is. The survey measures the "patient experience of care" to generate information important to "consumers." Put colloquially, it evaluates hospital patients' level of satisfaction.

The problem with this metric is that a lot of hospital care is, like pleurodesis, invasive, painful and even dehumanizing. Surgery leaves incisional pain as well as internal hurts from the removal of a gallbladder or tumor, or the repair of a broken bone. Chemotherapy weakens the immune system. We might like to say it shouldn't be, but physical pain, and its concomitant emotional suffering, tend to be inseparable from standard care.

What's more, recent research suggests that judging care in terms of desirable customer experiences could be expensive and may even be dangerous. A new paper by Joshua Fenton, an assistant professor at the University of California, Davis, and colleagues found that higher satisfaction scores correlated with greater use of hospital services (driving up costs), but also with increased mortality.

The paper examined patient satisfaction only with physicians, rather than hospitals, and the link between satisfaction and death is obviously uncertain. Still, the results suggest that focusing on what patients want—a certain test, a specific drug—may mean they get less of what they actually need.

In other words, evaluating hospital care in terms of its ability to offer positive experiences could easily put pressure on the system to do things it can't, at the expense of what it should.

To evaluate the patient experience in a way that can be meaningfully translated to the public, we need to ask deeper questions, about whether our procedures accomplished what they were supposed to and whether patients did get better despite the suffering imposed by our care.

We also need to honestly assess our treatment of patients for whom curative care is no longer an option.

I had such a patient. He was an octogenarian, but spry, and he looked astoundingly healthy. He'd been sent to us with a newly diagnosed blood cancer, along with a promise from the referring hospital that we could make him well.

But we couldn't. He was too old to tolerate the standard chemotherapy, the medical fellow on duty told him. When I came into his room a little later he said to me, with a stunned and yearning look, "Well, he made it sound like I don't have a lot of options." The depth of alienation, hopelessness and terror that he was feeling must have been unbearable.

The final questions on the survey ask patients to rate the hospital on a scale from worst to best, and whether they would recommend the hospital to family and friends. How would my octogenarian patient have answered? A physician in our hospital had just told him that he would die sooner than expected. Did that make us the best hospital he'd ever been in, or the worst?

Hospitals are not hotels, and although hospital patients may in some ways be informed consumers, they're predominantly sick, needy people, depending on us, the nurses and doctors, to get them through a very tough physical time. They do not come to us for vacation, but because they need the specialized, often painful help that only we can provide. Sadly, sometimes we cannot give them the kind of help they need.

If the Centers for Medicare and Medicaid Services is to evaluate the patient experience and link the results to reimbursement, it needs to incorporate questions that address the complete and expected hospital experience. It's fair and even valuable to compare hospitals on the basis of how well they maintain standards of patient engagement. But a survey focused on "satisfaction" elides the true nature of the work that hospitals do. In order to heal, we must first hurt.[17]

CHAPTER 4

PRESENTING YOURSELF AS A NURSE

New scientific findings on how the brain works confirm that first impressions count. We all pretty much instantly judge books—and people—by their covers. In his book *Thinking, Fast and Slow*, the Nobel Prize–winning psychologist Daniel Kahneman describes what the latest brain science tells us about how rational we really are when it comes to making decisions.[1] The sad fact is that none of us is as rational as we'd like to think. That's because human brains, which evolved over millennia, are, Kahneman explains, "machines for jumping to conclusions." Many brain functions are beyond our control, and sometimes we'll "believe almost anything"—particularly if our beliefs are confirmed over and over again. With plenty of confirmation to help us, our brains function by framing everything that follows according to a first impression.

The great sociologist Erving Goffman described this kind of social framing in his book *The Presentation of Self in Everyday Life*. How one presents oneself, Goffman explains, contributes to the construction of social and professional reality. "When an individual plays a part," he wrote, "he implicitly requests his observers to take seriously the impression that is fostered before them." Goffman explores the kind of perfomances that individuals, like actors on a stage, deliver as they try to influence the perceptions of others. Individuals constantly make what Goffman calls "definitional claims" on one another. In order to be taken seriously, an individual has to "mobilize his activity so that it will express during the interaction what he wishes to convey."[2] If, during such interactions, individuals contradict, by their self-presentation, what they say they want to convey, then we have what Goffman calls a "definitional disruption."

To assert their "definitional claims" and avoid "definitional disruptions" most professional groups spend an enormous amount of time crafting a credible professional image. Physicians, for example, are explicitly socialized to play "a public role," as one physician educator told us. "Physicians have to make decisions in treating their patients and thus they have to appear credible and authoritative. We teach them how to do this."

Businesses spend millons on management consultants who teach their managers and staff how to create a "desired professional image." As the Harvard Business School professor Laura Morgan Roberts explains, "People are constantly observing your behavior and forming theories about your competence, character, and commitment, which are rapidly disseminated throughout your workplace. . . . If you aren't managing your own professional image, someone else is." Roberts explains that there are various strategies people use to create a "desired professional image." One she calls "positive distinctiveness." This involves "using verbal and non-verbal cues to claim aspects of your identity that are personally or socially valued, in an attempt to create a new, more positive meaning for that identity. Positive distinctiveness usually involves attempts to educate others about the positive qualities of your identity group."[3]

Nursing groups also invest time in highlighting the "positive distinctiveness" of nurses. The virtue script that we discussed in the previous chapter is an example of efforts to enhance public acceptance of nursing. During the second wave of twentieth-century feminism, nurse scholars like Patricia Benner adapted concepts, such as Mary Belenky's "women's way of knowing," to demonstrate that nurses were far more caring and holistic than physicians.

Over the past forty years, nursing managers and educators have promoted the "advanced practice" movement, in which they claim positive distinctiveness by differentiating the advanced practice nurse from the vast majority of bedside nurses. It has been asserted that advanced practice registered nurses (APRNs) are "critical thinkers" and "skilled decision makers" who are able to practice "autonomously" and are thus very different from (read, superior to) direct care nurses. Although nursing academics also claim that the advanced practice nurse is a caring, holistic practitioner, the positive distinctiveness of APRNs is primarily asserted through their identification with the highest-status professional group in health care. Because, like physicians, APRNs can diagnose, prescribe, and practice independently, they seem to be superior to direct care nurses, who are still mired in tasks that are supposedly dictated by physicians. Indeed, in the United States, with the advent of the new doctorate of nursing practice (DNP), which gives the title *doctor* to nurses in clinical practice, advanced practice nurses seem to distance themselves further from the majority of nurses.

Another way that nursing elites have tried to establish their positive distinctiveness is through the leadership discourse that is so prevalent in nursing. There is a "leadership" course in almost every undergraduate nursing program and "leadership" skills are highlighted in graduate programs as well. Nurse managers have morphed into "nurse leaders"; nursing schools claim that they are educating people not to be, God forbid, just a nurse, but to be leaders. In fact many schools of nursing, in the United States at least, now offer entry into practice programs that produce what are called "clinical nurse leaders." These programs are designed to attract either nurses who have been in practice for some time or students who have a four-year degree in another subject and want to switch to nursing. The American Association of Colleges of Nursing implies that these newly minted nurses are superior to normal graduates because the former are better equipped to "lead" their colleagues on hospital nursing units. This claim is made not because they have more practice experience, but because they are educated in such subjects as population health, health disparities, and the management of chronic illnesses and can lead in quality-improvement strategies.[4] Many nurses and some nursing organizations believe that emphasis on advanced practice and leadership will not only enhance the image of leaders, or APRNs, but of the profession as a whole.

Focusing on advanced practice or leadership has not, in fact, trickled down to improve the image of the vast majority of nurses but rather has enhanced only a small elite. Indeed, the very rhetoric of advanced practice suggests that experienced direct care nurses who may have been working for decades are not advanced but rather inferior, deficient, behind (all antonyms of the word *advanced*). These distinctions also serve to divide a profession that needs to be united if it is to change traditional public perceptions of nursing.

Nurses can unite in correcting inaccurate public perceptions of their work by taking advantage of the opportunities that are available when they present themselves to patients and families, physicians, other clinicians and health care workers, administrators, and the general public.

Without being self-conscious or artificial, nurses can be aware of the impression they are making. Since the health of patients depends on nursing, nurses can reaffirm this important fact by presenting themselves as experts in the health care setting. The most immediate way to educate the public about your work is to begin with those members of the public with whom you are in daily contact—patients, families, and colleagues. Introductions are golden opportunities for nurses to frame themselves as true professionals and clinical experts.

Introducing Yourself

Your introduction to the patient and to his or her family, or to a profesional colleague, is an important moment that has lasting consequences for you as an individual professional and for nursing as a whole. Because first meetings are so important to how our brains frame our beliefs, introductions should follow the form that professionals use when they present themselves and their definitional claims. Here are the elements:

> Your first and last name;
> Your title or function; and
> Usually a firm handshake (if meeting face to face).

For a nurse this would mean introducing yourself with your first and last name, informing the patient or family member that you are a registered nurse, and explaining your role in the patient's care. If there are no concerns about infection control, this introduction should include a handshake.

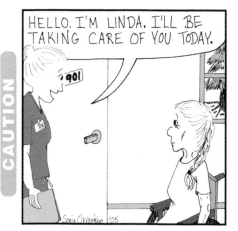

Sonia Oppenheim, www.familycomic.com

Introducing yourself this way will produce a very different response than simply saying, "Hello, my name is Joan," and leaving it at that.

A profesional introduction is particularly important today because nurses no longer wear starched white uniforms and caps. The lack of a standard uniform means that the public is deprived of obvious visual cues to figure out who is and is not a nurse. In most institutions in North America, nurses are identifiable by only their name on their hospital ID, which is often flipped over. Therefore what you say as you introduce yourself is critically important.

We recently spoke at a hospital in which hospital ID badges had on them only the following: "Sue, nursing," "Jim, physical therapy," "Joe, pharmacy." The CNO of the hospital had a badge that read, "Ruth, nursing." That was it.

The only people in the institution with name badges that had their last name and specific credentials were physicians. What does this say to the public?

Your introduction is your best opportunity to let people know that you are a nurse—a serious professional with important clinical knowledge. Being serious and professional is not synonymous with being distant and aloof. It simply means presenting yourself as a knowledgeable, expert caregiver. This is a presentation that tends to reassure patients rather than alienate them.

What's in a Name?

Many nurses complain that patients often confuse other health care workers with nurses. Many patients complain that they who don't know who is and who is not a nurse. This upsets them. Why? Because nursing has succeeded in convincing patients that nurses are to be trusted and they feel safer with a nurse than with other personnel. This is why it is essential for nurses to be identified as such. In many countries today, however, the convention is for nurses to introduce themselves with only a first name, as in "Hi, I'm Sally. I'm your nurse."

Sometimes the *N*-word might not get mentioned at all, as in "Hello, I'm Sally. I'll be taking care of you today," or "Hello, this is Jane from the VNA." In the United States and Canada, "I'll be taking care of you today" may be perceived by nurses as code for "I am a nurse." (In Australia and the United Kingdom, the code is "I'm looking after you today.") Unfortunately, the patients may not be in on the code and are thus at a loss to identify who is who in the clinical setting.

Sometimes it seems that when a nurse graduates from nursing school, she substitutes a blank space for her last name. The assignment board in a hospital might list the patient as "Mrs. Smith," "Mary Smith," or "Smith"; the physician as "Dr. Jones" or "Jones"; and the nurse as "Pat." A name badge might bear only a first name and sometimes not even an "RN." Or it might have a first name and then a last name initial.

When nurses answer the phone or call patients, they might introduce themselves as "Mary from Four South," "Jim from the emergency department," or "Pat from General Pediatrics." In this way, nurses present themselves as institutional property rather than as individuals or professionals. Some nurses construct an image of themselves as physicians' personal property by introducing themselves as "Janet, Dr. Wilson's nurse."

Lack of parity in the workplace is reinforced when nurses allow or encourage physicians to call them by their first names while they routinely address physicians by title and last name.[5] Some nurses and physicians communicate with each other on a first name basis. Usually, however, that happens when patients are not present. When the doctor and nurse enter the exam room,

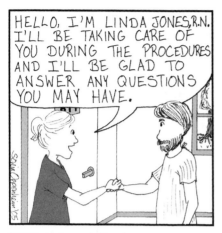

HELLO, I'M LINDA JONES, R.N. I'LL BE TAKING CARE OF YOU DURING THE PROCEDURES AND I'LL BE GLAD TO ANSWER ANY QUESTIONS YOU MAY HAVE.

Sonia Oppenheim, www.familycomic.com

the physician who was "Jim" in the hallway becomes "Dr. Smith." The nurse remains "Sally." The physician in such a situation may think that the nurse prefers it this way.

It's true that naming practices have changed as our society has become more informal. Nurses have told us that as recently as forty years ago, many institutions did not permit them to use their first names with patients. It was strictly "Miss Jones," or "Mrs. Jones." Today the tables have turned.

Some younger physicians avoid using the title *Dr.* and introduce themselves with their first and last names. However, in this situation, the patient understands through various other cues that the person presenting him- or herself is a physician. Even physicians who present themselves informally rarely leave patients confused about their professional role.

The kind of introductions that nurses now use deprives them of a full identity. It also reinforces a dangerous asymmetry of power that gives the impression that one group is clearly superior to another. When doctors call nurses by their first name and nurses call doctors by their last name and title, this is the equivalent of calling a child or servant by his or her first name but demanding that the adult, or master, be addressed formally.

Casting nursing as subordinate to medicine may not be the intention of nurses who use only their first names. "When nurses use their first names, they are doing it in the hope of showing the patient that they are on their side, that they are equals, on a par with, in the same shoes as, the patient," says nursing historian Joan Lynaugh. "Nurses generally are not seeking 'respect' from their patients, but some kind of identification with them. Indeed nurses are often taught to do that."

The question is, why aren't nurses seeking respect?

Recall that one of the four *R*s for RNs is respect.

The word *respect* comes from the Latin *spectare*, which means "to look." To re-*spectare* is to look not just once but once again, to see and to value. When we ask nurses why they call doctors by their last name in front of patients, even if they are on a first name basis with the physician, they invariably tell us that it's a sign of respect. Patients, they say, need to respect their doctors. In this case, the nurse asserts that respect resides in last name and title.

The question is, is using the doctor's last name and title about respect or about the reinforcement of hierarchical/patriarchal authority? When nurses call a physician with whom they are on a first name basis by his or her last name and title in front of a patient, they are asserting the physician's authority over the nurse, and the patient. Today, patient advocates almost uniformly argue for the patient's right to play a much more central role in their own care. Many patient advocates try to implement systems that will help patients question and, if necessary, even challenge their physicians and other health care professionals so that they, as patients, can make better decisions about their own health. As any number of scholars and researchers have noted, this is far from easy since physicians may subtly—or not so subtly—convey their displeasure at this reframing of the doctor-patient relationship. Dominick Frosch has done extensive research into patient participation in such decision making. In a 2012 study in *Health Affairs*, he and his colleagues reported that even some of the most affluent patients worry that asking questions and taking an active role in their own care will anger physicians and nurses, who will label them as "difficult patients."[6]

> When nurses allow physicians to call them by their first name in front of patients and in turn call physicians by their last name and title they are not merely underlining their own subordination to the physician. They are also reinforcing and even enabling traditional status hierarchies that disempower not only the nurse but also the patient.

When nurses allow physicians to call them by their first name in front of patients and in turn call physicians by their last name and title they are not merely underlining their own subordination to the physician. They are also reinforcing and even enabling traditional status hierarchies that disempower not only the nurse but also the patient.

"In the research we have done," Frosch explains, "it is clear that patients want to collaborate with physicians and the healthcare team. In spite of the rhetoric of patients being partners in their care, what patients encounter are a lot of obstacles. Because of this patients feel a need to adopt a 'good patient' role, which makes them reluctant to ask questions or disagree with recommendations because they fear that they will be perceived as questioning the authority or expertise of physicians, which will, in turn, mean they will not receive good care in future."

Considering how people are addressed in a consultation is very important, Frosch says. This includes not only how the patient is addressed but also how the nurse and physician are addressed. Anyone who insists on maintaining formality when addressing the physician—whether it be intentional or not—contributes to reinforcing the notion of the "good patient," that is, someone who is deferential to this authority. "By insisting on the use of formal titles, Frosch notes, "but only in reference to the physician, what we're really doing is maintaining a social distance. What you're reinforcing by this is not respect but deference on the part of the nurse and the patient. It signals to the patient that deference is what is expected and reinforces the sense patients have that partnership is not what they should expect in this encounter."

Frosch believes that changing formal titles would help pave the way toward true partnership. "Removing deference," Frosch is careful to point out, "does not equate to lack of respect for the expertise of the physician. The issue for patients is that they too want to be respected and they also want the decisions that are being made about their care to be respected. Patients have to live with those decisions and want to be a part of making them. They want to have a role in deciding what happens to them. Patients have a right and understandable desire to be involved in those choices."

This means that nurses must insist on parallel rather than asymetrical naming practices. As Frosch explains, if everyone is on a first-name basis this flattens hierarchies that can discourage patient participation in decision making. But if physicians—or anyone whom is called Dr. (which can include nurses with PhDs)—insist on last name and title, then everyone being addressed (i.e., patients, nurses, family members) should also be addressed by last name and title (Mr. Ms., Mrs.).

Introductions not only affect nurses's professional standing and patient empowerment; they also affect patient safety. It has become increasingly clear that patient safety depends on effective teamwork. Teamwork requires that each member of a team understand the identity, role, and function of the other members. To be a member of a team people must know who you are and how to find you. How do you find Sue, the nurse? Or Sue, who's taking care of Ms. Jones today? It is essential that nurses state their full names and roles and functions with their colleagues as well as with patients.

Your Turn

Go around your workplace and note the asymmetrical naming practices. For example, do the appointment secretaries refer to the physicians as Dr. [Last Names] but the clinical nurses and nurse practitioners as just "Nancy" or "Janice?"

This mandate to identify oneself is now embedded in the new safety methodology called SBAR (Situation, Background, Assessment, Recommendation). SBAR is being taught and used in hospitals and other facilities and is now taught in many nursing schools. The point of SBAR is to ensure that each team member will have sufficient information about whom they are communicating with and what they are being asked to do. The SBAR technique avoids the confusion that would be produced by the following kind of dialogue:

> *Nurse calling physician*: Hello this is Four South. I need a change in pain medication for Mrs. Smith.
>
> *Physician*: What? Who is this? What do you want?

With SBAR, the dialogue would be as follows:

> *Nurse calling physician*: Hello, this is Nurse Jean Jones. I have been taking care of Mrs. Smith, a sixty-five-year-old patient who has just had a total hip replacement tonight on Six South. She has been experiencing a great deal of pain for the past five hours. Her blood pressure is elevated, as is her heart rate.

This kind of exchange of information and role clarification not only ensures that important data is shared so that informed decisions can be made; it also reduces traditional status imbalances that jeopardize patient safety because higher-status people ignore information from and the concerns of those they perceive to be of lower status. For this reason, many patient-safety advocates, including physician safety advocates, advise fellow physicians to use first names in critical settings such as the operating room. Why? Because as has been demonstrated in aviation and other high-reliablity industries, it's a whole lot easier to tell Joe or Joan that he or she is about to make a terrible mistake than it is to tell Dr. Green or Dr. Collins.

A nurse can quickly establish context by introducing her- or himself with *both* a first and last name, explicitly stating that she or he is a registered nurse, and briefly explaining her or his role in the patient's care.

An opening such as "Hello, this is Ruth Miller, the nurse practitioner with urgent care. I understand you are running a fever. Can you tell me what your temperature is and when you began to feel ill?" would establish that context more than this: "Hello, this is Ruth from the health center. You called about wanting to talk to someone about how you feel." Similarly, "I am Janet Jones, a registered nurse who works with Dr. Wilson" conveys a different message from that of "I'm Dr. Wilson's nurse."

Resurrecting Nurse *as a Title*

Nurses say that one obstacle to parity with physicians is that they don't have a title like *Dr.* But nurses do have a title. It is *Nurse*. To us, it's a word with dignity that could and should be used to reassert nurses' professional identity.

Nurses could ask those physicians who prefer to be addressed as "Dr. (Last Name)" in front of patients, to please address them as "Nurse (Last Name)" in the same setting. Similarly, when nurses refer to each other as "Nurse (Last Name)" they show professional courtesy for each other and indicate to physicians and patients that they expect professional acknowledgment.

Use of the title *Nurse*, does not have to be stilted, nor need it jeopardize nurses' sense of closeness with their patients. Once the precedent has been set, you can move to first name communication with a patient or a physician if you choose. Just as a physician might be "Dr. Jones" in one situation and "Joe" in another, nurses can be flexible according to the situation. At the moment, the conventions of many workplaces give nurses no flexibility at all—only a first name. This is why, as the nursing educator Elizabeth M. Grady puts it, nurses must insist on symmetrical titles and naming practices with physicians.[7]

Interactions with patients should also include such symmetrical naming practices. If the doctor insists on being "Dr. Wilson," then the nurse should be "Nurse Jones" and the patient should be "Mr./Ms. (Last Name)."

A Canadian nurse's description of how she approached a resident for pain medication illustrates how the absence of such an identity sets nurses up for failure. The nurse said she began the phone conversation with the resident by saying, "This is Seven North. I need an order of . . . " The resident responded angrily to being bothered while he was busy with a patient. He asked for the nurse's name. Diffidently she gave her full name. He got her name wrong. She did not correct him. He said he'd get to her request later. She did not try to establish a time frame. He never did write the order. She never called him back.

This physician may well have been a difficult case. But the nurse, for her part, did not make a professional presentation or stand up for herself or for the patient who needed her care. She did not give her name and title. She did not specifically state her patient's condition and what she needed. The nurse became so intimidated that she could not negotiate an agreement with the doctor to attend to her patient's need in a reasonable amount of time. She did not, as nurse Crystal Lindaman advises, "set a tone that assumes that compliance is inevitable."[8] She did not persist. She did, however, instruct this young physician that he need not accord nurses professional courtesy.

In workshops, we have sparked some vehement opposition when we've urged nurses to use both their first and last names and to adopt the title *Nurse*. Some nurses assert that nurses should use *only* their first names for these reasons:

1. First names make patients feel that nurses are more approachable than physicians. Patients want nurses who are on "the same level" as they are.
2. Patients don't want to know nurses' last names. In fact, it's too much to ask patients to remember the last names of their nurses.
3. Patients don't need to know nurses' last names to respect nurses and value what nurses do for them.
4. "Nurse Adams" makes people think of "Nurse Ratched."
5. It's dangerous for nurses to have their last names known.
6. It's an invasion of privacy if patients and families know nurses' last names.
7. Even if it is a good idea to use last names and a title, it is too difficult to change established cultural practices within an institution.

Are these assumptions correct? Let's examine them.

1. *First names make patients feel that nurses are approachable.* Nurses have good reason to try to counter the distancing or brusqueness that characterizes some physician-patient encounters. Many nurses initiate reciprocal first name interactions with patients to ease patients' fears, lower their defenses, and facilitate communication. This ability to establish closeness within a professional context is one of the great qualities that nurses bring to patient care.

Many nurses believe that the use of first names helps to create and protect one area where they can claim superiority in any doctor-nurse comparison—the ability to establish intimacy with patients. Nurses often feel that in their struggle for recognition they can't win the knowledge (number of years in school) competition with physicians, and they can't win the status competition, but they can easily win the intimacy competition. They might fear that a more formal self-presentation will erode their greatest strength.

But does connection really depend on a first-name-only introduction? Do patients respond more candidly to nurses because they use only their first names? Or do they respond to nurses and trust them because nurses spend more time with them than do doctors, because nurses really listen to their

> "Patients don't want a friend, they want a nurse with knowledge and skill. A really good nurse will establish the context for a relationship. She or he will communicate to a patient: 'This is what I do. This is what you do. This is what I know. I will make sure everything is all right for you.'"
>
> —Nursing historian
> Joan Lynaugh, interview

concerns without frequently interrupting, because nurses respond effectively to these concerns, and because nurses know how to *be with patients as well as do things to them?*

In other words, does connection reside in the lack of a name and title, or does it reside in genuine affect, attentiveness, and empathy?

For those physicians who insist on maintaining their authority over patients, using just their last name and title is not the primary way they distance themselves from patients. Those that distance themselves do so by failing to listen, by interrupting what Arthur Kleinman calls patients' "illness narratives," by focusing on diseases to the exclusion of the human beings who bear them, and by abandoning patients when their illnesses can no longer be cured or when they have repaired a particular organ.[9]

A common rationale for using only first names is that this introduction puts nurses "at the same level" as that of their patients. Laudably nurses do not want to patronize or disempower their patients. But to be at the same level as the patient is to be frightened, anxious, and even ignorant about the care and treatment the patient needs. Surveys indicate that what patients really want is competence and expertise from nurses.

It's the expertise of nurses that makes it possible for them to do one of their primary jobs—rescuing patients from potential harm such as through falls, urinary tract infections, medication errors, bedsores, or other mishaps.[10] Even the health maintenance and disease promotion work that nurses engage in is a form of rescue. How can nurses do this if they don't have knowledge and insights that their patients lack?

2. Patients don't want to know nurses' last names; patients can't be expected to remember the last names of nurses. Maybe, maybe not. Some patients might be interested in and capable of remembering a nurse's full name. Others may not care a whit. By the same token, many patients may not be especially interested in, or capable of, remembering the last names of physicians they encounter in a busy health care setting. Nonetheless, it is important for nurses to make the point that they have a last name and, like physicians, are individuals rather than part of an undifferentiated mass. Even the patient or

Your Turn

Think about the encounters you have in your personal life. If someone calls you at home and says, "Hello, I'm Joan from Bank of America," what mental compartment do you put them in? The one reserved for consequential people or the one marked "forgettable and disposable"?

family member who cannot remember the last name will register that their nurse has one.

Erving Goffman noted that institutions enforce obedience and conformity by ritually stripping inmates or initiates of the clothes, hairstyles, and private possessions that give them a sense of identity. "The most significant of these possessions is not physical at all. [It's] one's full name." More than any other, Goffman asserted, that loss forces the inmate to suffer "a great curtailment of the self."[11] Historically nurses have been at risk for exactly this kind of institutional depersonalization.

Just as physicians are usually known to nurses by their full names, nurses should be distinguished as individuals by their first and last names, and not, as one physician put it, as "Maureen in the yellow angora sweater." Besides, there are patients as well as colleagues who do want to know a nurse's identity to be assured that they are speaking to a qualified professional. The first name–only convention also makes it harder for individual nurses to receive credit for their work. We recognize that the way nurses are treated in some workplaces causes them to be defensive and to anticipate being singled out for blame more than for credit. But lack of a last name rarely protects a nurse from the former and may deprive her or him of the latter.

For example, one woman we know was impressed with the performance of the nurses at an outpatient surgery center where her mother had a basal-cell carcinoma removed. The nurses identified a potential heart problem that physicians had overlooked and suggested that her mother make an appointment for a cardiac evaluation. When, three weeks later, the cardiologist described a previously undiagnosed heart condition, the woman was once again impressed by the nurses' clinical astuteness. She wanted to write a letter to the hospital administration to commend their actions. But who were these nurses? They did not introduce themselves with last names. Only their first names appeared on their name badges. The woman felt she could not send a letter with just the first names of these nurses. So the nurses never experienced the positive credit they could have gotten and surely deserved.

3. *Patients don't need to know nurses' last names to respect nurses and value what nurses do for them.* "They don't care what my last name is. All they need to know is that I'm Susan and I'm there to help them through their delivery," a labor and delivery nurse insisted. "It doesn't matter what they call us, patients value us for what we do," a student in an advanced practice nursing program argued.

These comments are illuminating. Hopefully patients do value nurses for their contributions to care and recovery. But patients can value their nurses while simultaneously assigning them a lower status in the health care hierarchy.

If nurses introduce themselves by their first names only, they are asking to be regarded as nonprofessionals because that is the conventional way that nonprofessionals present themselves. Restaurant servers, garage mechanics, and others who introduce themselves with their first names certainly can and should be respected and valued for the work they do. But they do not have the responsibility for defining their work and their place in the workplace in the same way that nurses do.

When members of the largest health care profession opt out of the standard professional greeting, they risk communicating that they do not regard themselves as professionals or on a par with the other professionals.

4. *Nurse Adams = Nurse Ratched.* In many of the seminars, nurses eventually agree that calling themselves "Nurse (Last Name)" may be a good idea. But then they argue that patients will automatically associate "Nurse Adams" with one of the most heinous literary portraits of a nurse—Ken Kesey's sadistic Nurse Ratched from the book and movie *One Flew over the Cuckoo's Nest.*

Nurse Ratched was a terrible character. But why assume that juxtaposing the title *Nurse* with any of the millions of last names nurses have will instantly evoke this evil character?

Many younger people have never even heard of Nurse Ratched. But let's say someone does associate Nurse Adams with Nurse Ratched. So what? A knee-jerk response does not indicate that this is a fixed and total image of any nurse who uses her title. If millions of nurses adopted the title *Nurse,* it would quickly become normal.

5. *Potential danger.* "I will not take any more risks," an emergency department nurse declared heatedly when the subject of introductions came up at a workshop. "I'm already in danger. People come in with weapons and sometimes they go berserk and hit us." Other nurses contend, "If they know our

last names, they might stalk us. They might follow us home." Whenever the use of last names is discussed, many nurses argue that the personal safety of nurses depends on concealing their last names.

We do not take the subject of personal safety lightly. We are aware of the vulnerability that women, in particular, could experience in dealing with strangers. Health care workers *are* often verbally or physically attacked. The very nature of nursing work puts nurses in close contact with people who may be violent or mentally disturbed or who misconstrue caring as a sexual invitation. According to United States government Bureau of Labor Statistics data from 2006, "the healthcare sector leads all other industries," in the rate of non-fatal assaults on health care workers that lead to lost days at work. In 2011, the Bureau reported eight RNs had been fatally injured at work between 2003 and 2009.[12] Because personal safety is so important, it merits a thorough evaluation. Nurses must protect themselves and be protected from physical danger to the greatest degree possible. The question is, does the use of a nurse's last name subject her to additional personal risk?

Emergency nurses point out that attempted or actual physical assaults by patients are not unusual. The emergency nurse quoted above indeed is "already in danger." She works in a hospital with inadequate protections. People carrying weapons are able to enter the facility, and the protocols for controlling physically aggressive patients apparently are nonexistent or not implemented.

We asked this nurse whether nurses and physicians are attacked at random in this facility, or whether attackers deliberately single out a particular clinician. She said that physical violence was directed against anyone who was around. She said it made no difference whether the staff member's last name was known or not. Still, she was adamant. She would never use her last name at work because she already was exposed to diseases such as tuberculosis, human immunodeficiency virus (HIV), and hepatitis and to physical attack. Her last name would add one more layer of vulnerability, she insisted.

This nurse was so terrified that she couldn't perceive the illogic of her position. She was hoping for some kind of magic to protect her—if they don't know who I am, maybe I'm safe.

We're concerned that some nurses are relying on an ineffective measure. If a nurse works in a situation in which disclosing her last name to certain persons could be dangerous, of course she must behave accordingly. But nurses and other health care workers must go to the source of the problem when their institutions are failing to provide proper security. They must find out from their professional associations and other groups what systems are effective and require their own institutions to adopt such measures.

One serious question in this debate is whether nurses belong to a special endangered class. When we've discussed this with nurses, several have suggested that it would be easier for a person to harass or stalk a nurse if her last name were known. But just how much safety does last name anonymity confer? If a patient is disturbed enough to harass or harm a nurse, couldn't he just follow her home after work? If someone is determined to find you, they will.

As female reporters we have covered volatile situations and violent people. We've experienced our share of danger. For those who deal with the public, irate customers or clients come with the territory. But teachers, police officers, lawyers, judges, journalists, stockbrokers, and therapists—a few of whom have been threatened and killed by deeply troubled people—simply do not have the option of jettisoning their last names. As a professional, it's standard practice to use one's whole name.

There are precautions that can be taken to reduce risks. It might be prudent to limit the amount of personal information given to a patient. Having

Minimizing the Chances of Violence in Hospitals

The National Institute for Occupational Safety and Health makes these recommendations, among others, for minimizing violence in hospitals:

If your workplace is understaffed, raise the issue with management. Point out that understaffed, overcrowded hospital workplaces are at higher risk for violence, particularly during meal times and visiting hours.

Watch for signals that threaten violence, like expressions of anger and frustration, pent-up body language, signs of substance abuse, and presence of a weapon.

Behave in ways that help diffuse anger, such as appearing calm, caring, unthreatening, and acknowledging the other's feelings.

Be alert and vigilant and don't isolate yourself with a potentially violent person.

Make sure you have an exit strategy or possibility.

Remove yourself from the situation.

Call security for help.

Alert management to the problem. Insist on security devices such as cameras, good lighting, escort services, and workplace design that restricts public access to certain areas[13]

an unlisted home phone number is an option. Employing a firm tone of voice and assertive body language can be effective in setting boundaries. Studies on violence in the workplace suggest that the best preventions are good security systems, instruction to employees on how to identify potentially violent people, and conflict resolution strategies and practices.

In many health care systems, patients and families—and staff—feel stretched to the limit and may respond with abusive language or behavior. In this context, it could be wiser for nurses to use the title *Nurse* and their last name when introducing themselves instead of using their first names. This technique can establish distance while the nurse ascertains whether the patient presents a danger to her. If she feels comfortable with the patient, she can move from title/last name (Nurse Smith) to first name whenever she wants, as in "Please call me Susan."

You can always move from distance to closeness, but it is much harder to move from closeness to distance. Health care workers are at risk for violence because they have so much interaction with the public. But we have found no studies that suggest that nurses are particularly at risk because they are nurses. Except in special cases, the anonymity that comes from using only a first name provides minimal, if any, physical protection but considerably lessens nurses' agency and status. For nurses, who have long fought for professional legitimacy, demoting themselves to nonprofessional status is a big price to pay for something of dubious value.

6. *Giving one's last name to patients is a violation of the nurses' right to privacy.* When we suggest that nurses use their last names, some students and working nurses reply that this violates their right to privacy. As one student put it, "If patients know our last name, then they can call us up and ask us questions at home if they want to."

Another nurse cast it in terms of unwanted attention: "We don't want our patients to know our last names. It's not an issue of professionalism, it's a privacy issue. A few years back, we had to wear name tags with our first and last names. Some male patients developed crushes on nurses and looked up their names and addresses in the phone book. There are a lot of creepy people out there and I know several nurses who were called at home for a date or even approached at their front door by an ex-patient."

While this nurse is correct in asserting that "there are a lot of creepy people out there," she is wrong to believe that concealing one's last name is not a professional issue. If nurses are to be accepted as professionals they must fulfill a central tenet of professionalism, which is to be responsible for one's practice and accountable to one's patients. The American Nurses Association Code of Ethics states, "Nurses are accountable for judgments and actions taken in the course of nursing practice, irrespective of health care organizations' policies or providers' directives."[14]

Nurses have a right to privacy but not anonymity. "How can you be held responsible for your practice if patients don't know who you are?" asks medical sociologist Ross Koppel. "When you become a professional you take on responsibility for your practice. You can't be anonymous and be a professional." To insist on a form of anonymity, Koppel argues, violates the entire process of professional licensure. "A professional is licensed not as Suzy or Bob. A professional is licensed as an identifiable adult—Susan Smith or Robert Jones."

The claim to anonymity also contradicts the patient bills of rights posted in hospitals and other health care institutions that explicitly grant patients the "right" to know who is taking care of them. We find it ironic when nurses argue that they are so vulnerable that patients don't have the right to know their last names, because the vulnerable party in the nurse-patient transaction is usually the patient. It is also the patients' private lives that are routinely exposed to the nurse. Nurses know patients' first and last names, their addresses, their personal data, sometimes their financial information, and embarrassing secrets about them. When nurses insist that they have a right to conceal even their name from patients, we wonder how they can then ask for the patient's trust.

7. *It's just too difficult to change cultural practices within an institution.* It certainly is difficult to change cultural practices if nurses unwittingly reinforce them. That's why it's important to start deconstructing deferential naming practices right now.

Many nurses say they would like more recognition and egalitarian treatment in the workplace. But they may be habitually enforcing an atmosphere of reverence and subordination to physicians. Decoding and altering naming

If patients do find out your home phone number and call you to request information, why interpret this as a violation of privacy? It may be a compliment. It suggests that you have important information or insights they are seeking. If you don't want to talk to patients at home, you can refer them to the appropriate resource or tell them you would be glad to talk to them during working hours.

If a patient appears on your doorstep and harasses you, it's imperative that you notify the police and the hospital.

practices ought to be a part of nursing education so that new nurses will not reinforce the idea that physicians are better than they are.

When we counseled nursing students in Philadelphia to insist on being called Ms., Mrs., or Mr. if residents and interns want to be referred to as Dr. in front of patients, one student demurred. "But he's a doctor," she responded, "and I'm just a nursing student."

"So what?" an older African American student countered. "I do it all the time. I just walk up to them, put out my hand to shake theirs and say, 'I'm Mrs. Smith. How are you?'"

We have noticed that African American nurses often are more sensitive to naming practices than are their white colleagues. There is a reason. It wasn't so long ago that African Americans were purposefully addressed only by first names, by nicknames, or by insulting titles such as *boy* for an adult man or *auntie* for an older woman. This naming system was used to keep an identified population in a subordinate social and economic position. Stopping this practice was one of the goals of the civil rights movement of the 1950s and 1960s. There was great resistance in some areas to adopting a more respectful form of address, namely, one that used honorific titles and last names, because the change would prompt and symbolize an elevation in status. We should not forget the courage it took to press this issue and the significance of the change.

To apply these hard-won rights to nurses might not be as daunting as some nurses fear. An older nurse in one seminar explained that she would like to be on a first name basis with the physicians she worked with, but feared that these young doctors would be offended if she called them by their first names. The instructors suggested that she pretend to arrive at work and say to the doctor, "Hi, Tom, how are you?" She replied that she was terrified that Tom would chastise her. The instructors countered that if "Tom" responded that way, the nurse should continue to use his title, but ask him to call her "Ms. (Last Name)."

She rehearsed at home until she felt more confident. One morning she went into work and said, "Hi, Tom, how are you?" Without batting an eye, Tom replied cheerfully, "Fine, how are you?"

The system of deferring to doctors, even when they may not want such treatment, can be quite entrenched. "I keep telling the nurses I work with to call me Emily," one physician we know says. "Some nurses say they can't bring themselves to call me by my first name. So then they call me Dr. Emily." Nurses are not alone in having to sort through the significance of various forms of address.

We decided some time ago to establish ground rules before participating in panel discussions or radio or television programs. We ask the host or moderator how they will address panel members who may be physicians, PhDs, or nurses.

Your Turn

List ways that nurses can identify their professional credentials in introductions and everyday practice. Be creative.

If the interviewers say they will refer to MDs and PhDs as Dr., then, we insist, they must refer to us as Ms. and to the nurses as Nurse or Ms. or Mr. If the hosts plan to call us by our first names, then, we tell them, they must address and refer to the MDs and PhDs by their first names also. We know that any disparity of address cues listeners to take our knowledge and insights less seriously than those of another expert, particularly one with a *Dr.* title. We feel that our messages about caregiving are too important to be overshadowed by traditional messages about status and hierarchy.

Two nurses attended one of our workshops in Victoria, British Columbia, in Canada. One of the nurses thought we were crazy to insist that nurses introduce themselves with their last name and title. The other thought we were right and suggested they give it a try for a day. Both nurses said they liked the results of the experiment. They felt better about their own work and patients seemed to view them with greater respect and asked them more questions.

Their badges, however, read, "Sue—Nursing." They went to an office supply store and ordered badges with their full names and *RN*. First the badges were a conversation piece, then they caught on. The manager ordered new badges for the entire unit.

Looking like a Nurse

Even though we write about current health care issues and contemporary nursing, we've learned the hard way that editors might illustrate our articles with an image of Florence Nightingale, with or without her lamp, or an old hospital-school photo of student nurses in their aprons and caps. Now we inquire about the illustrations well in advance of publication.

Both the lay public and nurses seem to find nostalgic images compelling. And why not? These images are the icons of nursing. Images of contemporary nurses at work usually require a caption to identify the subject as nursing.

Now freed from the laborious upkeep of starched uniforms, nurses must provide new visual cues to their identity to deal with the familiar patient lament "You can't tell whether the person coming into the room is a nurse, an aide, a

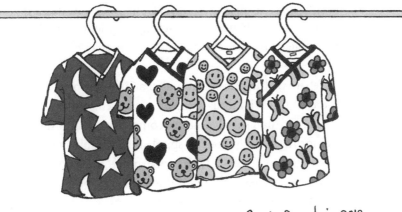

Sonia Oppenheim 2012

Sonia Oppenheim, www.familycomic.com

housekeeper, a technician or what." Because of the confusion, you also can't tell if a hospital unit is understaffed.

When patients express these concerns, you can be sure that they want to know who the nurses are and that what they consider to be an un-nurselike appearance makes them anxious. An elderly couple we know wrote a letter to the administrator of a Boston teaching hospital complaining that there was no way to identify the nurses because everybody in the institution looked "slovenly."

Perhaps this couple had antiquated expectations about how nurses should look. Nonetheless, the issue is serious. As one woman going in for a colonoscopy told us, "I was not at all reassured to have a woman in her fifties, with long hair, wearing scrubs with hearts plastered all over them come and introduce herself as Patti, the nurse. When I was settled in, another nurse came up to me. She was wearing neat slacks and a neat shirt, her hair was carefully coiffed, and she introduced herself with first and last name, told me she was a registered nurse, and exactly what her role was in my care. I wanted to grab her arm and ask her not to leave me. Her demeanor conveyed so much competence and knowledge."

Patients in our increasingly informal society find it unnerving not to know the professional or occupational identity of the myriad people who saunter into and out of their rooms. The formality of the traditional uniform had the effect of making hospital nurses—who often were very young—look older and more professional. In contrast, much of the clothing being marketed for today's nurses—many of whom are middle aged—is very informal, even girlish, in tone.

Pediatric nurses might consciously choose teddy bear smocks as a way to put their young patients at ease. But what impression does this clothing convey in a setting where maturity (irrespective of one's age) is an essential qualification? A nurse in this garb may believe she is telling a patient to not be afraid of her, but she is also suggesting that the patients and her colleagues should not take her seriously.

There is a big debate within nursing about what an appropriate nurses' uniform would be today. A celebrity designer, commissioned by a New Jersey hospital, found it was harder than she thought to come up with affordable, stylish, functional apparel for male and female hospital staff. As amusingly recounted in the *New Yorker* magazine, the stuff that one nurse took out of her scrub pockets—pen, notepad, tissues, scissors, adhesive tape, beeper, phone, and stethoscope—wouldn't fit into the "horizontal pockets, which were crucial to the line of the coat" that the designer came up with.[15] Standardization of dress is another hot topic. There is considerable debate about whether nurses should adopt standardized dress at all, apart from what a uniform might look like. But to us, that is not the issue. More important is the need to adopt a *style* of dress that assists nurses' efforts to be treated more professionally. Some nurses feel that lab coats and solid-color scrubs fit the bill. A badge or pin that gives the wearer's full name—minus the hearts and smiley faces—and that clearly identifies her or him as an RN is essential.

Some hospitals are rethinking the wisdom of having the equivalent of a come-as-you-are dress policy. The Hospital of the University of Pennsylvania decided it would mandate that nurses stop wearing silly-looking scrubs and all wear navy-blue scrubs. Over a period of a year, chief nursing officer Victoria Rich and the nursing department governing council led an effort to enlist nurses in this uniform change. Although many nurses were initially unhappy with the prospect, they were eventually convinced to make the change.

In Canada, the Association of Registered Nurses of Newfoundland and Labrador and the Newfoundland and Labrador Nurses Union are working to make it much clearer to patients who is and who is not a nurse. One way they are doing this is by encouraging registered nurses to wear a unique identifiable uniform.

Such efforts are supported by research findings that patients are confused by the indistinguishable cast of characters trooping in and out of their hospital rooms and that they want to be able to identify their registered nurse. In fact, in recent studies, most older adults prefer that nurses wear not dark scrubs but white ones.[16]

The issue of uniforms concerns us. We note that we respond more positively to people whose attire seems more professional. As we said above, brain science is beginning to confirm that such responses may actually be hard wired in how we as human beings relate to one another. Obviously cultural differences influence our perceptions, but the fact that costume affects perception seems to be universal.

What other people wear affects how we perceive them. It turns out that what we wear may also affect how we perceive ourselves and act. Psychological researchers have come up with the term "enclothed cognition" to describe "the systematic influence that clothes have on the wearer's psychological processes." Adam Gallansky at Northwestern University pretested subjects and discovered that medical lab coats were associated with attentiveness and carefulness. In one of Gallansky's experiments, subjects were assigned to wear a lab coat that was described as a doctor's lab coat. In another, subjects were assigned a lab coat that was described as a painter's coat. Other subjects simply saw a picture of a doctor's lab coat. Those subjects who wore the lab coat described as the doctor's increased selective attention compared with all the others.[17] In another study, students who wore street clothes caught fewer errors than those who wore a doctor's coat.[18]

This new field suggests that what nurses wear is not a trivial matter. When nurses wear uniforms that are perceived of as professional, they will not only be treated more seriously but also these uniforms may heighten their own professional self-esteem and behavior.

Who's a Girl?

There are other means by which the agency of nurses is undercut. The most common offense in everyday interactions is the use of the word *girl*. The son of an elderly patient tells the nurse manager that his mother needs help. The nurse manager wants to assure him that a staff nurse will soon be there and says, "I'll get one of the girls to help her." Through her word choice, she is diminishing the professional standing of nurses.

The word *girl* has various meanings and connotations. The sociolinguist Deborah Tannen, author of the best-selling book *You Just Don't Understand: Women and Men in Conversation*, told us that *girl* (or *lady*) has traditionally been used as a euphemism for *woman* because this last term, in some cultures, carries the unacceptable suggestion of sexuality, age, or both. So your eighty-year-old grandmother might tell you that she is having lunch with the girls and mean it as a compliment. We might refer to our best friends as "girlfriends." An African American woman might say to her friend, "Girl, let me tell you . . ." A husband might say to his wife, "How's my girl?" In these settings, the word conveys closeness and affection.

However, in the workplace, the word *girl* connotes standard dictionary definitions: a female child, an immature or inexperienced woman, a daughter, a female servant, a female sweetheart.

Do patients want a child to take care of them when they are sick? Do nurses want to be thought of as maidservants or sweethearts or young unmarried women? Just as forms of address were a major focus of the civil rights movement, one of the goals of the women's movement was to stop the routine use of the term *girl* to describe grown women.

Some might argue that men use parallel terminology. In fact, they don't. According to what Tannen told us, men use *boy* in a stylized way, as in "old boys' network" (which emphasizes the power of older males) or "night out with the boys" (which conveys the idea that men will temporarily put aside their adult responsibilities). Men don't use the term in a generalized way or in a professional setting. Has anyone ever heard a physician tell a patient, "I'll get one of the boys to come in for a neuro consult"?

Today a male physician probably wouldn't dare call a female physician a girl. Nor would a female physician refer to another female physician as a girl. When *boy* is used in a professional setting, it is overtly demeaning. Similarly, if a nurse uses *girl* to refer to nurses' aides or other health care workers—some of whom may be people of color—they risk sounding not just condescending but racist.

For all these reasons it is essential that nurses in the workplace cease using the word *girl* to refer to other nurses or to other adult workers. Instead, when referring to an RN colleague, one could simply say, "I'll ask my colleague for help," or, "I'll ask another nurse for help." And when referring to an aide or other health care worker, "I'll ask one of the aides to help you."

Body Language and "Presence"

Now that interdisciplinary teamwork has become central to patient safety, health care professional education, and health care delivery, it's critical for nurses to reflect on how various traditional behaviors enhance or defeat their ability to function as equal members of the health care team. In the aviation industry, a "high-reliability industry," crew members are team trained to be team leaders and team members. First of all, being a member of a team means that you are identifiable. It also means that you inquire about decisions or concerns, advocate for your point of view, and appropriately assert your views. Nurses need to learn to do this not only for patients but also for themselves. If they cannot advocate for themselves and be taken seriously as professionals, how can they advocate effectively for their patients?

Just as seemingly innocuous words and phrases can communicate volumes about nursing, so too can gestures, postures, physical arrangements, and actions.

Consider the following examples:

1. In one HMO, the physicians, male and female, usually shake hands with patients when they greet them. The nurses rarely do.

2. Nurses at one East Coast medical center point with pride to their strong nursing department and their collaborative relationships with physician colleagues. At this hospital, nurses round with physicians each morning and insist that they communicate their concerns as equal members of the health care team. Professionals from other facilities frequently visit to examine this collaborative model in action. We notice on one unit, however, that nurses and physicians arrange themselves in a stratified way to discuss cases. The medical students and residents stand against the wall in a hospital corridor and the attending faces them. The nurses stand behind the attending, craning their necks to hear what she is saying. The attending never turns to them, even when they have something to contribute to the discussion. The nurses never move in and stand next to the medical students and residents.

3. A nurse needs to talk with a physician about a patient. She finds the physician in the waiting room engaged in a conversation with another physician. The nurse stands quietly next to them. The physicians continue to talk without acknowledging her presence. Eventually the nurse shrugs and walks off, muttering that she'll catch the physician later. About an hour later, one of the physicians comes up to the nurses' station, where the same nurse is talking with several of her colleagues. Without apologizing, the doctor interrupts the nurses with a question. They immediately stop their conversation and the nurse responds politely.

4. A physician does a thoracentesis on an elderly woman with lung cancer while her daughter holds her hand. When the physician finishes, he starts to pick up the debris from the procedure. "Oh, let me do that," the nurse who is assisting says, reaching past him and commandeering the cleanup job.

5. A nurse calls a physician to clarify an order. She begins the conversation by profusely apologizing for "bothering" the doctor and ends by once again begging forgiveness for calling him.

What do these scenarios communicate? What do they teach physicians, nurses, and the public about the status and roles of RNs and MDs?

1. By opting out of the traditional handshake, the nurses are communicating that their role is not as significant as that of the physicians. No matter what the nurses say about themselves in the introduction, their failure to assert their individual presence through physical contact suggests that they prefer to be more in the background.

A firm but cordial handshake is an essential part of a professional introduction and provides the opening for nurses to state their names and credentials. When meeting a patient, a nurse can simply extend her or his hand, shake the patient's hand firmly, make eye contact, and say, "I'm Bill Jones, RN," or "I'm Nurse Jones," or "I'm Bill Jones, a registered nurse."

2. Nurses claim to be equal collaborators in patient care. But by standing behind the attending, the nurses collaborate in entirely another way. They construct a configuration that makes them look like spectators. The physicians have arranged themselves so that they converse with each other. When a nurse tries to contribute to the conversation, her hesitant speech conveys what she seems to feel, that she does not have a rightful place in this discussion, a point that is reinforced by her physical location.

Nurses on rounds could intersperse themselves among the physicians (rather than positioning themselves in the background) and speak up with authority when they have something to say. Nurse managers in teaching hospitals should be particularly alert to this kind of placement pattern. (When we pointed this behavior out to the nurse manager on the unit, she told us that she hadn't noticed it. She observed the nurses' placement at morning rounds. Yes, she agreed, we were right. From then on she made sure that nurses arranged themselves among the interns with some in front of rather than behind the residents.)

3. Nurses are undermined in their assertion that what they have to say to physicians about patients is as important as what physicians share with each other. In this case, the physicians' communication not only took precedence but also shut out the nurse. As in the second example, nursing is positioned outside the circle of influence. The nurse assents to this interpretation by shrugging and walking away. And when the physician interrupts her and her colleagues an hour later, by answering immediately she reaffirms that what the physician needs to know is much more important than what she and her colleagues are discussing.

The nurse could politely interrupt the physicians and state her business. And when the physician barged in on their conversation, the nurses could politely but firmly ask him to wait a moment until they finished consulting about a patient.

4. This scenario goes to the heart of the stereotype of nurses as handmaids to physicians. In this case, the physician, by cleaning up after himself and the nurse, communicates that he does not see the nurse as a maid. But the nurse becomes anxious about collegial treatment and rushes to reaffirm the traditional definition of the nurse—even though she might well have protested,

or at least complained later to her peers, if the physician had ordered her to clean up. By taking over the cleanup, this nurse is communicating a stereotypical job description of nursing to the doctor, patient, and family member.

In this case, the nurse could let the physician clean up after himself (as he had started to do).

5. When nurses or others apologize to a physician because they are asking the doctor to simply do his or her job, this immediately reaffirms asymmetrical power relationships. In conversations with physicians, nurses and other members of the health care team should never begin or end a conversation with an apology. A "thank you" is fine, but an "I'm sorry," not.

In the Canadian province of Newfoundland and Labrador, the Newfoundland and Labrador Nurses Union (NLNU) is conducting a three-year project to bring clarity to the value and role of the registered nurse in the health care system. As Debbie Forward, president of the NLNU explains:

"The public and stakeholders like CEOs and CNOs of health authorities and politicians do not have clarity about what specifically a registered nurse brings to the health care system. As nurses we have not told stories that articulate our value. Nor do we tell them by what we wear and how we present ourselves to patients.

"Our members have told us that they feel invisible and that they feel the role of the registered nurse may be fading away as health systems try to replace us with patient care assistants and licensed practical nurses. To address this we decided to do more than a six-week media PR campaign. We are launching a three-year campaign to bring clarity to the role of the registered nurse. We will be helping our members tell stories about what they do but we will also be encouraging them to present themselves professionally, with their first name, last name, and title *registered nurse*. Right now people identify themselves with their first name and sometimes with the term *nurse*. But that could be an LPN, a licensed practical nurse, not an RN. We have to start using professional introductions if we want the public to be clear about our value.

"We will also be asking them to consider a unique identifier for nurses in the workplace—that is, nurses should all wear the same-color uniform. There are several reasons for doing this.

"One is professionalism. Nurses say they want to be valued for their knowledge and expertise, yet we do not dress professionally. It's hard for someone to look at you and believe you have expertise when you're wearing balloons or teddies.

"Another reason is because patients are totally confused about about who does what in the health care system. They can't tell who is a registered nurse, an LPN, a PCA (patient care assistant), a housekeeper, porter, lab tech, or even social worker. Only physicians can be identified. Patients don't like this. They want to know who is who and who does what.

"Finally, when everyone looks the same, it's very easy to replace nurses with LPNs or PCAs because we all dress alike. Too many decision makers think they can replace an RN with an aide or LPN and there is no problem with that. If we want to convince the public that replacing one RN with two PCAs is a problem, people have to notice that the RN is missing in action. Right now, when we all wear the same uniform, a hospital can replace two RNs with two PCAs and no one will notice because there are still two bodies at the bedside and they both look the same. Today RNs can be replaced and no one will know they are gone. If we don't make these kinds of changes and we are replaced then we have no right to complain about it."

The ways in which nurses introduce themselves and the the attire they wear constitute both "private" interactions and "public" communications that convey information about the status and agency of nurses. Paying attention to self-presentation does not require a personality transplant and definitely does not mean that nurses have to turn themselves into unapproachable authoritarian figures. As British sociologist Celia Davies suggests, the choice need not be limited to either the authoritarian male professional model or the passive, dependent female role. She recommends "reconstructing" a model of professionalism appropriate to the needs both of the sick and of the largely female nurses who care for them. This new model of professionalism could be constructed around the concept of "meaningful distance," which "acknowledges that there will be a commitment and emotional response, but seeks to avoid over-identification on the one hand and under-involvement on the other."[19]

In other words, by asserting their agency in their self-presentation, nurses need not worry that projecting a professional image will make them seem distant or feel self-conscious, false, or stilted. Instead, nurses will be presenting a strong image of themselves, one that calls forth responses that are respectful of them as nurses and as human beings.

CHAPTER 5

TELL THE WORLD WHAT YOU DO

After a recent talk we gave, a nurse in the audience raised her hand. Why, she wondered, did she have to worry about explaining her work to the public? Wasn't that the job of her national nurses' association? They were the ones with the influence. She was, she said, "just a nurse." How much could "just a nurse" do?

The answer is, a lot.

Recall our discussion in chapter 1 of the "publics" with whom nurses are in contact. Think for a moment about how many people a nurse comes into contact with each day just at work. Consider a bedside nurse in a hospital.

Let's say the nurse has from four to twelve patients that she or he is in contact with. Most patients come with family members and friends. Let's give each patient two family members and two friends who visit. Now each "patient unit" consists of five people. So, on a daily basis, just counting patients and families and friends of patients, the nurse is connecting with or relating to some 20 to 60 people.

To be conservative, let's say the nurse works three days a week. Over the course of a year, she or he will work some 150 days. Since some of the patients will be in the hospital for a few days, we can subtract, say, 30 days from the 150, which gives us 120 days. If we multiply 120 by either 20 or 60, we get a range of from 2,400 to 7,200 people whom our "just a nurse," comes into contact with each year while caring for patients. There are other contacts in the workplace as well. The nurse interacts with other nurses, nursing assistants, administrative staff, physicians, and other personnel. These professional contacts can be added to the numbers.

So far we have estimated only workplace contacts. Nurses themselves have friends, family members, people with whom they attend church, sports events, political meetings, and social events or encounter in other settings. Now we have increased one nurse's contacts dramatically. What if we multiply "just a nurse's" contacts by the number of nurses in any given city, state, region, or country? There would be millions of contacts.

The question that thus arises is, what do nurses make of the "public relations" opportunities that present themselves with these contacts? Do nurses view exchanges as solely intimate and private, or do they understand that, while engaged in acts of professional practice, they can also have a significant impact on how patients and others view the role of nurses and nursing in our health care systems?

Life presents nurses with countless conversational openings to talk about nursing. Not every nurse will be called by a reporter from the *New York Times*, but nurses constantly speak with small publics who ask what they do or

A medical-surgical nurse who had participated in a major nursing conference called the hotel bellman for help in getting her bags to the airport shuttle bus. As the nurse and bellman were walking to the elevator, the young man turned to her and remarked, "The people here aren't ordinary nurses, are they?"

Intrigued by the question, the nurse asked what he meant. "Well," he said, "I've been walking through the exhibit area and there are all these fancy medical machines and equipment. 'Ordinary' nurses don't use such complicated equipment," he stated confidently. "This must be a conference for chiefs."

Without skipping a beat, the nurse replied: "This *is* a conference for ordinary nurses. We use all kinds of sophisticated medical equipment and medications when we take care of you. Ordinary nurses *are* the chiefs of patient care in hospitals."

Another nurse told us about an incident that occurred when she flew into Rochester, Minnesota, for a conference at the Mayo Clinic. On the way into town, her cab driver proudly boasted about Rochester's medical reputation. "We have some of the best medical care in the world," he said. "The best doctors and researchers are here. People come here from all over the globe just to see them."

She listened and then gently reminded him that he forgot an important part of the health care team. "All of these great doctors," she told him, "wouldn't succeed without great nurses. You must remember to tell your next passenger about that too."

who make a comment about nursing. Sometimes these comments contain erroneous information that needs to be corrected. Other times, the comment may give you an opportunity to advance someone's knowledge about your profession. Working with patients on a daily basis provides the nurse with many educational openings.

> Life presents nurses with countless conversational openings to talk about nursing. Not every nurse will be called by a reporter from the *New York Times*, but nurses constantly speak with small publics who ask what they do or who make a comment about nursing.

Patient Talk

Each time a nurse walks into a patient's room to take a vital sign, administer a medication, help a patient with an activity of daily living, or answer a question, she or he can convey a world of skill and knowledge. Given nurses' concerns about patient confidentiality, educating patients about what they are doing as they are caring for them represents a perfect opportunity for nurses to convey an accurate picture of nursing. Many nurses, however, do their work in silence. Even in conversation they don't tell the patient what they are doing and why they are doing it.

Consider the following examples:

- A nurse walks into a patient's room to take his blood pressure or listen to his lungs. She makes a notation in a chart or on a computer and walks out.
- A nurse talks to a postsurgical patient about her pain. He shows the patient the smiling/frowning faces on the pain scale card and asks her to identify what she's experiencing. Fine, the nurse says. He makes a note and comes back later with pain medication.
- A nurse is caring for a patient who had delivered a baby the previous day. She notes that the patient has not got up to walk. She asks her to get up and walk and offers to help her out of bed.

What's missing in these exchanges? What's missing is any hint that the nurse is doing something that requires clinical knowledge. What could the nurse say in these situations?

Scenario One: The nurse says: Hello, Mr. Smith, I'm here to take your blood pressure because I want to make sure it's within normal ranges and that nothing is going on that we need to follow. (Nurse takes blood pressure.) It's a little

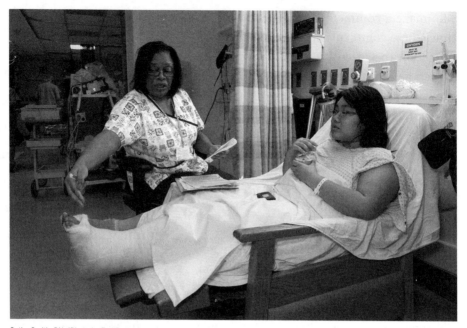

Cathy Smith, RN. (Photo by Earl Dotter.)

high. That could indicate . . . I'm going to keep an eye on that and consult with the physician about changing . . .

Alternately: Hello, Mr. Smith. I just want to take a quick listen to your lungs because I want to make sure they are nice and clear. (Listens.) I hear a little crackling in your left lower lobe. I'm going to keep an eye on that.

Scenario Two: The nurse approaches his postsurgical patient and says: Hello, Ms. Jones. I'm here to assess the level of your pain because we really want to keep any pain well managed. It's not a good idea for people to tough it out when they're in pain because pain can limit your ability to recover. (Shows the pain scale card. The patient points to a face that indicates moderately high discomfort. The nurse and patient discuss the level.) Ms. Jones, I'm going to consult with the physician, and then I will give you medication to make you more comfortable. Keeping on top of this will help your recovery.

Scenario Three: Mrs. Miller, I'm Nurse Sarah Burns. I see that you had your baby yesterday and you're doing really well. Have you taken a walk yet? No? I am here to make sure you do that because walking keeps your blood circulating effectively. Inactivity can lead to the risk of a blood clot. So let's get you up and get your blood moving. Okay? Hold on to me if you feel any dizziness.

Some nurses are concerned that if they explain why they are doing what they are doing, they will frighten the patients. We now know, however, that helping patients to understand the risks they face while helping them to prevent or manage problems effectively may actually relieve the patient's anxiety. People who are in hospitals or other health care settings know that these places can be dangerous and that there are risks involved in any treatment. It's better to prepare people to deal with difficult or unusual situations, so that they feel assured that they are being cared for and so that they can participate in their own care and act more effectively on their own behalf.

More to the point, explaining what you are doing and why you are doing it conveys critical information about what a nurse knows. It indicates that nurses understand the significance of the signs and symptoms they observe and that they assess them to create a plan of care and to enhance the clinical team's understanding and ability to deal with the patient's condition and needs. This counters the notion that nurses are uncritically following doctors' orders and collecting information and data that the doctor alone pieces together. As the health care system focuses more on collaborative practice and teamwork, patients and the public need to know what the nurse does on the health care team.

We've just shown how you can talk with patients to influence their perception of nursing. Patients' families represent another public. Say you are taking care of a patient who has just had a stroke. His daughter comes to visit while you are feeding the patient. You can do your work silently. Or, while you are feeding the patient, you can explain to him and to his daughter the significant aspects of what you are doing. It isn't necessary to deliver a dissertation on the four phases of swallowing. But it may be useful to explain that you are assessing the patient's gag reflex and why that is important. In describing this, you are teaching the patient and his daughter not only how he can eat safely but also that nurses have lifesaving knowledge.

To many people, the more domestic activities of nursing may seem simple or trivial. They may even wonder why it takes an educated person to do them. This is an opportunity to enlighten them. Explain why activities such as feeding, bathing, toileting, walking, or turning patients can be some of the most important things a nurse does.

Many people confuse complex nursing activities with kindness or niceness. For example, the mother of an artist we know had a brain tumor and underwent surgery to remove it. The artist explained to us that the nurses were so "nice." They were very attentive, talked kindly to her mother, and took advantage of every opportunity to "chat with her." She was surprised to learn that the nurses were doing much more than she or her mother imagined, such as tracking her mother's intracranial pressure, making sure her mother didn't develop an internal bleed, checking her temperature to make sure she didn't have a wound infection, and engaging in myriad other lifesaving activities. "I had no idea," the daughter said.

When nurses display their knowledge and clinical skill, many patients respond with what they think is a compliment, as in "My goodness, you know so much, you could be a doctor!" That displays of knowledge provoke surprise and such a response indicates how little patients understand nursing and how thoroughly they have been trained to think that physicians own clinical knowledge. The kind of patient talk we recommend could have a big impact on expanding the view of patients and their families and friends.

Be Prepared to Take Advantage of Openings

If you were asked to do a presentation on nursing at your church or to talk about health care on a local television show, you would take time to prepare your remarks. The more spontaneous communication opportunities that regularly come your way also require preparation. Although they don't come in the form of an invitation, these openings are nevertheless quite predictable.

For example, someone at a party asks you what you do. You respond, "I'm a nurse." The other person doesn't know what to say. "Oh, how nice," she mutters politely and then goes on to a different subject.

On hearing that you are a pediatric nurse, an oncology nurse, or a hospice nurse, an acquaintance responds, "That must be so depressing. How can you stand working with sick children, cancer patients, dying people?" To someone outside health care, anything that has to do with sickness, vulnerability, and death may appear to be draining and unbearably depressing rather than enriching and rewarding.

Other conversational openings may come in the form of jibes that seem to overtly devalue nursing. One nurse recounted that she was talking to a businessman about her work as a nurse practitioner. "So you've gotten out of the bedpan business," he retorted.

Another told of a man at a cocktail party who asked, "Why did you become a nurse when someone as obviously intelligent as you could have been a doctor?"

An Australian nurse was the only RN at a dinner party with a number of professional men and women. At the dinner table, one of the guests turned to her and said condescendingly, "So why are you doing nursing? To do a nice bit of caring?"

A student nurse told us she often goes out with a group of friends that includes medical students. Over dinner, those friends who are in business or law address their questions or comments to the medical students and never ask her questions about what she's learning and doing in nursing school.

Such experiences are demoralizing. Their frequency can leave nurses speechless, so angry they want to scream, or, worse, inured to it so that they just shrug.

Being prepared to respond constructively is a better approach. To be prepared, you must be willing to acknowledge that situations like this are not going to miraculously disappear. Indeed, you can be really effective if you embrace even the most negative comments as educational opportunities. Be glad that someone has mentioned nursing. Consider your friends, relatives, or acquaintances as people requiring instruction and try to evince sympathy for people who are ill informed. Even the most disheartening comments about nursing usually stem from ignorance rather than malice.

This interpretation allows you to prepare yourself to take on the challenge of educating the public about nursing. If you don't correct a misimpression with an assertive comment, the person who denigrates nursing will, literally, have the final word on the subject.

When someone says to you, "God, how depressing it must be to deal with sick children or dying patients all the time," you can respond, "Sometimes it's sad, but it's not depressing. Let me tell you about my work so you'll understand." Then you can describe your work and the difference it made to those who benefited from your care.

If someone makes a crack about bedpans, you can respond the way one nurse practitioner did: she described what the contents of a bedpan can reveal about a patient's condition.

When a nursing student told us that his friends commonly respond to his choice of career with "So now you're going to be a butt wiper," we asked him how he responded. "Oh, I tell them we have other people to do that now." We suggested that this way of dealing with the derogatory comment actually validated the notion that cleaning a patient who has soiled himself is beneath the dignity of a nurse with a university degree.

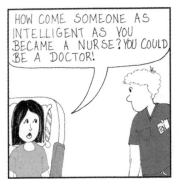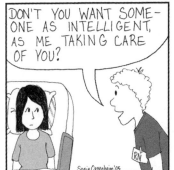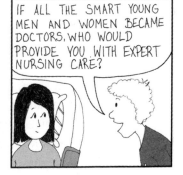

Sonia Oppenheim, www.familycomic.com

Why not tell your friends, we suggested, that cleaning someone can be one of the most important things a nurse can do? Tell them there might come a day when they will need a nurse who's educated enough to know that cleaning someone is a way to prevent all sorts of potentially catastrophic complications and who will do it without humiliating the patient. Tell them, "If you're ever flat on your back in the hospital, you better hope someone as smart as I am is there to wipe your butt."

Perhaps the most infuriating question you'll get is "Why did someone as intelligent as you become a nurse?" Or for students, "Why aren't you in medical school instead of nursing school?"

We have thought a lot about this question. We used to advise nurses to explain their choice and illuminate how nursing differs from medicine. We still believe that is an essential part of any response. Now we feel that the erroneous assumptions embedded in the question must themselves be challenged too.

The question "Why did you become a nurse; why didn't you become a doctor?" is simply illegitimate. When we tell people we're journalists, no one asks us why we didn't become poets. When doctors tell people what they do, no one asks them why they didn't go into bioengineering instead. They ask them what their specialty is and what their work is like. When a bright young man says he is in medical school, he's asked what he wants to specialize in, not why isn't he going into a different health profession altogether. Today, when a woman announces her decision to become a doctor, she's viewed as a representative of the advancement of women.

Not so with nurses. An interesting social disconnect takes place when an intelligent woman or man is a nurse or announces an intention to become one. Rather than being viewed as pioneers expanding the definition of masculinity, male nurses or nursing students are often viewed as peculiar, while female nurses or nursing students might be regarded as having made a retro choice. Nurses can change such attitudes by the way they respond to comments and questions.

Instead of telling people, "I became a nurse because I want to care for people," you might calmly reply, "You know, if you asked me what I do as a nurse, and let me describe it to you, then you would understand why I chose to become a nurse instead of a doctor." Or, if you're a student, you might say brightly: "Why don't you ask me what I want to do as a nurse; then you'll understand why I'm going to nursing school and not medical school. I plan to work with geriatric patients and help them stay independent longer."

In social situations, when people find out you're a nurse and say nothing or say, "Oh how nice," that is an opening. You can direct the conversation with a few engaging questions and comments like "Do you know much about nursing?

Today, with greater attention to teamwork and patient safety, public awareness of the profession is really important."

The Australian nurse could have said to the condescending dinner guest, "I certainly hope that if, God forbid, you ever have cancer, an experienced oncology nurse will be there to give you that 'bit of caring' that might save your life."

Learn to Accept Thanks

Nurses have the opportunity to explain their work when a patient expresses gratitude for excellent nursing care. Think about the last time a patient thanked you. How did you respond? Did you accept the acknowledgment? Or did you say, "Oh, it was nothing," "I didn't do very much," or "It was just my job"? A lot of us rely on this conversational tack when we are complimented. But for nurses it has consequences.

When nurses say, "Oh, it was nothing," the danger is that people will believe them. And if "it"—nursing work—is "just a job" or "not very much of anything," the logical conclusion one draws is that nurses are nothing special. Why then should the public worry if nurses are replaced with aides or, as so frequently happens today, with untrained family members who are expected to act as surrogate professional nurses in the home? If nurses do little or nothing, why should the public support additional resources for nurse staffing, education, and research?

An alternative response to gratitude can highlight the content of nursing care. A woman tells you, "You were so great. You helped my husband to cope with his diabetes." This is your opportunity to respond, "Thank you. I was pleased to take care of your husband, to teach him how to take his medication, and to help him learn how to alter his diet. If you have any further questions or needs please talk to me about them."

We talked with oncology nurses in Rhode Island about the tendency of nurses to trivialize their own work. Phoebe Fernald, an oncology clinical nurse specialist, approached us afterward. She said nurses' difficulty in saying, "Thank you," and "You're welcome," in response to compliments and gratitude struck a chord with her. "It's scary how automatically pat answers come out of our mouths," she said.

Fernald gave an illustration. She had recently helped family friends navigate their father's illness and death from cancer. At the calling hours before the funeral, the family thanked her and told her how much they appreciated what she had done. And what did she say? "Oh, I didn't do very much at all."

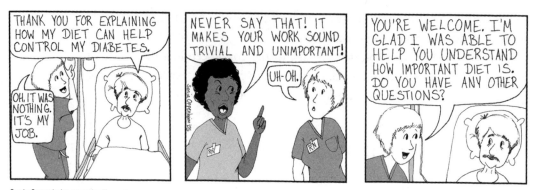

Sonia Oppenheim, www.familycomic.com

"But when I think about it," Fernald told us, "I did a lot. I took time to listen to them. They needed to talk about their pain and hurt. They needed to talk about their concerns—whether they were doing the right thing, choosing the right treatments; and when he no longer wanted more treatment, they needed to know that was okay too. They needed confirmation that they were making the right choices. And they needed it from someone who was an expert. [Fernald initially said, "From someone who they perceived to be an expert," but changed her wording when we reminded her that she is one.] When patients thank us, they are thanking us for our expertise and our skill in caring. When we say, 'Oh, it was nothing,' we're denying that expertise and skill."

When we suggested that Fernald could have said, "You're welcome. It was a privilege to be able to help you," she responded, "That would not be a dishonest answer. It was a privilege."

Don't Suppress Your Enthusiasm

As every nurse knows, affect is important in establishing a connection with patients. It is no less so when talking with members of the public. Don't be afraid of appearing engaged or emotional when you tell your stories. Let your eagerness, enthusiasm, and commitment to nursing be reflected in your voice and body language. When nurses speak with passion and conviction—rather than in cautious and passive tones—they convince the public that nurses are important professionals who cannot easily be replaced.

When you are discussing changes in the health care system that cause harm, don't be afraid to express your moral outrage. As long as you're not shrill or out of control, expressing profound concern is appropriate and justified. Similarly, don't be afraid to show your sorrow or grief. If you are telling a story about patient care that brings tears to your eyes and a catch in your throat, don't be embarrassed. As long as you don't give the impression that your work overwhelms you with grief and sadness, those who listen to you will be impressed with the depth of your feelings and your commitment to your work and patients.

Respecting Patient Confidentiality

When nurses are encouraged to talk about their work, they often worry that to do so will violate patient confidentiality. This is a pressing concern in school and the workplace. The importance of patient confidentiality is clearly stated in the International Council of Nurses Code for Nurses: "The nurse holds in confidence personal information and uses judgment in sharing this information."[1]

In the United States, the Health Insurance Portability and Accountability Act (HIPAA) of 1996 established a "privacy rule" that prohibits revealing "individually identifiable information. . . . The definition of individually identifiable information includes any information that relates to the past, present, or future physical or mental health of an individual, or provides enough information that leads someone to believe the information could be used to identify an individual."[2]

In Canada, various provinces have enacted and updated similar privacy laws. In many countries, clinicians and other health care workers may not reveal any patient information without the patient's consent.

It is critical for nurses to understand that these patient privacy laws do not mean they cannot talk about their work with patients at all. One labor and delivery nurse, for example, told us, "I can't go home and tell my husband and children that I just helped a thirty-five-year-old woman deliver a healthy baby. That would violate patient confidentiality." Nurses who work in rural areas may feel that they cannot talk about what it takes to care for patients who have had heart attacks because someone in their community who had a heart attack will think the nurse is talking about him or her.

Do you think these assessments about privacy are accurate?

They're not.

Respecting patient privacy and confidentiality does *not* mean you cannot talk about your patients. It means you can't identify patients, use their names, or reveal details about their care.

> It is critical for nurses to understand that these patient privacy laws do not mean they cannot talk about their work with patients at all.

According to nurse-writer Teresa Brown, who writes about nursing for a broad public audience:

> The rules about HIPAA are actually pretty easy to navigate. HIPPA says not that patients won't be able to recognize themselves in writing, but that other people will not be able to identify them . . .
>
> When I write for the *New York Times,* a twenty-five-year-old male patient with a new diagnosis of acute myelogenous leukemia might become a "young man with a newly discovered blood cancer." Similarly, a breast cancer patient with metastatic disease to the brain and bone can be described as a "patient with cancer that spread."[3]

As Brown points out, you can change details that might reveal the identity of patients or talk about a generic patient. When you describe a particular case as an example of your work, you can explain that you've altered some facts to protect your patient's privacy but that the essence of the story remains. In many instances, patients have similar problems and experiences, and unless you give specific identifying details, there will be no way that anyone can determine who your patients are. Your listeners aren't concerned with the name, age, or address of a particular patient. They're interested in what a nurse contributes to quality patient outcomes.

A nurse at an East Coast hospital had been interviewed for a Sunday magazine article about the emergency room. A photographer from the magazine called to arrange a photo shoot. The photographer had permission from the administration to do the shoot and wanted the nurse to appear in the article with patients. The nurse's manager told the photographer that the nurse would have to ask the patients if they would agree to be photographed.

But the manager didn't leave it at that. She kept harping on the need to prevent any violation of patient confidentiality. The photographer said the manager made the nurse so nervous that he, the nurse, didn't even want to approach patients to ask their permission. Finally, after much prodding from the photographer, the nurse asked several patients. As many people would have been, they were delighted that they might have their picture in the magazine and instantly agreed. By this time, however, the nurse had become so anxious about the photo shoot that he stiffened every time the camera clicked. None of the pictures were usable. The photographer was frustrated. She said she had never had such a bad experience on a photo shoot. Much to the chagrin of the hospital administrators, who were courting good publicity, this hospital and the people in it did not appear in the magazine.

An exaggerated fear of violating patient privacy is often a way that nurses silence themselves and each other, as the previous example illustrates.

We believe that professors of nursing, nursing managers and administrators and members of professional nursing organizations must teach nurses not only what they can't say but also *what they can say*. This effort is critical because, unlike physicians, nurses are susceptible to interpreting privacy rules as a muzzle that prohibits any statement about patient care, even something like "I checked the patient's blood pressure, temperature, and respiratory rate."

Some nursing organizations are working to clarify these misunderstandings. For example, in Canada leaders of the Newfoundland and Labrador Nurses Union (NLNU) and the Association of Registered Nurses of Newfoundland and Labrador (ARNNL) are helping their members to be able to talk about their work even in sparsely populated or rural areas where everybody seems to know everybody else.

Siobhainn Lewis, executive director of the ARNNL, and Mary Prideaux, vice president of the NLNU, came up with an example of a narrative that would not violate patient confidentiality: "As a cardiac nurse I closely monitor patients who are hospitalized for problems like Congestive Heart Failure [CHF]. I know from experience that patients with cardiac problems like CHF are at risk for shortness of breath. I can tell quite quickly when a patient is experiencing shortness of breath even before taking their blood pressure and respiratory rate. I can tell by just looking at them. If I walk into a room and see a patient bent over the bedside table, that tells me they may be having problems. If their color has changed, that's another indication. If they aren't speaking in full sentences, and if they are using their accessory muscles in their neck and shoulders to help them breathe, these are signals that tell me to take immediate action."

Dealing with Your Fears

Many nurses have told us they are afraid that they will make mistakes if they talk about their work. They say they fear being misinterpreted or that they will provoke an angry response. Some nurses worry that talking about their work might mean that they're exploiting their patients. Some are concerned about generating conflict or controversy, being fired, or being viewed as disloyal to their institutions. Others feel that they are "just a nurse," not

> We believe that professors of nursing, nursing managers and administrators, and members of professional nursing organizations must teach nurses not only what they can't say but also *what they can say*.

important enough to talk either about nursing or broader health care system issues. Perhaps nurses' worst fear is that nobody will care.

These are serious concerns.

Nurses have been convinced that they aren't either knowledgeable or important. Thus the "just a nurse" mantra. We are distressed when we hear nurses put down their own knowledge, accomplishments, and expertise. No nurse is "just a nurse," even one who has just got out of nursing school. Even novice nurses know a great deal more than most people about health and illness, and about broader health care system issues. It's important for all nurses to counter this notion.

As for the fear of making mistakes, we all need to recognize that despite our best efforts, we are vulnerable to making mistakes when we speak or write. When we use facts and statistics, it is important to ensure they are correct. If you are concerned about an argument or tone, run it by a trusted colleague who is knowledgeable about the issue.

At the same time, be realistic. Many mistakes can be rectified. In fact, mistakes are very useful, if you try to learn from them. Some points may be debatable rather than right or wrong. Indeed, much of the information about nursing that you might convey to individuals and groups will represent your perspective and experience as a nurse. Others nurses may have different perspectives, but it doesn't mean that yours is "wrong" or "mistaken." Your experiences and ideas are just as valid as anyone else's.

It is also important to recognize that no matter how much you learn, no one ever has perfect knowledge. Try as you might, you can never reach a point where it is guaranteed that you won't make a mistake. If you are waiting for that day before you speak up, you will be silent forever.

Far from exploiting patients, nurses who talk about their patient care are actually reassuring patients that they are in the hands of people who care about their work.

Worrying about how others will respond to one's comments is normal. But none of us can control the responses of others. The moment one opens one's mouth to tell a story, share a feeling, or express an opinion, one loses control over how it will be received. The more people you speak to, the more you can be sure that someone will misunderstand, misinterpret, misconstrue, disagree, feel betrayed, or just tune out. This is a fact of life. Just as it does not deter most of us from talking to our friends, acquaintances, or coworkers, neither should it deter us from speaking to a wider audience in person or through the media.

Sometimes nurses are afraid to make their concerns known because they may generate conflict. That may be difficult for some nurses to cope with. After all, for decades, the mandate of nurses has been to conceal conflict within health care institutions or to try to manage and smooth over conflict with patients and families. This is reflected in the comments nurses have made at our workshops. "I'm afraid of getting into a situation of 'one side against the other,'" one nurse said. One nurse wrote us a note that stated just how dangerous she believes conflict is; "I'm afraid of causing conflict/chaos."

Seeing controversy and conflict solely as stations on the road to chaos obliterates the constructive role of disagreement. Reluctance to risk disagreement hampers intellectual and professional development, not only for individuals but for a whole profession. One editor of a nursing journal feels that "conflict phobia" among nurses is curtailing rigorous intellectual debate about nursing. She says that she solicits critiques of articles in her journal to enlarge the discussion of important issues. But instead of critiques, she receives mostly innocuous commentary that fails to engage the issues. "I think even highly educated nurses are too afraid that they might offend someone," she told us. "So they just give a very tame response."

The oft-stated yearning that nurses should "speak with one voice" can be interpreted as a wish for total safety. In one voice there is no disagreement, thus no risk, and ultimately no story. Waiting for all three million U.S. nurses and the millions of other nurses throughout the world to speak with one voice is a perfect recipe for self-silencing.

Exposing System Problems

When you begin to talk about what you do, this often leads to discussion of the conditions under which you work. Many nurses today are very concerned about the impact of their working conditions on their health and well-being, job satisfaction, and ability to provide safe patient care. Invite nurses to talk and some may want to talk primarily about the obstacles they face in doing their job safely and effectively. We believe it is very important for nurses to publicly discuss patient care and safety issues. After all, the meaning of nursing and nursing advocacy includes not only caring for the patient but also attending to the context in which the patient receives care.

Some nurses are afraid to expose system problems because they do not want to be disloyal to their institution. Nurses have told us they don't want to publicly discuss serious problems because they don't want to harm an institution whose mission, if not its actions, is a worthy one. They worry that public exposure will rupture relationships in their workplace and in a community they value.

Claire Fagin, dean emerita of the University of Pennsylvania School of Nursing, is sympathetic to those who feel they face this dilemma. Fagin and others point out that institutions tend to be far more resilient than nurses may believe them to be and that exposing serious problems may strengthen institutions rather than weaken them. "I always advise nurses to go through channels before they expose any serious system problems," Fagin says. "But if you get absolutely nowhere, it's important to determine your bottom line. Is your bottom line loyalty to your institution or is it to protect patients? The bottom line has to be to protect patients."

A more pressing concern is the worry that if you reveal what's going on within your institution, you will be disciplined or fired. How do you use your voice and agency and protect yourself?

In the United States, the First Amendment does not protect freedom of speech in the workplace. Indeed, in most workplaces, nurses are what is known as "employees at will," who can be fired for "no just cause." There is, however, one exception to the restriction on freedom of speech in the workplace and that covers what is known as "protected concerted activity." Under the National Labor Relations Act, if employees act together, in concert, to raise an issue that is connected to wages, hours, and working conditions, they have some protection against management retaliation. This is one of the many reasons that nurses join unions: belonging to a union means that nurses can engage in protected concerted activity and can take on efforts to impinge on their ability to speak about their concerns to the National Labor Relations Board.

Nurses in the United States who don't belong to a union can also gain the protection of the National Labor Relations Act if they make sure to raise issues with at least one other RN or employee. So if you are raising an issue (either within your institution or publicly outside it) you need to make sure that you have safety in numbers, even if it's with only one colleague.

Before taking action, it's important to document concerns and try to raise them within the institution involved. If nurses are not represented by a union, they could consult with the staff of a local or national union that represents nurses, or they may want to consult with an attorney who specializes in employment law.

When nurses stop being silent and talk about their work, the public listens. The story of Barry Morley, an Australian critical care nurse, is a dramatic example.

In 2002, Morley; his wife, Kate Simpson, a clinical nurse; and their fourteen-year-old daughter, Grace, took a vacation trip to Bali. The Morleys' twelve-year-old son had died three months earlier, and the family was in mourning.

All three were in their hotel room on October 12 when around 11 P.M. they heard an explosion. A second explosion blew the roof off their hotel, extinguished the lights, and shattered the windows. They rushed outside. Bloodied and wounded people began streaming down a small lane to the hotel. These were the injured fleeing from the terrorist attack on Bali that killed 202 people and injured more than 400 others.

Morley and Simpson flew into action. They set up, in effect, a field hospital, recruiting guests and the less severely injured to gather supplies and help treat those whose lives were at stake. They were confronted with massive head wounds, traumatic amputations, lung injuries, and severe burns. They bandaged wounds with strips of cloth torn from sheets, employed surfboards as stretchers, and wrapped chest wounds with plastic bags to prevent lungs from collapsing. Morley triaged the wounded at the bomb site and saved those he could while Simpson worked at the hotel. Young Grace consoled the dying.

Morley and Simpson were the only health professionals at the bomb site for almost five hours. Their knowledge, expertise, and actions saved dozens of people. Yet hardly anyone knew that Morley and Simpson were at the Bali bombing, much less what they did there. This is because, Morley said, they didn't want to talk about it. They worried about gaining status from other people's suffering. They also worried that other nurses would consider them boastful. When Morley gave a rare newspaper interview, he attributed what he and his wife did to "common sense."

Finally, about a year and a half after the incident, Morley realized that to tell his story was not to brag about himself but to illuminate the knowledge and skill of nurses. And he began to talk about his and his wife's actions. His nursing colleagues had nothing but appreciation for his decision to break his silence. The broader community responded with equal respect. He and his wife and daughter received the Order of Australia, the country's highest award. A scholarship was founded in the name of their late son, Ben, for members of the College of Emergency Nursing who are engaged in research and education in emergency preparedness and continuity management.

In an article he wrote, "The World Is Loud but Nurses Remain Silent," Morley entreated his colleagues to "be more vocal for the benefit of our profession, our society, and other societies." He argued that "Any event that affects the health and well-being of a nation or group of people should gain a public comment from the nursing profession" lest the public think that "nursing is ill-equipped to offer an opinion." In his article, Morley traced his own journey from silence to voice:

My wife and I were the only health professionals at ground zero when those two massive explosions occurred. My wife and I assisted in the retrieval of victims from those night-clubs, set up a triage point 120 meters away and began front-line management. We personally treated over 55 victims, 25 of whom were critically injured. On our return to Australia we were interviewed and asked how we managed to be so resourceful. The first time I was asked this question, I answered rather poorly saying, "It was all just common sense really." The fact is there was nothing common sense about it at all. Our response was remarkable and life-saving, and reflected years of critical care nursing expertise.

Through trial and error of subsequent interviews we now take the opportunity to express the incredible expertise that one gains over a career in nursing and also feel compelled to express political opinion. It's highly important for us as humans and as nurses to state our belief that violence, whether perpetuated by an individual or a government, is a solution for nothing. We believe that violence merely serves to exacerbate the original problem. I ask you as my peer; is Iraq more stable, is the threat of terrorism now gone, now that our country has participated in the war upon that nation?

It is not correct for nurses to view such events as non-nursing issues and thus, although important, as not a part of the core issues that nurses discuss or upon which we make political comment. Where issues affect the health and well-being of a nation or group it is incumbent upon us to form an opinion and voice it publicly . . . It is the public voice of nursing that increases our capacity to hold a greater share of power in shaping policy and public opinion.

I am concerned less about the fact your opinion may differ from mine than I am that you and other colleagues have nothing to say at all. Be vocal, express your opinion publicly and within professional journals. Nursing must start to talk before it can expect to be heard."[4]

CHAPTER 6

CREATING ANECDOTES
AND ARGUMENTS

Anecdotes that nurses relate about their work and arguments they make to explain their role in the health care system help people to understand and appreciate the nature of nursing and the agency of nurses. Telling stories also helps nurses feel more self-confident and appreciative of the work that many consider to be "routine" or "just part of my job."

Research on the value of storytelling and narrative confirms what we have seen in our lectures and workshops: storytelling is a powerful way to counteract the negative voices that have long told nurses (or women, or other marginalized groups) that they are not as important or valuable as dominant groups. This socialization has convinced many nurses that they are "just a nurse," and that no one wants to hear about their work. Such devaluing voices can be insidious. We hear this negative chatter even when we think we have tuned it out of our minds, and we may be influenced by it in ways we do not consciously understand.

In his book, *Whistling Vivaldi: And Other Clues to How Stereotypes Affect Us*, psychologist Claude Steele describes the pernicious influence of what he calls the "stereotype threat." He explains that when people know they belong to a group that has been socially devalued, they tend to underperform in situations in which they feel that the "stereotype threat" is salient.[1] For example, women math whizzes do less well on math tests when they think that the test is one that judges women's math ability. Because social prejudices hold that women are inferior to men when it comes to math, women who otherwise perform admirably underperform on tests they think pit them against men. Similarly, white athletes underperform when they think they are being judged against black athletes, who are supposed to be superior to their Caucasian counterparts. Although Steele does not deal with nurses in an environment dominated by doctors, the message is clear: if you live in a sea of stigmatization, you may be affected by it even while being unaware of how deeply you are affected. According to Steele, one way to counteract this tendency involves storytelling, or what he calls "narrative intervention." A narrative that focuses on "positive success and engagement" can "interrupt an otherwise negative recursive process."[2]

We have witnessed the confidence-building impact of storytelling in the workshops that we have been conducting for more than two decades. Nurses who construct stories of their work that emphasize its important aspects begin to look different as they speak. They stand taller. Their body language announces that the speaker believes in her- or himself and that this is a person of whom you should take account.

Let us give you a concrete example.

We were leading a workshop on constructing anecdotes in a geriatric hospital. We asked a group of nurses to explain what they did. One of the nurses raised her hand and stood up. Although she had volunteered to talk, everything about her demeanor, from her barely audible voice to her hunched shoulders, shouted reluctance.

We asked her what she did with her elderly patients. "Well," she said, "I go in and check on them and sometimes even give them a hug."

We asked her to be more specific. She then explained what she was checking on—their mobility, signs that a chronic illness might be worsening, whether the patients were taking their medications correctly, whether they were well hydrated and nourished, any signs of increasing or encroaching dementia.

We then asked her about the "hugs." Is it important to touch or hug a patient? Unhesitatingly, she explained that a lot of people fear the elderly, as if aging were contagious, and they avoid touching elderly people. Many of the elderly suffer from social isolation. That little hug, she explained, is actually quite a big thing and can help temper the effects of social isolation.

Great, we said. Now construct an anecdote that includes that detail, especially the part about the basis for the hugs. She did. What surprised us were not the words coming out of her mouth, but her demeanor. As she stood in front of her colleagues telling a more complete story than the first one, her posture shifted, her shoulders relaxed, and she seemed to gain a few inches in height. Doubt and diffidence in her demeanor was replaced by a look of self-confidence and self-assurance.

Perhaps you already stand tall and just need help to formulate a story. Or you may yearn to stand taller. Wherever you are on the continuum, constructing anecdotes and arguments will enhance your value of your work and encourage others to see it in a different light.

To begin constructing your anecdotes or arguments, think of an incident from your work that would help someone understand nursing. Do not try to describe all of nursing or your specialty. If you start out saying that you are going to tell people what geriatric nursing is, for example, you are unlikely to get to the compelling details like the ones given above. Most likely you'll wind up with dull generalities instead of a story.

> Silence any internal voice expressing doubt about the value of nursing such as in "They would think it's ordinary." What is ordinary to you may be extraordinary to the listener.

No Such Thing as a "Little Thing"

Just as television hospital dramas hook us with specifics about diseases and patients, you can advance public understanding by describing in detail the concrete, routine nursing activities that make a difference to patients, their families, and the public. Silence any internal voice expressing doubt about the value of nursing such as in "They would think it's ordinary." What is ordinary to you may be extraordinary to the listener. It's your job to show why these ostensibly ordinary actions are important.

Ignore any voices, internal or external, that encourage you to describe nursing work as a "little thing." Having observed nurses in action for years, and noting the complexities of keeping patients safe, we conclude that there is no such thing as a "little thing" when it comes to the care of the sick. The "little" act of turning a patient in a hospital bed, if not done correctly, can cause a patient to develop an excruciating decubitus ulcer that may cost thousands to treat. If patients do not walk after surgery or another treatment, they can develop a clot or pneumonia that could kill them. If caregivers do not listen to the sick or understand their needs and concerns, such patients can become depressed and lose the will to heal. Giving a patient a chance to talk is not simply a nicety; it has an impact on the patient's recovery. Instead of calling these actions little things, nurses need to explain why they are really very big things.

Make it Both not Either/Or

Many nurses are so focused on getting people to view them as caring and compassionate that they forget to talk about their medical and technical knowledge and skill. Instead of giving a holistic presentation of their work, they give a halfistic picture of nursing. Similarly, many frame nurses' caring as an individual attribute without taking into account that it stems from knowledge and experience.

For example, how many nurses in one specialty will tell you that they could never work in another? An oncology nurse says she could never deal with working with children. A pediatric nurse says he could never cope with cancer patients. A psych nurse says that working with the elderly would be impossible, while a geriatric nurse would have the same problem with psych patients. Veteran nurses constantly complain that students or new nurses focus only on getting the task done and not on the patient that the task concerns. This tells us that nurses' ability to be caring and compassionate is context and knowledge driven and not a result of individual attributes. Veteran nurses also tell us stories that confirm that compassion cannot be produced on demand but depends on skill and knowledge.

Nurse Katherine Harris described how this became an issue for her when her hospital reduced her hours in Labor and Delivery and she went to work in a rehab hospital taking care of ventilator-dependent patients. Before she reported to work, the temp agency gave her an orientation in the basement of its headquarters that consisted of a four-hour video.

When Harris reported to work at the long-term care facility, she was assigned to a floor for long-term ventilator-dependent patients. There Harris found bedridden patients who seemed to her to be in limbo between life and death. No one guided her through this maze of human suffering to explain who was in a coma and who was paralyzed but mentally alert.

At the sight of all these patients, she experienced wave after wave of sadness. She said she wanted to be compassionate and kind as well as competent, but she could be neither. "The people on the staff weren't concerned about me knowing how to talk to the patients or being comfortable with the kind of patients I'd had no experience with. All they wanted me to do was to put medications into the feeding tubes that were permanently inserted into their stomachs," she said.

No one taught Harris how to master what turned out to be a complex skill. "I had to figure out which meds I could mix together in their G tube. I had to look it all up because no one would teach me, and then people would get upset because I was so slow. No one helped me. Not the managers or the other nurses. It seemed like because they'd been doing it for so long, they assumed everybody knew how to do it."

Harris found the experience frightening and depressing. "There was no time for me to get answers to even the most basic questions. When I asked a question, people were very short with me." Harris said that after only a few hours she felt utterly defeated by the whole experience. "I felt really sad and scared for everyone—for me and for the patients I was supposed to care for. When I went in there, I thought I could learn how to communicate with these patients and be kind. It was something I would have liked to learn how to do but the place didn't allow me to do that. I was surrounded by fences of mean people and so after a few shifts I said, 'Forget it.'"[3]

To ensure that nurses will have the kind of education and entry into practice that they have been fighting for for years, they must clearly explain, as Nurse Harris did, the connection between education and compassion.

Highlighting one aspect of your work doesn't mean that you have to negate other parts. In one workshop we gave, we asked nurses to explain the difference they make in patient care. An oncology nurse wrote the following: "People may think the most important part of being an oncology nurse is inserting an IV, accessing a port-a-catheter, administering anti-nausea medication, or infusing chemotherapy. This is not true. The part of my job that makes the greatest impact is educating a patient to take care of himself safely and efficiently at home."

This nurse was suggesting, probably without even realizing it, that inserting an IV, accessing a portacatheter, administering anti-nausea medication, and infusing chemotherapy are not important. How could that be true? If the IV isn't inserted correctly, the toxic chemotherapy agents will infiltrate into the skin and could cause a burn that might require a skin graft. If the portacatheter isn't accessed safely, the patient could develop a catheter-related infection that could kill him. If the patient doesn't get adequate anti-nausea meds, she could be hospitalized for dehydration and malnutrition and possibly die. And if the chemotherapy isn't infused correctly, the patient will not experience a remission or cure and could die. Death or a hospital admission is at the end of everything this nurse described as somehow not as important as educating a person to go home.

By explaining what she does and why she does it, the nurse can convey the value of all she does, as in this rewrite: "As an oncology nurse, I administer chemotherapy by carefully inserting an IV into the patient's vein to deliver the solution. If the patient has a portacatheter that has been surgically implanted as a conduit for the chemo, I access it using a sterile technique to prevent a potentially fatal catheter-related infection. I monitor the infusion of the chemotherapy to make sure it is correctly done. I also make sure the patient takes anti-nausea medication because it helps the patient tolerate the chemotherapy and prevents dehydration or malnutrition from nausea and vomiting. One of the other big things I do is teach the patient how to care for him- or herself safely at home."

How to Construct Anecdotes about Your Work

Here are steps to help you to create an anecdote that is full of detail and compelling to your listeners:

1. Paint a picture
2. Avoid using jargon
3. Use facts and statistics
4. Paint yourself into the picture
5. Paint the whole picture

Paint a Picture: It Was a Dark and Stormy Night . . .

Begin by setting the scene. Stories unfold with characters doing something in a given time and place. Think of an experience you've had in your work that would draw us into your world. You will want to give details about the place and time and the patient(s), but you are going to alter them if necessary to protect the identity of the patient(s). You can tell your audience right off the bat that you changed things to protect your patients' privacy, but that the story you are telling is a true representation of what you do as a nurse. Include the "telling details" that spark the layperson's interest and convey the complexity and tone of what you do and the environment in which you do it. Here is an example of scene setting from a story by the transplant nurse Jo Stecher that appeared in a longer version in *When Chicken Soup Isn't Enough*:[4]

> I came to work that morning and had two patients in our transplant unit. One was a young fellow about 22 year old who had received a liver transplant about 48 hours previously. While I was doing my morning head to toe check of him, I found that he was very sleepy. He wouldn't respond when I talked to him and he kept his eyes closed. When he did try to talk to me he was mumbling.
>
> I knew all this was problem. As an experienced transplant nurse, I know that when you give somebody a liver and it works, they're not jaundiced. They're alert, they're perky, they're eating and talking and walking the halls.

In this scene setter, the nurse sets up the time and place, introduces us to the characters (altering the details if necessary for privacy), explains the problem at hand, and does it in such a vivid way that we want to know what's going to happen next.

Reflect Clinical Judgment

Your anecdote should also reflect the fact that you use clinical judgment when engaged in patient care activities. That's what Jo Stecher does when she continues her story:

> This young man was doing none of that. So I checked all his vital signs, his blood pressure, pulse, temperature. Everything was absolutely where it should have been at that point in time. When I looked at his urine it was getting a bit dark amber colored. The quantity, the output, was fine, but it had gotten darker. I did his morning lab work and everything was fine.
>
> But I was worried. As the shift progressed, he became more lethargic, more sleepy. I did another set of blood work on him and it started to document that life in his liver was deteriorating. His urine was now a thick brown sludge that was basically unmeasureable."

Judith Donnelly, who works in a telemetry unit at a New England hospital, was taking care of a heart patient scheduled for surgery the next morning. That night the patient called for the nurse because he was experiencing shortness of breath. As Donnelly checked him, she found what she had expected: he had fluid building up in his lungs and was sitting up to breathe more easily. His condition was stable, but his heart rate was somewhat elevated. Donnelly asked the secretary to get a med order and began preparing the appropriate medication.

Then the patient said urgently, "Can you help me? I have to have a bowel movement."

Donnelly turned to the secretary and said quietly, "Call a code."

"Code?" the secretary replied.

"Now," Donnelly said.

When the code team and the resident arrived, the patient was still "normal." Suddenly his heart rate dropped to thirty, and he began losing consciousness. The code team went to work. After the patient was stabilized, the resident asked Donnelly, "How did you know?"

She told the resident the patient said he needed to move his bowels.

The resident understood, but we didn't. Donnelly explained that the patient would not have had that urge under the circumstances unless something was happening with the vagus nerve. This nerve both affects the heart rate and stimulates the bowels. The patient's urgency was the tip-off that his heart rate was about to drop.

As an experienced nurse, Donnelly said she acted on her own "gut feeling" about what this patient needed.

> To illuminate your clinical judgment in your anecdotes, you need to describe what you are doing and explain why you are doing it.

This nurse clearly knows her stuff. She is making minute-by-minute, life-transforming decisions based on her knowledge and skill and years of experience.

Explaining that you are working from your store of knowledge is important. Nurses mention that they try to reduce the anxiety that patients feel in the alien environment of the hospital. For example, perioperative nurses say that one of their main tasks is to help manage the anxiety of surgical patients. However, they might not explain that anxiety can lead to complications for the surgical patient. For example, it elevates a patient's blood pressure and that can cause problems during surgery and recovery. Patients who are calmer have an easier operative and postoperative course and less pain. If you leave out such facts, you risk depicting yourself as a nice person rather than a knowledgeable clinician who does things for specific reasons.

To illuminate your clinical judgment in your anecdotes, you need to describe what you are doing and explain why you are doing it.

Nurses might say, "I took the patient's blood pressure and temperature and listened to his lungs." This doesn't tell us what the nurse is looking for and why his actions are knowledgeable and consequential. The simplest way to convey this is to use the word *because*. "I took the patient's blood pressure because I wanted to make sure he hadn't developed any internal bleeding after surgery. I checked the patient's temperature because it can indicate the presence of infection. I listened to his lungs to determine whether there were signs of pneumonia."

This helps people to understand why vital signs are considered *vital* and not *trivial*.

Depict Your Knowledge as Internalized

In painting a picture of your work, be sure to show that your actions are guided by your own expertise. Sometimes when nurses tell stories, they make it sound like all they are doing is following orders. Starting a sentence with "I had to . . . " gives that impression.

"I had to take his vital signs every four hours."

"I had to call the doctor to get the order for pain medication."

"As JD's assigned nurse, I had to follow the hospital protocol for attempted suicide patients, which included . . . "

Nurses have explained that they talk like this because their work is dictated by doctors' orders and institutional protocols. This explanation suggests that nurses are in a uniquely subordinate position.

In fact, all professionals follow protocols or guidelines. When doctors prescribe a drug or perform a procedure, they are following protocols. When actors perform in a play, they use the words a playwright wrote and follow the directions of the director. For most professionals, protocols or guidelines become part of the structure in which they do their individual work with their own agency. Neither the actor nor the doctor feels required to say, "I had to do what so-and-so told me or what the protocol recommended." They are more likely to say, "I did thus and so." When nurses use language that elevates protocols or orders above their actions, they depict themselves as puppets controlled by external sources of knowledge and judgment.

Nurses can counter this impression by simply describing what they did:

"I took his vital signs."

"I consulted with the physician about the patient's pain medication."

"As JD's nurse, I did what we do to protect all suicidal patients, which included . . . "

Nurses can depict themselves as either more or less dependent on physicians as shown in the following responses to a patient's questions:

"I have to ask the doctor."

"I will consult with the doctor."

We advise nurses to use the words *consult, discuss,* and *confer* when talking about conversations they have with physicians and other members of the team about patient care issues and concerns. Avoid formulations like "I don't know; I'll have to ask the doctor" or "I have to get the doctor's order." If you have recommended a treatment or medication, make sure your story includes this fact, as in "I knew my patient was in pain. I consulted with her physician and suggested that she give the patient some pain medication. I administered the medication and made sure the patient was no longer in pain."

In Jo Stecher's story, it is clear that she is a functioning member of a team and that her ability to work on the team is dependent on her knowledge, which she shares with the attending surgeon:

"Lou, look this young guy's in liver failure. His liver has failed." I presented the data supporting this conclusion. I explained that the patient was going into a hepatic coma, becoming encephalopathic. He was filling with poisons that his transplanted liver was not able to detoxify. Because I had been a transplant nurse for over eight years, I determined this even without doing any neurological testing, although we certainly did that.

Indeed, his blood work was reflecting a failed liver. The other liver lab values reflected that too. So did his urine. The brown sludge in his urine was bile that the liver was not utilizing properly. (Usually you excrete your bile in your stool, which is why your stool is brown.) The fact that his labs were normal in the morning was meaningless because they changed rapidly over the course of the shift.

"We have to put him back on the list to get a new liver," I told the surgeon. "We're wasting time by not being proactive."

Avoid Jargon

In communicating with the public, distinguish between what one says to other health care professionals and what one says to laypeople. Avoid jargon that makes your story incomprehensible. One type is "medical-speak" in which medical terms and abbreviations are used without translating them into ordinary language or explaining them.

Anecdote Makeover by Nurse Midwife Ruth Johnson of Massachusetts

Gobbledygook version

"As a nurse midwife, I am the guardian of the birth process and partner with a woman to make sure she has a healthy baby. As wise and understanding professionals, we team with women to help them access supportive networks that will help navigate this important life transition."

Makeover

"Certified nurse midwives care for women throughout their pregnancies, deliver babies, and monitor mothers and babies after the birth. Women cared for by nurse midwives are less likely to have a cesarean section, an episiotomy, or a baby admitted to the intensive care nursery than those managed by physicians. In addition to caring for childbearing women, nurse midwives provide primary health care to women—annual physicals, Pap smears, contraception, testing and treatment for sexually transmitted diseases, hormone management, and treatment of urinary and vaginal infections. Our patients range from young women having their first exam to older women looking for a professional who can help them to negotiate midlife changes."

For example:

"My patient suffered from a short run of ventricular tachycardia, and my intervention saved him from the ultimate negative patient outcome."

"My patient was admitted from the ED with fulminating pulmonary edema. Opening PA pressures were 58 over 28, with a wedge of 30. O_2 sat was 84 percent and her ABGs showed a P_O2 of 82. She was in sinus tech with frequent runs of multiform PVCs and her SVR was 2400."

Would a non-nurse get it? Any of it? Probably not. A non-nurse would, however, understand the following:

"My patient had an irregular heart rhythm, and my quick action saved him from dying."

"My patient had too much fluid in her lungs. Her oxygen levels were low, and she had many irregular heartbeats. She had difficulty breathing and could have died suddenly. So I acted quickly to reduce her fluid volume and gave her morphine to help her relax."

Another version of jargon is "nurse-speak." This is academic/nursing theory/caring discourse that creeps out of nursing schools and professional organizations and into ordinary conversation. We hear it in our seminars when we ask nurses to pretend that we are reporters interviewing them about their work.

"What do you do?" we asked a volunteer in one seminar.

"I'm a nurse practitioner," she said. "I deliver primary health care services. I do skilled assessment. I'm a patient educator and a patient advocate."

On another occasion, an oncology nurse stepped forward. She described her work with women on high-dose chemotherapy who experience premature menopause: "I do symptom assessment, I monitor the effect of chemotherapy on ovulatory function, and I do patient education."

Another participant explained, "Unlike physicians, nurses deliver holistic care. As a nurse midwife, I am the guardian of the birth process and partner with a woman to make sure she has a healthy baby."

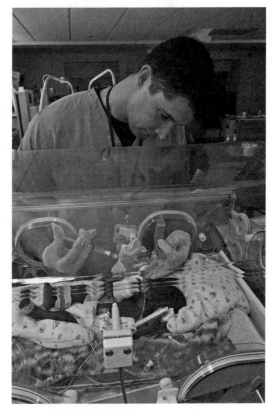

Steve Delp, RN. (Photo by Earl Dotter.)

Other nurses might know what this means. But these descriptions don't show what these nurses do, what problems their patients have, and why nurses' work is consequential.

To kick the jargon habit, remind yourself that you are presenting a picture to someone who is unfamiliar with your workplace, with nursing practice, and with medical and nurse-speak.

Use Facts and Statistics

A great way to bolster your arguments and descriptions is to use a few choice facts and statistics. These enhance your credibility. When you read useful studies or find relevant statistics in a journal article, news report, or other document, jot them down for future use. If you are preparing to speak to a community group about prevention of infectious diseases, to testify at a legislative hearing about a funding measure for nursing education, or to talk to a journalist about the implications of a new patient care study, go online and check out material that will be relevant to your topic.

For information on restructuring and working conditions in health care facilities, two reports by the Institute of Medicine (IOM)—*Keeping Patients Safe: Transforming the Work Environment of Nurses* and *Nursing Staff in Hospitals and Nursing Homes: Is It Adequate?*—are full of useful statistics.[5] IOM reports on medical errors and injuries also have data that nurses can use to tell compelling stories.[6]

Such studies document that in the care of the sick and vulnerable, "small things" can be enormously important. For example, if you're a medical nurse, you could use facts and statistics to show the significance of giving a patient a bed bath. Explain that when you are bathing a patient, you are looking for signs of skin breakdown like a little red spot on the hip or heel that could turn into a bedsore. Explain that it could become a crater-sized decubitus ulcer that goes all the way down to the bone.

According to studies, about 11 percent of hospitalized patients under the age of seventy are at risk for bedsores. When patients are between seventy and eighty-nine years old, the risk jumps to 54 percent. Treatment of bedsores costs from four thousand to seventy thousand dollars in the United States. Bedsores are largely preventable with good nursing care (and hospitals are penalized in reimbursements if their rate of bedsores and other patient maladies is high). If nurses have the time to properly bathe patients, to turn them, to make sure they're well nourished, and to clean them if they are incontinent, this goes a long way toward preventing pressure ulcers. The United States spends $1.3 billion on pressure ulcers each year.[7]

Facts and statistics can be integrated into an anecdote about the role nurses play in preventing deep vein thrombosis (DVT) and pulmonary emboli. The latter is one of the most catastrophic consequences of immobility following surgery or during a hospital stay. When patients don't walk, blood pools and stagnates in the legs, and a clot could develop. A piece of the clot could break off and travel into the lungs, where it could lodge in the pulmonary artery, shutting off the supply of blood to the heart and causing instant death.

Without proper prevention and action, 20 percent of patients who have had major surgeries might suffer from DVT and 1 to 2 percent might have a pulmonary embolism. Nurses evaluate which patients are at risk for DVT, help them to walk or do leg exercises in bed, make sure they have pressure stockings or other specialized equipment, and monitor for symptoms of DVT or pulmonary embolism.

In preventing such complications, nurses save money as well as lives. The average cost of treating a three-month episode of DVT is twelve thousand dollars for the medications alone.[8]

Useful Statistics Drawn from Medical and Nursing Studies Done in the United States

- Fifty-eight percent of adverse events that resulted in lengthened hospital stays and disability were due to preventable errors. Drug complications were the most common type of adverse event, followed by wound infections. Most of these adverse events led to disabilities lasting less than six months, but 13.6 percent resulted in death, and 2.6 percent caused permanent, disabling injuries.[9]
- Bacteremias (an infection that occurs when bacteria get into the bloodstream) account for 10 to 20 percent of hospital-acquired infections. Each episode of bacteremia adds an average of $2,836 to a hospital bill.[10]
- Urinary tract infections (UTIs) account for 40 percent of hospital-acquired infections.[11] Each episode of a UTI adds $676 to a hospital bill.[12]
- Studies show that when nurses work longer than twelve-hour shifts, or work more than forty hours a week, the risk of making an error (most are medication errors) increases significantly.[13]

Paint Yourself into the Picture

When nurses tell stories, they tend to highlight the contributions of other health care professionals while often obscuring their own. Although physicians admit that patient care is a collaborative affair, in public they often give the impression that patients' survival or recovery depends on physicians' efforts alone. As nurse and organizational consultant Elizabeth Grady has explained, nurses seem to have difficulty acknowledging the "I" in the "we," whereas physicians more often have trouble finding the "we" in the "I."[14]

For example, Susan Sweeney, an emergency nurse at a level-one trauma center in Rhode Island, told us a moving story. A beautiful nineteen-year-old man was brought into the emergency department following a car accident. He was dead on arrival. But the injuries that killed him were all internal. He looked perfect on the outside.

When his mother saw him, she refused to believe he was dead. He was just sleeping, she insisted. See, she said, calling to him to awaken him, his hand is moving. He's in a coma. He'll recover.

Nurse Sweeney and her colleague, a trauma physician, recognized that the woman was in shock and needed a great deal of attention. Sweeney assessed the situation and recommended against medicating the mother because it would only delay what she inevitably had to recognize—her son was dead. Nurse

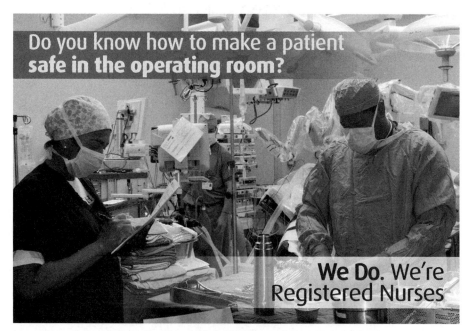

An example of an effective advertisement for patient safety in the OR. (By Suzanne Gordon; photo by Earl Dotter.)

Sweeney spent more than an hour working with the mother to help her deal with her denial and grief.

But when Susan Sweeney initially told us the story, she described the care of the mother solely as a group effort. We asked her to clarify who did what. Did both she and the trauma physician spend an hour with the mother?

No. She explained that early on the physician left to do other work and that she was the one who stayed with the distraught mother.

It was Nurse Sweeney, in fact, who cared for the woman. It was Nurse Sweeney, in fact, who recommended a treatment plan and carried it out. It was Nurse Sweeney who worked with the mother until she was able to be taken home.

Finally, Nurse Sweeney let us see what she did. If she hadn't included herself in the picture, how would we know the important and humane work that nurses do?

Paint the Whole Picture

In your anecdotes and arguments, create a full and rich view of nursing practice. Contemporary nurses have a tendency to focus on the psychosocial and emotional aspects of the care they provide to the exclusion of the medical and technical knowledge and skill they employ.

When we ask nurses why they counterpose the technical and medical with the psychosocial and emotional, they tell us two things. One is that their nursing school professors have told them to focus on what is unique to nursing and that gets defined as the emotional attributes the nurse brings to her or his work. Describing the technical and medical would lead them into activities that are in the physician's domain, they say.

For example, the physician has ordered the chemo and the anti-nausea meds that an oncology nurse would administer. This narrow view ignores the reality that the work of most people is directed by someone else. As journalists, for example, we might be assigned a story, told whom to interview, and be given a word limit and a deadline. We may be operating within parameters, but we absolutely bring our own knowledge and skill to carrying out the assignment. What matters is not who orders the treatment or action but who knows how to do it. In the administration of chemotherapy, doctors don't and nurses do.

Don't assume that your listeners will go along with descriptions that denigrate skills to elevate caring, as did this emergency nurse who proudly asserted, "As ER nurses, people don't value us for our technical wizardry, but for what we give of ourselves to our patients." If we were in an ER with something serious, we'd go for the technical wizardry first, as would most patients.

The ER nurse could have said, "People really do value us for our technical wizardry when they are in an emergency situation and also appreciate what we give of ourselves to our patients."

Makeovers

In constructing your anecdotes, the idea is to get the basic information into draft form first and then shape it to make it more effective. One way to test the anecdote's effectiveness is to tell it to a non-nurse or to a nurse who isn't familiar with your field. The first versions of anecdotes are often diffuse and unclear. This is okay because the rough draft is a starting point. In workshops we've worked with nurses to refine their stories. Her is an example of a first draft (version one), and a makeover (version two).

Oncology Nurse Anecdote

VERSION ONE

Recently, I took care of a patient in the hospital who was diagnosed with cancer. One of the things I did that was important as a nurse was take the time to listen to the patient's concerns and needs. I saw him for a period of two days while I was on my shift. When I went into the room, I would reintroduce myself and take the time to ask how he was and to inquire about his needs. One of the other things I did was provide a daily bath. The patient was unable to bathe himself and required full assistance. While I did the bath, I took the time to make sure his skin wasn't broken down and that he received the care he needed.

I washed the patient's hair and brushed his teeth. One of the other things I had to do was provide the patient with medications. He didn't know a lot about the medications. He didn't know their names; he didn't know why particular pills were being given. He didn't understand why the doctor had changed his medication. I took the time to explain to my patient that his pain was being managed by the medication he was receiving and to explain that he needed to tell me if he wasn't comfortable.

In this anecdote the nurse recounts some aspects of her care. However, the picture she paints is just a sketch. We don't know what kind of cancer the patient has or why he is in the hospital. We don't understand the importance and complexity of pain management. We don't see the medical and technical activities she undertakes to keep the patient safe. We are left with the impression that the nurse is a well-meaning person who is solicitous of her patient. One might conclude that she could be replaced by someone equally attentive but less educated and skilled and therefore less expensive.

Version Two

I was taking care of a patient, Mr. R, who had esophageal cancer, cancer of the tube that passes food from the mouth to the stomach. This is a serious diagnosis with an 80 percent mortality rate. Mr. R had surgery two days previously to remove part of his esophagus and reattach the remainder to his stomach. He was in a lot of pain and was very anxious about the chemotherapy he would eventually receive.

One of the things I did was manage his pain. Pain management is a critical nursing activity. Pain is not simply experienced at the emotional level. Unmanaged pain creates changes at the cellular and tissue level. We know that unmanaged pain retards healing and can even lead to death. Patients who are in pain don't walk and can develop deep vein thrombosis. They don't cough and are at greater risk for pneumonia. Some patients reject pain medication because they think that toughing out pain shows strength of character. When such patients are asked if they are in pain, nurses know that they might say no, while the expression on their face or their body language says yes.

It's important to monitor the effectiveness of patients' pain medication and stay ahead of the pain. You want to make sure they are always comfortable.

Mr. R was not able to eat. He was being fed intravenously. I monitored his fluid intake and urine output to make sure he wasn't becoming dehydrated or malnourished.

I was also concerned about the risk of pneumonia, so I listened to his chest every four hours for any abnormal sounds. I checked his temperature every four hours for any signs of infection. I checked his respiration and took his blood pressure. One of the risks of this surgery is internal bleeding. I needed to make sure his blood pressure was within the normal range and that he was not bleeding internally, which can lead to cardiac arrest and death.

I listened to his concerns and reassured both him and the family. I didn't just care for him. His wife was at his bedside and was worried about what was coming next in his care.

In version two, the nurse fills in the blanks. We now understand that she is dealing with a very sick patient who has a range of emotional, medical, and technical needs. We understand the intricacies of pain management and why vital signs are so significant. After hearing this nurse describe her work, the listener would understand the complexity of that work and why we need nurses and not nurse substitutes at the bedside.

Three Anecdotes or Arguments

We urge every nurse to have at least three anecdotes or arguments ready to use when openings occur. These aren't designed to make you feel better about your work or to share incidents with your closest colleagues. They are intended for various publics, all of which could have a bearing on support for nursing. They should address the concerns that ordinary people—or policy makers, politicians, journalists, businesspeople, or even health care administrators—have about health care or the health care system. They should show how the work of nurses makes a difference to patients.

What subjects could you address? What health care issues do people worry about?

Research and news coverage suggest that people are worried about medication errors and injuries. They don't want to leave the hospital or clinic sicker than when they came in. They don't want a wrong limb or organ removed. They don't want the wrong medication or a drug overdose.

They probably assume that it's the doctor who is responsible for protecting them. It would likely be news to them that often it's the nurse. How many people, for example, know that in one study, 86 percent of medication errors that were caught were caught by nurses, not by doctors?[15]

Administrators and policy makers are under pressure to both cut costs and enhance patient outcomes and satisfaction. If you are addressing this audience, highlight how your work saves money and improves patient outcomes. Nurses often fail to tailor their stories to public concerns because they are so accustomed to talking "insider baseball" to one another.

Some nurses believe that the primary mission of the nurse is to concentrate not on illness but on health, which may be defined not just as the absence of disease but as a broad spectrum of human functions. As the nurse theorist Mary Parsee defines it, nursing is about "human becoming."

Others believe that nursing is about helping patients to develop self-care, or about delivering holistic care, the latter of which often refers to a focus on psychosocial issues. Others avoid talking about "tasks," preferring "critical thinking," and "skilled decision making." Nursing professors and leaders, in an effort to define nursing as distinct from medicine, might urge nurses to eschew "medical" terminology in their descriptions in favor of a nursing vocabulary that renames many health care activities.

Whatever the nursing theory, philosophy, concern, or dogma, attempting to describe nursing to the public in terms of abstract concepts constricts nurses' ability to communicate effectively about their work. When it comes to getting the four *R*s, nurses (like physicians) will be measured on the basis of their actions and clinical outcomes. In the public arena, concrete description trumps philosophy every time.

Tailoring Your Anecdotes for Various Audiences

Once you have three all-purpose anecdotes handy, you can tweak them to appeal to specific audiences. To do this, ask yourself, What people are you talking to? What are their concerns and interests? What arguments, facts, or ideas will move them?

For example, if the oncology nurse who told her story were talking to a high school class, she might punch up details about the cutting-edge technology that she uses and monitors. At a community meeting, she might emphasize the part about how cancer nurses manage pain and debilitating symptoms. If she were jumping into the debate about end-of-life care, she could discuss how she would help this patient if his treatment were not effective and he faced difficult choices about continued treatment or hospice care. If she were talking to a group of hospital administrators or politicians, she must address their concerns about costs and highlight how her actions save money by preventing complications, readmissions, or expensive futile treatments.

You may be able to reshape one anecdote to address various issues, or you may need several different anecdotes to illuminate aspects of nursing that most people aren't aware of, such as the following:

- Nurses prevent costly complications and medical errors.
- In teaching hospitals, nurses teach physicians and physicians in training.
- Nurses contribute to medical cures and to medical diagnosis and often recommend the medications doctors prescribe.
- Nursing care saves money and lives and lessens suffering.
- Hospitals are nursing institutions. People aren't admitted to hospitals unless they need nursing care.
- Nurses are the first clinicians a patient sees in an emergency department. It's the triage nurse who decides how quickly the patient needs to be seen, where, and by whom.
- Nurses play a critical role in patient safety.

Never Put Down Another Nurse

When you're constructing your anecdotes or arguments, be careful not to elevate your own work or field of nursing at the expense of other nurses. The practice of putting down other nurses is common within nursing to the detriment of the profession.

Nurses with baccalaureate or graduate degrees sometimes insist they are "professional" nurses, not "technicians" or "technical" nurses. For instance, a nursing director at a major teaching hospital stated in a conversation with a medical sociologist that operating room nurses are "technicians," not "real nurses." Although she may not have realized it, she was speaking to a "public," an influential one at that. As it turned out, her views reflected badly on her rather than on the OR nurses.

Such remarks could boomerang because the public has its own perception of what is valuable. Studies indicate that most patients and members of the public value technology and technique and want a nurse who is competent in these areas. The word *professional* is recognizable code within nursing, but not outside it.

Labeling has also become a problem as advanced practice nurses (APNs) gain more attention. Nurse practitioners (NPs) and certified nurse midwives (CNSs), among others, sometimes try to differentiate themselves from staff nurses by insisting that they are APNs, NPs, and CNSs, but not RNs. One nurse practitioner described a NP-operated primary care practice to a *New York Times* reporter as an example of how NPs were "moving nurses into the twenty-first century," inadvertently implying that direct care nursing is mired in the past.[16]

Nursing has many points of entry into practice, and nurses understandably want their particular work and skills to be noticed. You can explain your work without making a derogatory comparison with other nursing work. It is inaccurate and undermining of nursing to suggest that staff nurses don't use critical thinking, don't make clinical decisions, and aren't capable of handling authority and autonomy.

Rather than insisting, "I'm an NP, not an RN" (which is factually incorrect), an NP or other APN will gain more mileage by simply explaining what she or he does.

If someone asks, "Are you an RN?" the accurate answer is, yes, advanced practice nurses are RNs who work in specialized areas.

Similarly, staff nurses should avoid casting aspersions about the authenticity of academics and nurse managers. Just as managers should not attack unionized nurses as "unprofessional," unionized nurses should avoid formulations like "He's not a 'real nurse,'" "She's just one of those 'pumps and pearls nurses,'" or "She no longer has the 'heart of a nurse.'" There is a difference between noting that an administrator, manager, or academic researcher no longer engages in clinical practice and making ad hominem arguments. Debating positions is a better strategy than questioning who is a "real nurse."

Nurse Education Anecdote

Many nurse educators in the United States believe that a baccalaureate degree should be required for entry into nursing practice. Although a university degree is mandated for nursing in a number of countries, the demand to produce nurses faster and more cheaply means that this educational standard is often attacked. Nurse educators must effectively explain why nurses need higher education.

Here is a U.S. nurse educator discussing why nurses should have a four-year degree:

VERSION ONE

Nursing is very complex work. Today, rapidly expanding clinical knowledge and mounting complexities in health care mandate that professional nurses possess educational preparation commensurate with their diverse responsibilities. Nurses are professional, not technical, workers. Nurses mobilize critical-thinking skills and judgment in their clinical decision making. They are holistic caregivers who must use this judgment to individualize care to each patient and must also educate and advocate for patients. Any trained monkey can learn to monitor the equipment on an ICU or take a temperature or blood pressure, but only a professional nurse can use her critical thinking and assessment skills to deliver holistic care to a patient.

Here are some of the problems in this argument. It's a grab bag of nurse-speak that fails to show what nurses need to know to do their work. It demeans the activities involved in much of nursing and, by extension, the people who do it. Even if some activities are delegated to a less educated caregiver, do nurses want to suggest that a nurse's aide is less than human? By using this riveting image, a credible speaker with a PhD has linked the activities of nursing with lesser primates. Try erasing *that* from listeners' minds. On the face of it, it's an inaccurate metaphor because a monkey could not be trained to monitor patients on the ICU and take vitals.

VERSION TWO

Nurses work with complex high-tech equipment, toxic medications, and invasive treatments, and with patients—in hospitals and in other settings—who are sicker than ever before. In urgent situations, they need to make snap decisions that have life-and-death consequences. To rescue patients from preventable complications and to help them survive and thrive, they need to know pharmacology, anatomy, and pathophysiology, among other subjects. Because nurses work with vulnerable human beings who are often anxious, frightened, and irritable and sometimes angry, they must have a foundation in psychology and communication. It takes time and financial resources to produce a nurse with the education and skill necessary to take care of today's patients.

Here is a checklist for assuring that your anecdotes are compelling and effective.

Anecdote Checklist

1. Does your story paint a picture?

☐ Would a non-nurse find your story interesting?
☐ Does your reader or listener see you at work?
☐ Do you include *critical details* that show the reader or listener what you do and why it is important?

2. Is your story jargon-free?

☐ Do you translate complex terms into lay language?
☐ Do you decode your work for the listener or reader?
☐ Are you using language appropriate to your audience?

3. Do you bolster your argument with facts and statistics?

4. Do you paint yourself into the picture?

☐ Do you use the voice of agency?
☐ Can the reader or listener see what you are doing and what your role is?
☐ Is your clinical knowledge and judgment evident?

5. Do you paint the whole picture?

☐ Do we see the full range of your nursing activities—medical and technical, emotional and social, and body care?
☐ Do you focus only on the psychosocial?

- ☐ Do we understand why vital signs are vital?
- ☐ Is the nurse's intelligence, curiosity, and decision making evident?
- ☐ Does your anecdote refute traditional stereotypes about nursing or inadvertently reinforce them?
- ☐ Does your anecdote help us understand the significance and *consequential nature* of nursing work?

Part II

Communicating with the Media and the Public

CHAPTER 7

HOW THE NEWS MEDIA WORK

Although most people don't think of Florence Nightingale as a whistleblower, lobbyist, or media maven, she was all three. Throughout her long career, Nightingale maintained a dynamic relationship with the media of her era to get her views across to the public.

It was the press that drew Nightingale's attention to the poor treatment of British soldiers in the Crimean War. William Howard Russell, the first British war correspondent to file dispatches from the front, reported in the *Times* of London that cholera and other enteric diseases—not artillery fire—were responsible for hospitalizing 20 percent of the British expeditionary force. Because of abominable hospital conditions, these soldiers were more likely to die than survive. While France provided nurses to care for its sick and wounded soldiers, Great Britain did not.

When Nightingale learned of this, she contacted her friend Lord Sidney Herbert, the secretary at war and the person in charge of wartime finances and supplies. In November 1854, after extensive negotiations, Nightingale embarked for the Crimea with thirty-eight nurses. During her stay there, she used the popularity she gained through newspaper accounts of her activities to lobby for money to finance her efforts. When she encountered military, medical, and bureaucratic recalcitrance, she got much of what she wanted in part by threatening to inform the press of opposition to her cause.

After she returned to England, Nightingale used every means to improve military and civilian hospitals, to provide home care for the sick poor, and to give respectable women paid work outside the confines of the Victorian household. One of the first health care statisticians, she used research findings to bolster her arguments. Nightingale also collaborated with a notable female political writer, Harriet Martineau, who was then a columnist for the *Daily News*.

As Lois Monteiro writes, "Nightingale contacted Martineau when her attempts to pressure reform in the Army in 1857–58 were going too slowly; she turned to public opinion as the pressure source." In 1858, Nightingale sent Martineau a "private reading" copy of a report she had produced on army reform. Over the years, Nightingale continued to feed Martineau information for the latter's columns. Martineau's book *England and Her Soldiers* grew out of the two women's working association.[1]

After Nightingale, nursing's major advances continued to be won through individual and collective advocacy. Nursing's earliest struggle was "the effort to distinguish trained nurses from everyone else who purported to care for the sick," says nursing historian Joan Lynaugh. "It involved the insistence that nursing work required education and standards." This campaign took place from roughly 1860 to 1915. Finally, according to Lynaugh, the idea that "there is a distinct thing called nursing" requiring a distinct education achieved worldwide acknowledgment.

"Efforts to bring about significant change require coalitions that have a purpose, leaders who won't give up, and public activity," Lynaugh asserts. "They grow out of the awareness that the only way you can achieve anything is to connect your own little world to other worlds in which people share your views, at least about one particular issue." Today nurses have unprecedented power to connect their world to others' to explain what nurses know and do and to articulate their views on issues of public concern. To be influential, nurses must be aware of what issues are timely and how they can connect their point of view to these issues. With the web and social media, there are many avenues for staying on top of current developments and there are many opportunities to enter into the public discussion.

Even though social media can be very effective in mobilizing people for specific goals, nurses still need an ongoing presence in coverage by news organizations. The reason is that the public still relies on the news media for information. According to Pew Research Center reports, people are spending more time than ever with the news, and the way they access it is increasingly through the Internet and through digital devices.

A Pew Research Center report in 2011 found that 50 percent of the people surveyed read newspapers or newspaper websites at least once a week, perhaps reflecting that newspapers tend to offer a wider array of local information than does television. While public distrust of the news media was at an all-time high, news organizations were more trusted sources of information than many other institutions, including government and business. People surveyed had a favorable view of the news sources that they use. Fully 62 percent of those surveyed said their main news sources get the facts straight.[2]

News media reports, irrespective of how consumers access them, are "mediated" by journalists, editors, and producers who decide what is newsworthy or of interest to their readers, listeners, and viewers. Journalists receive an overwhelming amount of material from interested parties. It is up to them, along with their editors and producers, to decide what is credible and worth passing on to their readers and viewers. Because of this, journalism offers a threshold level of credibility that can be lacking in social media postings and the grab bag of information on the Internet.

Unlike most blogs, which have no mechanism to verify the accuracy of their content, news reports usually receive some fact checking and editing, which hopefully sorts out fact from fantasy. North American newspapers tend to distinguish between factual reporting and analysis and opinion.

In order to maintain their credibility, journalists who cover health care have a lot to keep track of and therefore need legitimate sources who can evaluate and explain what is going on. They keep lists of experts they have consulted in the past. Thanks to Internet search engines, reporters can come across new sources of information that they might never have thought of. Since reporters these days are reachable via e-mail, most expect to hear from people with knowledge about the issue at hand.

Historically journalists have been far too narrow in defining who is and is not a credible source. Prior to the second wave of the women's movement and to the civil rights movement, neither women nor minorities were usually considered to be "legitimate" sources of information. It took the force of two mass social movements and several decades for women and minorities to penetrate the pages and broadcasts of traditional news media. Nurses can, and must, continue to broaden the media's view of who should be consulted about health care issues. Nurses can further this expansion by establishing their own expertise on the web, by becoming viable sources for those tackling important issues, and by providing ample feedback on coverage.

Even though the web has lowered the barriers that nurses have traditionally encountered in getting public attention, one thing remains the same: nurses must be willing to use all existing communication tools to communicate with the public about their work and to contribute their expertise to discussions of issues that pertain to their work and to health care in general.

The Broad Scope of Health Care Coverage

To advance the type of communication we have been discussing, we are primarily concerned in this chapter with how the news media report on health care,

The Difference between Advertising and Journalism

Advertising and public relations communications are referred to as "controlled" communications because they are under the control of the corporations and organizations that create and pay for them. Advertising and public relations campaigns represent vested interests. Their purpose is to directly influence what people buy, do, or believe.

The goals of advertising and public relations are different from those of journalism. This is why pharmaceutical and health products companies, despite spending enormous amounts of money on advertising, still make a full-fledged effort to get favorable mention in the news and to avoid negative coverage. News stories can carry the imprimatur of truth, while advertising is expected to be taken with a grain of salt.

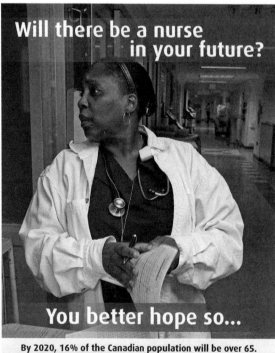

An example of an effective advertisement for the future of nursing. (By Suzanne Gordon; photo by Earl Dotter.)

how these reports can be useful to nurses, and how nursing can be a bigger part of news coverage. When we speak of the news media, we are referring to the practice of journalism. Whether the specific medium of communication is newspapers, magazines, radio, television, or the Internet, the role of the journalist is "to find, gather, organize, explain, interpret, and disseminate the news, ideas and opinions of the day to an ever-increasing audience," and to do so with accuracy and fairness.[3]

By definition, journalism is a dynamic process. The name itself derives from the Old French *jour* and *journal*, meaning "day" and "daily." The timeliness of journalism is also captured in the word *news*—something that is "new."

Advances in communication technology have sped up the time factor even further and have led to an intermingling of media. Print reporters are on TV and radio. Many have their own blogs, and some tweet regularly. TV stations have websites. Newspapers increasingly have TV broadcasting outlets on site. A search engine such as Google compiles reports from various national and international media. Still, the function of the journalist is to give people the information they need to make informed decisions as citizens and, increasingly, as consumers.

News Media Coverage of Health Care

Those who wish to influence the news must first monitor it. The easiest way to do this is to choose one or two news outlets, check them regularly, and have them alert you when there is news on subjects that interest you.

Not all news outlets are equal. We subscribe to the *New York Times*, although neither of us lives in New York. The reason is that the *Times* is a serious and influential news organization with comprehensive coverage from around the globe. It employs some of the best journalists in the world, who explore significant issues in depth and in context. Such information is key to understanding the complex world we live in. The *Times* does enterprise and investigative reporting on many issues, including health care.

Like other news organizations today, the *Times* is multimedia. Its content appears in its printed editions and on its website. The two are not identical, although most of what appears in the paper is available on the web. The digital *Times* likewise has coverage, such as regional news, that does not appear in all the printed newspapers. The *Times* website also carries extensive commentary from readers, blogs, and even videos. It is possible to challenge the news organization's coverage and to correct inaccuracies via the website.

Some things on the *New York Times* site can be viewed for free, but full access requires a subscription, something more news organizations are requiring to support the work of their news staffs. We consider a subscription a good value because free access to high-quality news reports and archives is not readily available by surfing the web.

We have signed up to receive an e-mail alert whenever the term *nursing* is the subject or appears as a major component of a *New York Times* article. We also follow *nurses* through Google Alerts, which draws from a large selection of news reports and blogs. The advantage of Google Alerts, or alerts from other aggregators such as Yahoo or Facebook, is that they cast a very wide net and include reports from foreign countries.

A similar way to keep in touch with subjects that interest you is via RSS (Really Simple Syndication). You can subscribe to updates on various subjects from news sites and have them organized on an RSS feed reader such as

Google Reader. You can also set up a feed reader through a browser like Firefox or through a mail program like Microsoft Outlook. Increasingly people set up feed readers on digital devices. The advantage of feed readers is that your subscriptions are consolidated in one place. This avoids having your e-mail inbox clogged with incoming links to websites. In addition to these possibilities, you can check out various nursing websites for postings of timely news stories and comments.

One can *unsubscribe* to information to avoid being overwhelmed. With the explosion of content, it may be just as important to focus one's attention as it is to keep abreast with current events.

This is why we have chosen the *New York Times* as our primary source of news. Other U.S. news organizations that go beyond the superficial are National Public Radio and *The PBS NewsHour* television program on PBS (Public Broadcasting System). We want to follow disinterested sources of information, meaning we look for news organizations that do not have a vested interest in the outcomes of its coverage. News aggregators on the web draw information from myriad outlets, some of which might have a monetary interest in what they cover and what they omit. Some aggregators have business arrangements that might influence their content.

By staying abreast of coverage and by noticing how news is organized, it is possible to identify openings for nurses to participate more fully in public debates and to put their expertise on display.

Health care coverage has various facets. Some journalists specialize in certain aspects of health care such as health care policy or medical research. Others may be generalists who do stories that pertain to health care from time to time.

Health care news, like other news, is categorized. These categories often influence the manner in which the story is presented. For example, a health care development might appear as the following:

- breaking news
- policy news
- business news
- research news
- enterprise reporting
- trend story
- human interest feature
- op-ed or editorial

Here are some health care stories that we followed in the *New York Times* that have a connection to nursing practice, even if nursing is not explicitly mentioned.

Breaking News

Although the term is applied to almost everything, *breaking news* implies that something of consequence has just happened that people will want to know about. There is no doubt that this was an accurate description of the horrendous event that occurred in Tucson, Arizona, on January 8, 2011, when a gunman shot and killed six people and wounded fourteen others. This story was treated as breaking news internationally because

- The gunman apparently targeted and then shot a prominent member of the U.S. House of Representatives, Gabrielle Giffords. Other victims noted immediately were John M. Roll, the chief judge for the United States District Court in Arizona, and Christina Green, a nine-year-old child.
- The circumstances were shocking. The congresswoman was speaking with constituents about Medicare and reimbursements on a Saturday afternoon in a supermarket parking lot when the gunman opened fire.

With web platforms, news organizations continually update their stories as reporters gather more information. Early on in the coverage it was not clear whether Giffords had been killed or mortally wounded. The *Times* as well as other news outlets ran a photo of Giffords being carried off on a stretcher.[4] Soon thereafter, the newspaper reported that she was in critical condition at the University Medical Center in Tucson.

Although there were multiple aspects to this story, the one that prevailed centered on Giffords's very serious head wound. Predictably it fell to a physician, Peter Rhee, medical director of University's trauma and critical care unit, to keep journalists, and the world, informed on Congresswoman Giffords's status. Rhee had a graphic way of phrasing things. He told the press that Giffords had been shot once in the head "through and through." Within four days of the shooting, the *Times* ran a profile of Rhee, in which, among other things, he described his enthusiasm for his work and remarked, "I am very good at what I do."[5]

Giffords's remarkable survival provided an opportunity, not only for Rhee, but also for Giffords's other physicians, nurses, physical therapists, and others who worked with her, to educate the public about brain function, medical treatment, and the kind of care that is needed in a case of such severe trauma. (It also offered an opportunity for nurses not involved with this case to describe the kind of work that nurses do under such circumstances. We say more on how they would do that in the next chapter.)

Except for passing references to "doctors and nurses," the medical reporting was highly physician centered in the days following the shooting. While

Times readers were given detailed accounts of Giffords's treatment by the medical center's top physicians, they were spared any indication that critical care nurses were also central to Giffords's survival. A singular description of nurses' work was given by Dr. G. Michael Lemole Jr. as Giffords was being prepared to be moved to the Institute for Rehabilitation and Research at Memorial Hermann Hospital in Houston. The *Times* reported: "Dr. Lemole said that Ms. Giffords had already begun 'aggressive' physical therapy in Tucson and that nurses took her to an outside deck Thursday, allowing her to look at the sunshine and mountains. Getting her into the sun, Dr. Lemole said, is important to re-orient her and allow her body rhythms to begin to return to normal."[6] From this we might conclude that the role of nurses working with critically injured patients is to wheel them outside for a bit of air.

Although the *Times* is a distinguished newspaper, it is no better than most at including nursing in its coverage or in signaling the significance of nursing actions when it does describe them. The example above the feeds impression that physicians have all the knowledge about what patients need and nurses mindlessly carry out orders.

In reporting on Giffords's transfer from Tucson to the rehabilitation hospital in Houston, the *Times* for the first time named a nurse who cared for Giffords. In the story, Nurse Tracy Culbert recounted an incident that occurred on the flight to Houston. Culbert said that she gave Giffords one of her rings after the congresswoman tried to touch it. "She took it into her hand and she was looking at it, turning it to see all sides," Culbert was quoted as saying.[7]

In the way that the story was constructed, the significance of that interaction—that the brain-injured congresswoman was aware of things going on around her—was not attributed to the nurse. Rather, it was a physician who made this point.

Health Care Policy News

Escalating health care costs are a big story in the United States and in many other countries. While other industrialized countries have some form of universal health care, the United States is unique in having the highest per capita costs in the world with only middling positive outcomes and millions of people with no or inadequate insurance coverage. Congress's passage of the Affordable Care Act, otherwise known as Obamacare, was the latest attempt to tame the beast with reforms that would extend coverage to more people, alter reimbursement standards, and require much of the population to buy health insurance. In 2012, the legality of the last provision was challenged before the U.S. Supreme Court.

To the surprise of many, on June 28, 2012, the Court upheld the consti-
tutionality of a key provision of the law that would impose a penalty on those
who do not obtain health insurance when the law goes into full effect. For
two or three days after the decision, the news media and various organizations reported and discussed the changes that would occur under the law. On
June 29, the *New York Times*'s lead editorial succinctly analyzed the judicial, legal, political, and health care implications of the court decision and summed up
its practical impact: "In general, the decision means that tens of millions more
Americans will have access to affordable health insurance and that reforms in
how medical care is delivered and paid for can be aggressively pursued to bring
down the cost of health care."[8]

The Business of Health Care

News organizations classify many activities that have an effect on health care
and eventually on nursing practice as business news. These include stories on
products and problems of companies involved with health care and medical
and biotechnology, Food and Drug Administration (FDA) decisions to approve
or disapprove drugs and medical devices, the financial ramifications of changes
in health care policies, and even employment disputes between nurses and hospitals or government payers. If big money is involved, it's likely to get slotted as
a business story. Other ramifications stemming from the same developments
might be covered as a trend story or human interest story.

News about drug approvals or recalls can have a big impact on a pharmaceutical corporation's bottom line and, in some cases, a big impact on the health
and expectations of the whole society. Such is the potential of Onexa, an anti-
obesity drug, developed by the pharmaceutical company Vivus. In early 2012,
an advisory committee to the FDA overwhelmingly recommended approval of
Onexa, reversing a previous recommendation two years earlier against approval. Immediately after the committee's positive recommendation, Vivus's shares
nearly doubled.[9]

Previous drugs to treat obesity have had a checkered history in terms of
limited effectiveness and negative side effects. With a third of Americans obese,
and another third overweight, new anti-obesity drugs on the market might have
major financial, health, and social effects, as well as an impact on patient care.
The same is true if such drugs later prove to be a health risk.

A study challenging conventional wisdom that electronic record keeping
would reduce health care costs was also reported as a business story in the *New
York Times*.[10] Based on research newly published in the journal *Health Affairs*,

the story said that "doctors using computers to track tests, like X-rays and magnetic resonance imaging, ordered far more tests than doctors relying on paper records." It raised the question of whether billions in federal spending to encourage doctors to embrace digital health records will generate the eighty-billion-dollar annual cost savings predicted by a RAND Corporation analysis. Drawing on a number of sources, the story explored the increasing role of electronic record keeping in health care.

A photo that accompanied the story showed nurses at Children's Hospital of Pittsburgh in front of a bank of computers. Although nurses are just as involved with electronic record keeping as are physicians, the story neither cited nor quoted nursing sources.

Business news sites are also the places to keep up on Johnson & Johnson's activities, such as the record $1.2 billion state fine levied in Arkansas against a subsidiary of the corporation for minimizing or concealing the dangers associated with the antipsychotic drug Risperdal. The story cited recent large fines against other drug companies for fraudulent sales practices and noted that these cases have had little effect on corporate share prices. Depressingly, it quoted a portfolio manager as saying, "Investors at this point have become inured to these large settlements. And you've seen it almost across all of pharma."[11]

Research News

Much of journalism is based on timely events. The election of a president, a jury's decision, a bank robbery, a bloody battle in a war—all these are events that get reported as timely news. But what about interesting things that are going on that don't just happen at a given time? These get into the news via a device known as a pseudoevent. A news conference to announce something is a pseudoevent. The thing being announced could have been going on for a long time, but the announcement of it at a given time and place is what makes it "news."

The publication of research findings in medical and other journals serves the same purpose. Researchers may have been working on a problem for years, but a study's publication on a certain date is what constitutes a news event.

Perhaps the bulk of health care news comes from studies in published journals. Health care news tends to swell midweek because the biggest medical journals, the *Journal of the American Medical Association* (*JAMA*) and the *New England Journal of Medicine* (*NEJM*), publish on Wednesday and Thursday, respectively.

Medical reporters monitor *NEJM* and *JAMA* and perhaps other journals such as *Circulation* and *Annals of Internal Medicine* for newsworthy studies and may receive alerts from them as well.

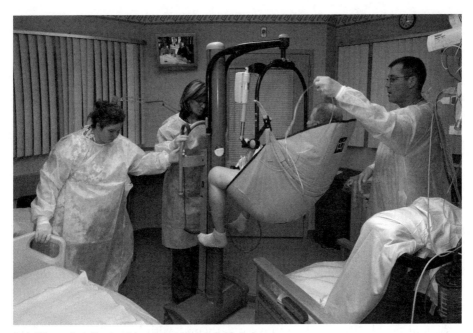

Safely lifting a patient with appropriate equipment. (Photo by Earl Dotter.)

A lot of these published findings wind up as brief capsule reports. But some prompt bigger stories or features. To write or produce them, reporters usually need more material than what is contained in the published study. The journals, which seek news coverage, are happy to accommodate them by providing additional resources on their websites. Some of this material, such as advance access to experts, and audio and video packages that can be used for radio and television reports, might be available exclusively to journalists and public affairs officers of medical institutions, but a remarkable amount is accessible to the general public.

In addition to being reported on as breaking news, medical studies are the basis for general or analytical pieces on illnesses, treatments, and preventive health measures. On Tuesdays, the *New York Times* has a science section that covers developments in all aspects of science, including biomedical innovation and research. Within the section is a subsection, "Health" that focuses more specifically on illnesses, treatments, and preventative health measures. Many of the stories are based on medical studies.

For example, the lead story in the *Times*'s health section for March 27, 2012, reported that there is renewed interest in research on aspirin because new findings suggest that aspirin might reduce the risk of many cancers and stop the spread of tumors.[12] It added that there is much uncertainty about what would be an effective daily dose and that caution is needed because aspirin potentially is a toxic drug. The article reported that more than forty million American adults now take a daily aspirin to prevent heart disease.

Other items in the section included an article on an experimental drug that works in a novel way to lower cholesterol, a physician's review of a book that deals with organ harvesting and brain death standards, and short articles on recent health research findings.

The *Times* health section has carried Jane E. Brody's popular column, Personal Health, for many years. Brody writes on a large number of subjects. Her column in the March 27, 2012, issue discussed widowhood from a personal perspective.[13] She wrote that in some ways, she found the second year after her husband's death harder than the first year. Even though she wrote from her own experience, Brody cited studies on the link between human relationships and healthfulness. Similarly, when she recounted the overmedication of her elderly aunt in "Too Much Medicine, and Too Few Checks," she delved into the research on what she called "a public health crisis that compromises the well-being of growing numbers of older adults."[14]

Reporters like Brody who write regularly on health issues "save string" on subjects they think will be newsworthy by keeping a file of journal articles, other materials, and the names of experts in the field. Brody is one of the few writers who has cited nursing research and who has quoted nurses who are experts in various fields.

The lead story in the health section sometimes is a piece by a physician or nurse drawing on an experience that is pertinent to health care. For example, Theresa Brown, RN, perhaps the most widely published American nurse, wrote a piece in early 2012 that described her interactions with a violent hospital patient titled, "Feeling Strain When Violent Patients Need Care."[15] Brown confessed that "with this patient I felt personally threatened—unsafe—which made me feel scarily distracted." She then used statistics from a 2011 American Nurses Association study to show that she was not the only nurse who felt at risk: some 34 percent of nurses cited "on-the-job assault" as one of their three greatest safety concerns. That percentage increased from a previous survey in 2001. Actual reported assaults of nurses on the job declined in the same period from 17 to 11 percent. But more than half of all RNs have reported being verbally threatened at work.

The publication of research findings can be timely enough even if a reporter happens on to it somewhat later than the publication date. This seemed to be the case with a front-page story based on a commentary that appeared more than a month previously in *Anesthesiology News*.[16] The *Times* story, "As Doctors Use More Devices, Potential for Distraction Grows," stemmed from the critical musings of Peter J. Papadakos, an anesthesiologist and director of critical care at the University of Rochester Medical Center, about how the hospital environment is changing for the worse. Papadakos lamented the "digital nightmare [that] is increasingly common on hospital wards" and warned that "we have almost no data on how electronic distraction affects worker productivity and dedication to repetitive tasks in health care."

The article that reporter Matt Richtel wrote for the *Times* either coined or picked up a term for this phenomenon that Papadakos did not use: "distracted doctoring." "Hospitals and doctors' offices, hoping to curb medical error, have invested heavily to put computers, smart phones and other devices into the hands of medical staff for instant access to patient data, drug information and case studies," Richtel wrote. "But like many cures, this solution has come with an unintended side effect: doctors and nurses can be focused on the screen and not the patient, even during moments of critical care. And they are not always doing work; examples include a neurosurgeon making personal calls during an operation, a nurse checking airfares during surgery and a poll showing that half of technicians running bypass machines had admitted texting during a procedure." The reporter sought information from a number of sources. One was a medical malpractice lawyer that represented a patient who was left partially paralyzed after an operation during which his neurosurgeon used a headset to make cell phone calls to family and businesses.[17]

Reporters are always looking for a colorful succinct quote that captures the point of the story. Richtel got one from Abraham Verghese, a physician, professor at the Stanford University Medical Center, and best-selling medical writer, who mulled over the pros of digital uses, and the cons, especially as they affect interactions with what he referred to as the "iPatient." "The iPatient is getting wonderful care across America," Verghese was quoted as saying. "The real patient wonders, 'Where is everybody?'"

Although the phrase *doctors and nurses* was used in the article, no nursing sources were cited and no nurses were quoted. Indeed the label "distracted doctoring" pretty much precluded nurses even though there are more nurses than physicians in hospitals presumably using a larger share of electronic devices than physicians. Nurses might breathe a sigh of relief at being neglected in such a story, but what that really indicates is that nursing sources are not seen as being essential in reporting on hospital-wide phenomena.

Trend Stories

The *Times* does a lot of reporting on trends in health care.

A front-page story, "Test for Hospital Budgets: Are the Patients Pleased?" described how hospitals are reacting to a new rule under the Affordable Care

Act in which Medicare would take patient satisfaction into account when re-imbursing hospitals. It was a significant story in several respects. It described a significant change that would occur if "Obamacare" were to go into full effect in 2014. It showed how a hospital could score high in clinical care yet be punished financially for lacking hotel-type amenities or even because it was situated in a part of the country (read New York City) where people complain more than those elsewhere.[18]

The reporter, Jordan Rau, captured this point in an anecdote about Pearl Schwartz, an eighty-eight-year-old patient at NYU Langone Medical Center, who described herself to the reporters as "a great kvetcher." Schwartz described her nurses as "splendid, warm and kind," and said that her operation to receive a pacemaker went well. But, according to the report, she complained that "her sink was too small, she had to wait eight hours in the radiology unit for an X-ray, and no one brought her anything to read as she had requested."

The press has noticed that hospitals are hiring hospitality training consultants to improve the responses of the Pearl Schwartzes of the world. A *Times* piece on the financial growth of the Disney Institute, a consulting division of the Walt Disney Company, lumped hospitals with other clients, such as an ice cream company, an airline, and a whole country (South Africa) that are paying to learn how to become "more like Disney," as the article put it.

It cited a Florida hospital as a Disney client that now employs a ukulele-playing greeter dressed in safari gear to welcome patients. It mentioned that the University of Iowa Hospitals and Clinics came under fire for a plan to spend $130,000 on Disney advice while laying off staff members.[19]

This story had "legs," as they say in the news business., Nurses and nursing unions complained that they were being "scripted" by consulting companies such as Disney and the Studer Group, both in Florida, and HCPro in Massachusetts to feed patients language that the patients might repeat to boost scores on customer satisfaction surveys.

Once an issue like this surfaces, reporters for various news organizations try to do their own story and seek out sources in their area to discuss it and provide anecdotal material. This is what Liz Kowalczyk did for her *Boston Globe* story "Nurses Balk at Bid to Guide Dealings with Patients."[20] Kowalczyk talked with spokespeople at health care institutions and consulting companies, who mostly denied that nurses were being scripted. Kowalczyk, an experienced health care reporter, clearly talked with nurses at various hospitals to get their experiences. She attributed such information to "nurses" and in one case to "nurses unions." But to make her story credible, she really needed to put at least one nurse on the record. She did so in the following way without mentioning the nurse's place of employment: "Ann Lewin, a nurse on a medical-surgical unit, said she felt like a 'Stepford nurse' and worried that patients would be suspicious if nurses were using the same phrases. She decided to continue 'to do what I've always done. Of course, I try to assess the patient and make sure they are comfortable.'"

One other important source for the story was Ellen B. Griffith, a spokeswoman for the Centers for Medicare and Medicaid Services, who provided perspective on the idea of prompting patients' responses to patient satisfaction surveys. Kowalczyk quoted Griffith's e-mail statement that read, "Hospitals are not permitted to attempt to influence or encourage patients to respond in a particular way. Efforts to help hospitals improve are permitted as long as these efforts focus on improving the actual care provided rather than simply encouraging patients to respond in a certain way to survey items through scripting or coaching by hospital staff."

Another *Times* story, "Chefs, Butlers, Marble Baths: Hospitals Vie for the Affluent," detailed how hospitals across the country are engaging in an "international competition for wealthy patients willing to pay extra, even as the federal government cuts back hospital reimbursement in pursuit of a more universal and affordable American medical system."[21] As an example of the trend, the story described a suite in a new penthouse wing at New York Presbyterian/Weill Cornell hospital that costs twenty-four hundred dollars a day and features bed linens by Frette, marble bathrooms, panoramic views of the East River, a menu of gourmet food, and a butler to wait on patients.

The reporter, Nina Bernstein, used descriptions and examples to capture the conflicts and consequences of hospitals' creating accommodations, such as the $3,784 maternity suites at Cedars-Sinai Medical Center in Los Angeles, to attract wealthy cash-paying customers. In one anecdote, a patient, Nancy Hemenway, pointed out that the luxury wing of New York's Mount Sinai Medical Center gets handpicked staff. "I have a primary-care physician who also acts as ringmaster for all my other doctors," Hemenway said. "And I see no people in training—only the best of the best."

Brian Katz, a surgeon at Mount Sinai, said that there are patients with Medicare "which pays physicians almost nothing . . . [who] will come up here and pay to enjoy five-star comfort."

The reporter sought out an expert, David Rosner, a professor of public health and history at Columbia University, to add perspective. "Every generation of hospitals reflects our attitude about health and disease and wealth and poverty," he said. "Today, they pride themselves on attracting private patients, and on the other hand ask for our tax dollars based upon their older charitable mission. There's a conflict there at times." Rosner also provided a personal anecdote that illustrated hospital inequality. He said that one of his graduate students spent two days on a gurney in terrible pain from herniated disks until

News Values

Timeliness: something just occurred.

Prominence: an "important" person, corporation, organization, or institution was involved.

Currency: the event is part of a larger continuing debate or discussion.

Impact: the event or issue affects a lot of people.

Conflict: individuals or groups are competing or fighting with each other.

Scandal or wrongdoing: the activities are unethical or illegal.

a dean intervened to get her moved from an emergency area to a room. "She hadn't even been given a bed pan," he said.

No nurses were quoted in this story.

Enterprise Reporting

Serious news organizations put time and effort into identifying issues that we need to know about because they can have a profound effect on us as individuals and as a society. The *New York Times* ran such a story in 2012 headlined "Generic Drugs Prove Resistant to Damage Suits." It revealed that because of a U.S. Supreme Court decision in 2011, generic drug manufacturers could not be sued for failing to alert patients about the risks of taking their drugs.[22]

The story used as examples two patients who each had a hand amputated after injections with an anti-nausea drug led to gangrene. One of the patients, Diana Levine, a celebrated professional violinist, received an injection of Phenergan from a physician's assistant to treat a migraine headache. The article reported that "her hand and forearm turned black and eventually had to be amputated. Reports had shown that the drug can cause gangrene if it enters an artery, especially if it is placed directly into the vein rather than injected into the muscle or through a diluted intravenous drip." A jury accepted the argument that although the label on the brand name drug warned that gangrene was a risk if the drug came into contact with arterial blood, the warning was not sufficient. The drug maker Wyeth was ordered to pay Levine $6.8 million.

This was a very different outcome from that of Debbie Schork, a deli worker in Indiana, whose gangrenous hand had to be amputated after an emergency nurse injected her with promethazine, a generic version of Phenergan. The Supreme Court's majority had ruled that because the generics manufacturers are required by law to use the same labels as those of the brand name drugs, they could not be held responsible for labels that failed to alert patients to problems. On this basis, Schork's suit for damages against the maker of the generic was thrown out of court.

The article pointed out that the nearly 80 percent of prescriptions in the United States are filled by a generic, so the Supreme Court's five-to-four ruling, which was split along ideological lines, could affect millions of people.

The reason this article might be seen as an example of enterprise reporting is that there was no new event to prompt this story. Rather the journalist used initiative to discover the consequences of a judicial decision.

The problems stemming from judicial, legislative and regulatory decisions are usually brought to the attention of journalists by interested parties such as lawyers trying to sue for damages and public or private interest groups. Then it is up to the reporter to get a full picture by collecting data and by speaking to parties on all sides of the picture. One of the unanswered questions in this case is whether clinicians had enough information to know how to inject the medication safely. A situation of such disparity that affects so many patients is likely to lead to follow-up reports.

Interestingly enough, another enterprise article concerning a generic drug—"A Cheap Drug Is Found to Save Bleeding Victims"—appeared farther back in the same section of the *Times*.[23] The article reported that the drug, tranexamic acid, has been demonstrated to slow hemorrhaging in trauma victims in a trial of patients in forty countries, and British and American armies have adopted it for the battlefield. Yet because the drug is cheap and manufacturers make little profit on it, it is used in very few civilian hospitals where it might save victims of car crashes, shootings, and other serious trauma. The article said that a spokesperson for the drug maker Pfizer, which makes an injectable form for hemophiliacs, declined to say whether the company had applied to the Food and Drug Administration for approval of trauma use.

This article is another link in ongoing examinations of how profits are pivotal in determining how patients are treated. According to the article, a recent study suggested that use of the drug in American emergency rooms might save the lives of up to four thousand bleeding victims a year. There was some indication that hospitals would phase in use of the drug.

Human Interest and Features

The news media followed Congresswoman Gabriel Giffords's remarkable recovery and rehabilitation and at various points did stories on her activities.

Feature stories on her were fairly frequent in the period between the shooting and her retirement from Congress. Feature stories deal with the "human" side of events and offer an opportunity for nurses to express their expertise. But that didn't happen much in the coverage of Giffords. In many stories, physicians were the experts and nurses the providers of sentiment.

Giffords's family, in their conversations with reporters, depicted the congresswoman as being alert, involved, and even in charge of what was going on. No doubt, it was important to them to show her as capable, given that she still had obligations as a U.S. representative. As part of this depiction, there were episodes in which Giffords appeared to be taking care of the nurses rather than the other way around.

This happened in piece by Jaimee Rose, an *Arizona Republic* reporter with unusual access to the Giffords family and the physicians and nurses who were involved in her care. In her article on Giffords's daily life, she included a nurse as a source of information on Giffords's activities: "She pushes a grocery cart up and down the hospital halls as therapy, focusing on using the correct muscles, says nurse Kristy Poteet, who has worked with Giffords since she arrived in Houston on Jan. 21. More therapy comes from games of bowling and indoor golf, Poteet says."[24]

Then the reporter put in an anecdote about the nurse that reframed the nurse as intimidated by her patient and in need of acceptance: "Sometimes, nurse Poteet gets nervous. She was nervous the first time she met her patient, but the worry went away 'right when I saw her, right when she looked at me. She grabbed my hand and rubbed my arm.'"

Editorials and Op-Eds

In major newspapers, the last two pages that face each other in the first section are generally reserved for editorials, letters, and opinion columns. The editorial page will be found on the left and the op-ed (for *opposite editorial*) page on the right.

Editorials represent the opinion of the news organization. They are written by editorial writers—staff journalists assigned to the editorial page—or by the editor of the page. Editorials usually have no byline because they are supposed to present the newspaper's opinion and recommendations rather than those of an individual. By concentrating on opinion, the editorial staff has a different function from that of the reporting staff and is separate from it. On a large newspaper, editorial writers might specialize in certain areas such as health care. Editorial writers have to be alert to breaking news and must understand the elements of complex issues. Their job, after all, is to write timely editorials that both summarize and take stances on these issues.

Newspaper editorials can have an effect in the community, particularly when they are well argued and call for specific policy or regulatory actions to deal with pressing problems. When editorial writers make policy recommendations, however, they do so in accordance with the editorial page's political philosophy. For example, in the United States, the *Wall Street Journal* is noted for editorials that are among the most conservative in journalism. They differ markedly from those in the *New York Times*, which tend to be more liberal. The *Times*, for example, has been supportive of Obamacare and the need for more extensive health care insurance coverage in the United States.

Letters to the Editor and Op-Eds

Most newspapers run letters to the editor, usually on the editorial page. Some accept op-eds from the public. Letters and op-eds are very good vehicles for nurses who want to influence the public discussion. We explore them in chapter 9.

Your Turn

Monitor the news sections. The first section of a newspaper usually contains a mix of national, international, and local "breaking" news. What makes these stories news? Are they based on an announcement, the release of a report, a hearing, a press conference, an event? Does the newspaper have a separate regional, metropolitan, or local section? What kinds of health stories appear there? Who writes the health-related news?

Monitor the business page or section for health news. How heavily does it cover the health industries in your area? Is this where stories on nurse staffing or on labor disputes appear? What have you observed that suggests opportunities for nurses to raise their public profile?

CHAPTER 8

REACHING OUT TO THE MEDIA

Many nursing organizations, nursing schools, hospitals, and other health care institutions have PR, marketing, or communication specialists working for them. Therefore, it may seem mysterious that nursing still ranks as the least visible health care profession. The mystery can be solved, however, by looking at what many of these PR practitioners are actually assigned to do.

"Internal" and "External" Communications

The primary goal of any organization is to serve and retain its members and to recruit more. Most nursing organizations expect their marketing and PR people to do more "internal" than "external" communication. Their mission is to enhance communication and the image of the organization with members and with others in the profession.

In a nursing school, for example, a communication specialist might spend most of his or her time putting out newsletters and promotional materials for prospective students and alumni. Duties might also involve promoting the nursing school *within* the university.

In a subspecialty organization, a PR staffer might put out an organizational newsletter, supervise the publishing of clinical journals and books, and help plan and promote conferences and conventions. However, the reality is that the vast majority of nursing organizations, subspecialty groups, and professional associations do very little "external" communication and outreach to journalists and to the public. They may produce policy statements or position papers on important issues and may even hire speechwriters and media trainers to teach officers how to speak in public, do interviews with journalists, and appear on television and radio. An organization might even invite journalists to a conference to speak about the how-tos of nursing coverage or a group of organizations may organize a conference about the lack of media coverage about nursing. Nurses may even create websites that analyze the content of media coverage of nursing.

These actions are self-limiting if the organization does not engage in consistent outreach to the media on pressing health care issues and help its members to speak out and participate in collective actions that will turn rhetoric into reality for nursing. An unintended consequence of not having an external communication plan is that it reinforces the silence of nurses. When nurses don't see members of their profession in the news, they might conclude that the media aren't interested in their stories and that nothing can be done to change that.

When we first began to write about nursing what struck us was that the profession seemed to carry on a cloistered conversation within the traditional organizational forms described above. What is striking as we write this third edition is that in the midst of a huge communication revolution, this insular conversation goes on almost unchanged—except it takes place in plain view for anyone who happens upon it. As we've examined nurses' use of media, both traditional and digital, we see that nursing discussions, no matter what their content, are usually intended to reach other nurses. While, nurses and their organizations help groups like Johnson & Johnson or the DAISY Foundation to describe, define, and promote nursing to some publics, they do little of it themselves.

Contrast this with medicine. Medicine engages in multidimensional communications aimed at various audiences to convince them to pay attention to and support developments in medicine and medical practice. We understand that nursing does not have the resources of medicine. Nonetheless it has many more bodies, and thus voices that could be raised and heard, particularly via the new media. While organized medicine is using newer communication technologies to enhance its older media strategies, nurses seem to use the new media mostly to share with one another their triumphs and frustrations with their work. This is different from communicating with non-nurse publics and does not constitute a viable "external" communication strategy. Internal communication activities do not get nursing into the news, nor do they necessarily raise the public profile of the profession.

This is why in this chapter we focus on using traditional and new social media to educate broad publics about nursing, nursing practice, and health care.

We begin with an interesting way that a nurse used new media to participate in an important debate about patient safety. Kathleen Burke, an orthopedic nurse at the University of California San Francisco Medical Center had learned via social media of an effort to gauge the effect of a new regulation issued by the U.S. Centers for Medicare and Medicaid Services (CMS). In 2010, CMS issued a rule that nurses must administer medications within a half hour before or after the time specified for their administration. If the medication was ordered every four hours and the nurse began administering it at 7:00 in the morning, then she had to administer it again within a 10:30 to 11:30 a.m. time frame with no leeway before or after that period. In response, the National Patient Safety Foundation used its Listserv to ask nurses what they thought of this new requirement. The question was whether nurses thought the rule was realistic and would advance the safety of patients. Nurses were asked to complete a survey and comment on the rule so that their responses could be conveyed to the Institute for Safe Medication Practice.

When Kathleen Burke, who's been a nurse for over fifteen years, heard about the requirement, she was quite concerned about nurses' ability to adhere to it. When she learned that there was a forum for nurses to speak out, she jumped at the chance and wrote the following:

Survey
Response

As a condition of participation in Medicare, the Centers for Medicare and Medicaid Services (CMS) in its Conditions of Participation Interpretive Guidelines, has made a requirement that scheduled medications be administered within thirty minutes before or after the specified time. To the outside observer, this rule seems quite a reasonable expectation—that a patient would receive a medication close to the time that it was scheduled or ordered. But from the perspective of a bedside nurse, this rule seems to have been devised by people who have little experience with the way nursing work is organized and who have had little direct observation of the work of bedside nurses. I am one of those nurses. I have the practical experience of frontline patient care that seems to have been missing when this rule was devised. So recently, when completing the Institute for Safe Medication Practice survey asking frontline nurses our opinion about this rule, I not only sent in my survey but also wrote the following short essay about what it's actually like to give out meds in a busy teaching hospital.

You asked: How does strict adherence to the thirty-minute rule create an opportunity for error? As a bedside nurse, I can tell you firsthand. But first, let me give you a little peek into what the process of medication administration looks like on my unit.

First, it is important to understand that many patients come into the hospital from home on multiple medications. I may very well be administering five to ten medications per patient (in addition to administering pain medication, antibiotics, managing IV lines, etc.) during my 0900 medication pass time. Second, medication administration does not happen in isolation.

Despite trying very hard to minimize interruptions during medication pass time, I nonetheless have to give out meds while attending to all my other responsibilities and demands for my attention. On a typical day shift I have four patients. Many times I must wait in line for access to one of two automated dispensing cabinets (we are a thirty-six-bed unit), especially during 0900 medication pass times. Then I must safely take out each medication while double-checking it against the electronic medication administration record (eMAR) for that patient.

After that, I must find any medication that is not stocked in the automated dispensing cabinet. These medications may be in any one of four locations: (1) the patient's individual medication cassette, (2) the refrigerator, (3) the other automated dispensing cabinet, or (4) the pharmacy (e.g., a missing medication). I must prepare a paper label for any medications that I need to draw up into a syringe. For IV piggyback medications, I must first mix them and then prepare a paper label.

Next, I travel down the hall with my eMAR and all the medications. Hopefully, when I arrive in the room, the patient is ready for me, water cup in hand, for his or her medications. I check the eMAR against the patient's armband and individually open each little packet of unit-dose medication. I do this while confirming and explaining to the patient the medication, dosage, purpose, and so on, and responding to any concerns or questions the patient may have. (I tease my patients that some of those little packets are "nurse-proof"—they can be so cumbersome to open.)

Hopefully, I make it from the countertop, where I opened all the medications successfully, to the patient without dropping anything or knocking over the medicine cup. Then I watch as my eighty-three-year-old patient takes *one* pill at a time ("Honey, I can't take all those pills at once"), while I cautiously survey her every attempt to reach her mouth, so as to catch any medications that may fall out of her hand or cup and into the bed sheets or down her gown. Then I stop and take her blood pressure before she takes her antihypertensive medications. Finally, I go back to my eMAR and document with my initials every medication I administered . . . and the *time.*

On to the next patient, right? Not so fast. The patient I have just so carefully watched as she puts pill after pill in her mouth needs to use the bathroom. Because she is an elderly postoperative patient with a knee replacement, I need to help her get up to use the bedside commode. This can take twenty minutes or longer. Of course, assisting my patient out of bed and to the commode is the perfect opportunity to assess the patient's strength, ability to follow commands, and scan and assess her skin, etc. But it also means that there is no way to get to the next patient within the time allotted.

I hope you are getting the idea that medication passes are time-consuming. Nurses are not administering medications to robots but to human beings. And during a med pass, my patients may express other needs that I cannot ignore at the time. I just gave you one very common scenario. Many more opportunities for distraction and interruptions to workflow occur that cause medication administration times to be delayed.

So where's the opportunity for error? There are many. One of the most prevalent is the time crunch and the level of frustration with the whole process of medication administration. This frustration causes distraction—one of the most frequent contributors to medication administration errors. The push to administer medications within the thirty-minute rule causes nurses to find workarounds . . . like pilfering another patient's cassette for a missing medication, documenting that the nurse gave a medication at 0900 (to keep in compliance and not get "caught" on audit) when it was really given at 1005, or withdrawing and preparing two different patients' medications at the same time to save time. Here's an example: Both patients are in a semi-private room. Why walk down the hall, back and forth, twice? Just bring Ms. Smith's meds and Ms. Rogers's meds to the same room at the same time! These are just some examples of a nurse's effort to "be in compliance" rather than do what is in the best interest of safety for the patient.

Giving nurses more flexibility for some medications and administration times, and educating us as to how and why these workarounds put our patients and our practice at risk, is the answer. And, wait, it might just be a good idea to talk to nurses before promulgating rules that make our jobs harder, more frustrating, and thus less safe for patients.

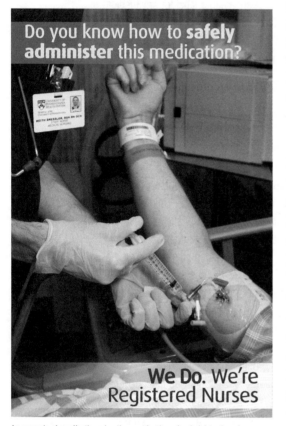

An example of an effective advertisement for the safe administration of medication. (By Suzanne Gordon; photo by Earl Dotter.)

When the Institute for Safe Medication Practice read Burke's story, they asked her if they could reprint it in their newsletter. Of course, she said yes and they did. This newsletter went out to many in the patient safety community as well as to regulators at CMS. Her story, combined with thousands sent by other nurses, convinced CMS to change their position and requirement. The new requirement allows nurses an hour before or after the specified time to administer medications. Burke's story helped change policy. It has also reached a larger audience by being included in a book about patient safety that was edited by Ross Koppel and Suzanne Gordon.[1] It is an example of how nurses can use their voices and participate in broad discussions that affect the world of health care.

The First Step: Deciding Whom You Want to Reach

It is important to define whom you want to communicate with so that you can determine how you will communicate. Consider how to reach the audiences or "publics" that you have in mind. If nurses are trying to explain a new protocol to the clinical personnel in their hospital, they might distribute a memo via e-mail. If patients with a particular illness need to know some specifics about self-care, nurses might prepare a brochure or sheet of instructions that can be taken home. They might buy or create a video

> **It is important to define whom you want to communicate with so that you can determine how you will communicate.**

that patients could watch when they come in for treatment. You might do a mailing to people in your neighborhood or community to advertise new services at your health care facility. You might also purchase newspaper ad space or commercial time on local television. You might send a notice about the program to a variety of electronic Listservs. You would most likely post the notice on your organizational website or even create a special website or Facebook page for such information.

At the same time, you might want to tell the public about some of these things via the news media. This means that you will have to convince intermediaries—journalists and television and radio producers—that your information is newsworthy, so that they will turn it into a story that reaches the public.

Before you pick up the phone or send out a news release, consider what audience you are trying to reach and which media outlets would be most effective.

Perhaps you would like people in your community to know about a nursing program that can serve them. In that case your best vehicle for communication might be community newspapers and websites.

Perhaps you will be rallying in front of your state or provincial capitol to support new legislation or regulations. You'll want as much publicity as possible throughout the state so that citizens can tell their political representatives to support your cause. Therefore, you will want to expand your efforts to the media beyond the capital. You'll want to get your advance press releases to newspapers, television, and radio throughout the region. If you're working with a PR professional, he or she should know whom to contact and how to distribute information. You can find out yourself by contacting the capital news bureau or pressroom.

Whether you are seeking a national audience or a local one, you will need an up-to-date media list with the e-mail addresses of journalists in your area who cover health care. Experienced PR specialists who work with nurses have contacts with the press. But whether you employ a PR person or not, nurses must establish and tend relationships with reporters and bloggers who can be helpful to them.

Introducing Yourself

You introduce yourself to the media by bringing them something that's newsworthy. An e-mail, press release, or phone call describing a newsworthy event or project can be your introduction. But how do you know if what you are doing is a story? Stand back and look at your work with some objectivity. Have you seen articles or television reports on similar topics? Have you seen a gap in the discussion that you can fill? Does your activity have some of the news values outlined in chapter 7? Is your issue relevant to the broader audience that a media outlet would reach? Can you present your work in a way that makes its value and relevance obvious? If your work is narrowly focused, ask yourself if it can be generalized. Is it poignant, dramatic, quirky, offbeat (as in man bites dog)? Does it fulfill a need? Does it challenge conventional wisdom?

Considering the newsworthiness of all sorts of activities and issues is a constructive activity for nurses inasmuch as the goal is to fully integrate nursing into health care coverage. Reaching out with a variety of events, activities, or innovations will make a broad range of nursing expertise more visible. It will open the door for nurses to become regular news sources on health matters far beyond those related to hospital working conditions. Professional organizations can broaden the public view of nursing by becoming as vigorous in promoting stories about nursing practice as collective bargaining groups have been in exposing threats to nursing and patient care.

Any research study or program on patient care is a possibility for a nursing angle. For example, research on patients' fear of being labeled "difficult" if they question their doctors and nurses is an apt subject for nurses to weigh in on. Coverage of "alarm fatigue," which results from too many computerized alarms, is an invitation to discuss how nurses are dealing with this phenomenon.[2]

Computerization in health care is an issue that has a nursing component that people should know about. For example, widely used "computerized physician order entry" systems are supposed to prevent errors that occur when doctors handwrite orders. However, these systems change the process of medication ordering. Isolated with his or her computer, the physician is more likely to enter orders without the input of nurses. The contextual knowledge the nurse has of patients—such as what drugs they are sensitive to, what has been tried and failed, and what doses of the drug are appropriate—is lost in the electronic ordering process.[3]

Opportunities

Be alert to your particular issues surfacing in the media. When the media focus on a dramatic or even sensational event, be prepared to jump in. Periodically an event—a tragedy, a new study, a court decree, a new law—catapults an issue to the top of the news agenda, where it receives intense coverage for a while. Nurses must take advantage of these openings even though some may be created by controversial or unpleasant events. In such cases, the press is looking for credible sources to present various sides of the issue. If you want your side to be represented, you need to be ready with appropriate spokespeople.

> "You can leverage awareness campaigns that already exist. February is Heart and Stroke Month. That's an opportunity to show what nurses do in this area. In May, maybe you can get a reporter to follow a nurse during Nurses Week."
>
> —Karen McCarthy, director of strategic communication for the Canadian Nurses Association

In many instances the kind of events that will propel an issue are predictable. If a blue-ribbon panel has been considering a particular problem or policy, most likely the media will cover its findings. Such groups make a point of packaging their reports in a media-friendly way. Journalists will report on a high court's decision in a controversial case. They usually know in advance when the court will hear the case. The agendas of legislative, policy-making, and regulatory bodies can be monitored to predict when news-making developments will occur. Journalists often get advance notice of when new research findings will be released. As members of a profession concerned with health care issues, nurses can stay abreast of these processes and be ready with their stories when the issue is about to crest again.

Focusing the Story

Pretend that you are the reporter trying to tell the story. You'll have to come up with something that can serve as a "peg."

Say you are a geriatric nurse practitioner who has initiated a program to release nursing home residents from physical and chemical restraints. Your work could be a timely and relevant story. One peg for a story could be how the health of the residents improved at a particular nursing home where this program was implemented. A research study that shows how this approach prevents suffering and saves money could also be a peg for a story.

Your Turn

Think of a story or two that you could pitch to journalists stemming from your work, institution, practice, research, or expertise.

How does it relate to a timely, important concern or event?

Try spinning the stories in various ways so that the same development can be connected to patient safety, health care financing, or treatment and care for specific groups.

For nursing, the point of outreach is to show, in a newsworthy way, how nurses understand patient needs, prevent problems, enhance public health, offer alternative policies, and meet contemporary health needs. It is not to get free publicity for your institution. Reporters will resist that kind of overture.

Unless you are working with a journalist who has demonstrated his or her knowledge about nursing, assume ignorance. The natural tendency of many journalists is to credit physicians with any improvement in health care delivery. That's why you'll have to highlight the nursing component of the story.

Assembling Written Materials

Reporters generally expect to see something written on the story you are trying to pitch. It makes their job easier and more efficient if they have something to read that gives the gist of the story.

Most of the time this is a brief e-mail, a news release, or both. Sometimes a news release will be more effective if backed up by research studies or news coverage that has appeared elsewhere. Reporters may pay more attention if they see that other journalists have found the topic newsworthy. However, they will be looking for their own angle.

If you are mounting a campaign you will want to e-mail materials to journalists or assemble a media kit that can be distributed via e-mail and also in hard copy if necessary. A media kit might contain some or all of the following:

- A press release or letter that piques the interest of the reader, briefly gives the facts, conveys a sense of immediacy, explains the relevance of the event or issue, and tells how to contact the people involved.
- A simple fact sheet that lists important points or background events or developments.

- A fact sheet that describes the organization or organizations sponsoring the event or involved in the issue.
- A "backgrounder" or briefing paper that gives in-depth information. If the backgrounder includes statistics or research data, the sources must be listed in a bibliography.
- Biographical sketches of the important players, including information on how to contact them.
- Copies of articles that have appeared in the press and brief descriptions and links to television reports and features that have been done on this or a similar topic. You could create a YouTube video on the subject; however, in general, it is more efficient for a journalist to sift through concisely written material than to take time to view videos.
- Copies of and links to pertinent research articles.
- A question-and-answer sheet that suggests and anticipates key questions and gives the answers.

News Releases

News releases are the primary tool for making contact with journalists. Journalists often claim they barely look at the scores of handouts that cross their desks or their computer screens. The reason journalists toss or delete the great majority of the news releases they receive is that the form is greatly abused by corporations peddling products and by organizations that indiscriminately crank out statements containing nothing remotely newsworthy. Many releases are poorly written, have no local angle to interest news outlets in a given area, and have no news elements. But when a release is informative and targeted properly, it can be effective in various ways.

A weekly newspaper, for example, might run an excerpt from or even an entire news release on programs of interest to the public or on people in the community. Most of the health service announcements in such publications and on their websites—a blood drive will be held, flu shots will be administered, a blood pressure screening clinic is operating—originate in news releases. So do many ideas that can be developed into good stories.

Larger news outlets, and radio and television news organizations, might use the information for an immediate story. They might cover an event because of a release. Reporters might hold on to a release for use in a future story. They might add the cited expert sources to their address book. Since journalists receive so many news releases through various avenues, they scan them rapidly, usually reading only the headline and the first paragraph.

If journalists don't see a peg for a story right at the beginning, you can be sure they won't spend their time wading around in your verbiage. Like the newspaper reader or the television viewer, they want to know what the story is right away. Then they can decide if they're interested.

Format

Even though many news releases are sent via e-mail and are posted on websites with splashy four-color designs, the form remains pretty constant. Observe the structure of the following news release.

News
Release

Nurses Long Work Hours, Scheduling Can Increase Patient Mortality

University of Maryland News, January 13, 2011

A new study has found that patient deaths from pneumonia and acute myocardial infarction were significantly more likely in hospitals where nurses reported schedules with long work hours.

The finding was just one of several revelations from a study of nurses' work schedules, patient outcomes, and staffing led by University of Maryland School of Nursing researchers in collaboration with researchers at the Johns Hopkins University School of Medicine.

The study is the latest in ongoing research on nurse scheduling and staffing funded by the National Council of State Boards of Nursing. In the current study, Alison Trinkoff, ScD, MPH, RN, FAAN, professor at the School and co-authors Meg Johantgen, PhD, RN; Carla Storr, PhD, MPH, RN; Yulan Liang, PhD; Ayse Gurses, PhD; and Kihye Han, MD, RN, shifted their focus from the effects on nurses in previous studies to patient well-being.

The team linked patient outcome and staffing information from 71 acute care hospitals in two representative states (Illinois and North Carolina) with the survey responses of 633 randomly selected nurses who worked in these hospitals. Their findings are published in "Nurses' Work Schedule Characteristics, Nurse Staffing, and Patient Mortality," in the January/February issue of the journal *Nursing Research*. Most U.S. hospitals use 12-hour nursing shifts exclusively, as opposed to eight-hour shifts, a trend begun during nursing shortages nationwide in the 1980s. "Although many nurses like these schedules because of the compressed nature of the workweek, the long schedule as well as shift work in general lead to sleep deprivation," says Trinkoff.

"Alertness and vigilance required for providing good nursing care depend upon having an adequate duration of quality sleep and rest," says Trinkoff, "and long work hours can impact the quality of nursing care and can increase the potential for error."

"Nursing work hours may also be increasing to compensate for decreasing physician work hours in hospitals because the medical profession has taken steps to limit the hours a physician in training may work, whereas nursing has not taken similar steps," says Trinkoff.

In the new study, the work schedule component that was most frequently related to mortality, along with long work hours, was lack of time off the job. Trinkoff and her colleagues previously found that lack of time off was also an important factor contributing to nurse injury and fatigue. Nurses need time off to rest and recuperate to protect their health and similarly, the lack of recovery time may affect performance on the job, she says.

"The finding that work schedule can impact patient outcomes is important and should lead to further study and examination of nursing work schedules," says Trinkoff.

In a previous paper, Trinkoff and co-authors reviewed evidence to challenge the 12-hour shift paradigm, which can result in sleep deprivation, health problems, and greater chance for patient errors. In another paper, they described barriers that keep nursing executives from moving away from the practice, and they offered strategies to help mitigate possible negative effects of 12-hour shifts. The strategies were based on the authors' extensive research, surveying, and experience in the nursing profession.

"Now that we have data that these conditions affect the public adversely, there is even more reason for providers in each hospital and clinic to look at the situation and find solutions," says Trinkoff.[4]

Components

A news release typically contains the following components:

1. *Letterhead.* Your news release needs a letterhead with your name or the name of your organization, mailing address, phone number, e-mail addresses, and web page location.

2. *Contact information* usually goes at the top of the release. After "Contact:" put the name(s) of the person or persons that a journalist can contact to verify the information in the release and to learn more. Be sure to give their e-mail address and phone numbers.

3. The standard news release identifies itself with the word NEWS or NEWS RELEASE written in large type at the top of the page.

4. Next a *release time* is given. Almost always you just type FOR IMMEDIATE RELEASE along with the date it was issued, which means the news organization can use the material as soon as it comes in or any other time. Some releases, reports, and studies will have an "embargo" date on them. This sort of release is intended to give journalists time to prepare their stories, but they must wait to publish or broadcast them until the specified time and date.

5. A *headline*, or tag line, goes at the top to catch the interest of the recipient. This is not the headline that the news organization will use. It will write a headline that fits its own format. Note the headline on the news release from the

University of Maryland. Like a news headline, it captures the point of the news release. It uses the present tense to convey not simply timeliness but urgency. Try to make your headline dynamic. Employ active verbs when possible. Your release should make as strong an assertion as you accurately can. This is not the time to fudge an issue.

The Lead

Never save the best stuff for last. Construct your news release like a news story—inverted pyramid style with the foundation for the story at the top. The first paragraph of a news story or news release is called the *lead*. Like the headline that preceded it, a good lead is a small story all by itself.

A summary lead is the most common type. It usually contains several of the five *Ws*—who, what, where, when, why (and sometimes how). It does it in one or two sentences.

- The "what" of the lead is the problem: in the University of Maryland release it is that patients are at risk of dying.
- The "why" in this case is the nub of the story: nurses' long work hours.
- The "who" refers to researchers at the University of Maryland and Johns Hopkins School of Medicine.
- The "where" is hospitals in Illinois and North Carolina that are representative of American hospitals. But the location of the researchers and the research sites is also important to the local media.
- The "when" is now.

When writing the lead (and the rest of the news release) don't be melodramatic or flowery. Write the way reporters do—in simple declarative sentences in the active voice.

The Body

Stick to the facts. Use direct quotations to introduce subjective material, opinions, or allegations. Get in a pithy quote as soon as possible. Quotations are essential to your news release because they allow you to inject "voice," opinion, vigor, and, sometimes, colorful language.

A direct quotation is a good way to make a strong point as experts did in the fifth and sixth paragraphs of the University of Maryland release.

Direct quotations for news releases are anything but spontaneous. The speaker herself might construct one or a PR person might write it with her or for her. But the quote is carefully tailored to deliver maximum impact and still sound like something the person would say. It should also be conversational and sound as though it was spoken rather than written.

Direct quotations must be attributed to the speaker. Inexperienced writers tend to put the name and the title of the speaker before the quotation. But unless the name is the most important element, advance attribution slows down the eye and lessens the impact of a dramatic or colorful quote. Look at the quotations in this book and at those in newspapers. You will see that the sentence often begins with the quote and finishes with the attribution. Also note the punctuation. In the United States, quotation marks go after the punctuation at the end of a quote.

The *Elements of Style*, by William Strunk Jr. and E. B. White, is an excellent, inexpensive source of information on grammar and style. This slim volume is a classic reference guide used by tens of thousands of students and writers.

A speaker is credible in a news release (or a news story) because he or she has expertise or authority. How is that fact established? By the person's title, position, work, and experience. Nurses often worry that being "just a nurse" is insufficient. For the working nurse, doing the work of nursing is precisely the credential that matters.

Note how the researchers are identified with their titles and academic credentials. By using the RN credential, they are emphasizing its importance to the subject matter. They are nurses who are authorities.

Be sure to highlight your nursing credentials when you are sending out a news release. In some instances PhDs let their institutions send out news releases with no explicit mention of their connection to nursing. Their name appears as Mary Smith, PhD, or as Dr. Mary Smith. This not only contributes to the invisibility of nursing; it actually risks giving medicine credit for nurses'

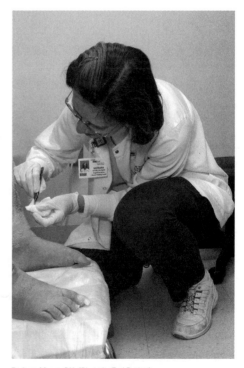

Barbara Myers, RN. (Photo by Earl Dotter.)

accomplishments. Although PhD nurses may feel strongly that they have earned their *Dr.* title, in this society they will generally be mistaken for physicians unless they make an extra effort to identify themselves as nurses.

When you are writing your news release, plan to spend about half your time on the headline, the lead, and the first direct quote. These are the most important elements, and it's reasonable to rewrite them until you have reduced them to the essentials. The rest of the release elaborates on the main points. For an inverted-pyramid-style release, you don't need a snappy ending. Just end before you start belaboring the points. Remember the release is designed to be a quick read.

Organizations often end their releases with a boilerplate paragraph that describes the function of the organization.

Here is a news release from the Registered Nurses' Association of Ontario:

News
Release

Provincial Task Force Action Plan Will Ensure Same Day Access For Patients, System Effectiveness, and Cost Savings

2012–06–28

MELISSA DI COSTANZO

TORONTO, June 28, 2012—A set of recommendations released today promises Ontarians improved access to quality primary care, system integration and effectiveness, and cost savings for the government and taxpayers.

The recommendations are contained in a provincial Task Force report led by the Registered Nurses' Association of Ontario (RNAO) with representatives from key organizations that work in primary care. RNAO launched the Task Force in February in response to the gross under-utilization of primary care nurses, and the belief that the sustainability of Ontario's health-care system depends on the success of primary care reform. "Our system is based on an illness model and we need to shift it to one that places greater emphasis on health promotion, disease prevention, and chronic disease management," says Rhonda Seidman-Carlson, president of RNAO, adding that "the full utilization of nurses is the key to our primary care success."

Primary Solutions for *Primary Care* lists 20 recommendations and ambitious timelines to maximize and expand the role of Ontario's 4,285 primary care nurses—Registered Nurses and Registered Practical Nurses—to eliminate the care gaps that prevent patients from receiving same day care and coordinated health system navigation.

The Task Force calls for its recommendations to be implemented in two phases. Phase one, to begin immediately, focuses on maximizing the current scope of practice of RNs and RPNs. Phase two, to be implemented over a two-year period from 2013 to 2015, looks at expanding the scope of practice for primary care nurses to further benefit patients and the health system.

Among the recommendations:

- The Ontario government immediately appoint a committee, co-sponsored by RNAO and the Ministry of Health and Long-Term Care, to roll out Task Force recommendations
- The government and LHINs issue immediate directives to employers to utilize RNs and RPNs to their full scope of practice
- Employers, educators, associations and nurses work together to ensure RNs are empowered to conduct a broad range of clinical assessments and interventions, health education, and chronic disease prevention and management
- Government and regulator work on legislative changes required to authorize RNs to prescribe and dispense medications
- Government and regulator work on legislative changes to authorize RNs to identify and communicate a diagnosis
- Government and regulator work on legislative changes to authorize RNs to order diagnostic and lab tests
- LHINs and primary care organizations utilize RNs to co-ordinate care and patient system navigation
- Employers, educators, associations and nurses work together to ensure RPNs are empowered to take leadership roles in evidence-based clinical and educational health programs

Primary care nurses work in Aboriginal health access centres, community health centres, family health teams, nurse practitioner-led clinics and physicians' offices. A recent survey revealed that only 61 per cent of RNs in primary care work to their full scope, with most saying they are capable of doing much more.

"Our research revealed that RNs and RPNs who work in primary care nursing aren't being utilized effectively. There is an incredible amount of untapped potential and we need to change that so nurses can do more for their patients and make our system more efficient," says Judie Surridge, co-chair of the Task Force and president of the Ontario Family Practice Nurses.

Doris Grinspun, chief executive officer of RNAO—who, along with Surridge, co-chaired the Task Force—says the leadership that resulted in Canada's first nurse practitioner-led clinic in Sudbury in 2007 and 24 NP-led clinics five years later is exactly what needs to happen now with primary care nurses. "We commend the Ontario government for the bold action it took to expand the scope of practice of nurse practitioners so they can fully serve the public. It has benefitted patients in spades. Now, we need to do the same with RNs and RPNs. If RNs can prescribe in the UK, why not in Ontario?" says Grinspun, adding that "the changes proposed in the report are long overdue, and implementing the recommendations will lead to higher satisfaction and better health outcomes for patients, improved system effectiveness, and reduced costs for taxpayers."

RNAO says the report's recommendations are in line with what the Drummond Commission concluded about Ontario's health system. Reiterating Don Drummond's assertion that expanding the scope of practice of nurses is one way to guarantee the sustainability of the province's publicly-funded, not-for-profit health system, RNAO is calling on the government, employers, associations, regulators, unions, and nurses themselves to act immediately on the Task Force's recommendations to benefit Ontarians.

The Registered Nurses' Association of Ontario is the professional association representing registered nurses in Ontario. Since 1925, RNAO has advocated for healthy public policy, promoted excellence in nursing practice, increased nurses' contribution to shaping the health-care system, and influenced decisions that affect nurses and the public they serve.

> Download a copy of the Task Force's report.
> Read what stakeholders had to say. (The names of politicians and health care professionals who could be interviewed were listed.)
> For more information about RNAO, visit our website at www.rnao.ca. Check out our Facebook page at www.rnao.org/facebook or follow us on Twitter at www.twitter.com/rnao.
> Marion Zych, Director of Communications, RNAO. Cell: 647–406–5605 / Office: 416–408–5605 Toll free: 1–800–268–7199 ext. 209 mzych@rnao.org.[5]

Accuracy

Make sure your news release is accurate. Check and recheck all the names and other proper nouns for correct spelling. Then have someone else proofread your release. It is astonishing how easily errors can creep in and not get caught. Your credibility could suffer if there are errors in your release. It is a maxim in journalism that if a name is incorrect, then nothing else is believable.

It should go without saying that a release must be honest as well as accurate. You are expected to present information from your point of view. However, you must not mislead, exaggerate, or distort the truth to build your case.

Broadcast Releases

Radio and television stations can use information in a standard news release to create a report, but they cannot broadcast it as is. If they are interested in doing a report based on the release, they will convert its essential information into a short, broadcast-style piece.

If your release is on an upcoming event, include an extra sheet with exact information on where and when the event will take place, as well as the names of participants on the scene who will be available for interviews.

For broadcast writing, simplify the issues. Write for the ear, not the eye. Use short sentences. Use colloquial language. Avoid hard-to-pronounce words. Don't use abbreviations. Follow a difficult name with phonetic spelling in parenthesis so that the reader will know how to pronounce it. Spell out numbers. By all means use participants as sources of information, but in most cases, paraphrase instead of quoting directly, for example, "Stella Smith is among the registered nurses who say a safe staffing law will improve the care of patients in area hospitals."

Distribution

There are times when you will want to broadly distribute a news release to news organizations. You might e-mail your release to all the news organizations in the area or, for a fee, get it onto a PR newswire that goes to news organizations. Even with widespread distribution, targeting is important. You will want to make sure that appropriate reporters get their own copy.

In some instances, it's better to contact just a few reporters. If you have a story that you think would be of particular interest to a certain feature writer, columnist, or writer who focuses on health policy issues or would fit the format of a television newsmagazine show, put your efforts into making a good match. Tailor your presentation to that reporter or media outlet.

Explain who you are and why your project might make a good story. If you are pitching to television, or planning to post videos, make sure you can provide good visuals, an interesting setting, and people who will appear on air to tell their stories.

If you are seeking attention for new research or for your participation in a health care campaign, don't make the mistake of thinking that a journalist will read your release just because it is on your website. Some journalists may check your website for news. But nursing organizations and institutions can't assume that journalists regard them, as they do some medical associations, as news producers that require routine monitoring. Even those journalists who pay attention to nursing advise nursing groups not to use materials posted on their website as a substitute for assertive outreach to journalists.

> If you are seeking attention for new research or for your participation in a health care campaign, don't make the mistake of thinking that a journalist will read your release just because it is on your website.

Helen Palmer, health correspondent for American Public Radio International's *Marketplace*, a national daily business program that frequently covers health care, explained to us: "I don't have time to check out websites on the off chance that there might be news on them, and I certainly can't check out websites that I don't know exist. Groups that have something to say need to find out who the journalists are they want to reach and make sure they let us know when they have something that is newsworthy.

"The California Nurses Association and the Massachusetts Nurses Association are very media savvy. They e-mail news releases. If I were looking for something on a nursing issue I'd be very likely to go to the California Nurses Association or the Massachusetts Nurses Association because they've made themselves known to me. If I wanted to track down a nursing issue or run something by someone on nursing, I believe they would find me a nurse who could talk to me on that particular issue."

Phone Calls

When you send a news release or a letter containing the elements of a news release, follow up with a phone call. You can't be sure the reporter has read his or her mail, paid attention to the specific piece, or even received it. That phone conversation will allow you to elaborate on the initial communication or present it if the release hasn't been read or has got lost. Don't call just to ask if the reporter received it. Use the opportunity to sell the story.

If you've made phone contact with the reporter before sending the release or letter, it is wise to have a written version before you so that you can make your points on the phone without getting flustered.

Getting through to a reporter is not always easy, but keep trying. Many news organizations have voice mail systems that act as fortresses. Try to get the direct extension for the people you want to reach.

Just as patients need advocates in the hospital, nurses need advocates in media institutions, as the following story illustrates.

A freelancer who writes for major media outlets received a press release and a follow-up phone call about a nursing program at a hospital she had written about in the past. Intrigued by the program, she called an editor at the city newspaper, offering to do a story on the program. The editor confessed she had received the same press release, but because she didn't know much about nursing, the release went into the wastebasket. She did, however, respond to the call from a journalist she trusted and assigned her to do the story.

Making the Clinical Workplace Work for You

As we have seen, many of the health care institutions in which nurses work do not promote nursing and won't unless nurses intervene. The media officers who work for hospitals and medical centers usually do an excellent job of promoting doctors and medicine. If a journalist needs an expert to bring him up to speed on urinary incontinence, for example, he might phone the media relations department at a medical center and ask to do an interview with an expert on staff. Almost invariably—even if the subject is one in which nurses have particular expertise—that authority will be a physician. In pitching stories and responding to requests from journalists, PR people at the institutions where most nurses work are often on automatic pilot. The flight instruction is, Find a doctor.

A veteran practitioner of medical center media relations suggests that the reasons for this are that most PR and marketing people in health care institutions begin and practice their work in a media culture that devalues nursing, and they develop their careers in institutions whose fortunes are viewed as being synonymous with those of the medical staff. The raison d'être of the PR staff, then, is to promote the medical staff.

Tony Swartz-Lloyd, who was the vice president of communications at Boston's Beth Israel Hospital for twenty-three years, says that many communication staffers view nurses as a quantitative, not a qualitative, variable in patients' hospital stays. "They understand that hospitals need enough nurses to keep the hospital running," he says. "They say there aren't enough qualified nurses, and that nurses are overworked and underpaid. But their understanding usually doesn't go beyond that. They can't tell you why having an individual, highly qualified nurse is important."

This, Swartz-Lloyd says, is very different from a PR staffer's understanding of physicians' work. "A PR person can easily explain why it's important to have a doctor who is skilled and qualified. They'll explain that if you don't have a good orthopedic surgeon, he could attach your left leg to your right."

But, he says, they don't understand that to patients, nursing is equally important. "They don't understand the consequences of nurses' not being able to do their work effectively or not being supported by their institutions. They don't get that you don't just want nurses there to 'answer the bell' but you also want them to do research and teaching and publishing and furthering their own education. This is a good thing, not a ducking-out-of-work kind of thing."

Communication specialists in medical centers also quickly get the message that doctors think anything interesting revolves around them. It's natural for marketing and communication people to absorb the attitudes that some physicians have about nurses. "Because medicine is a 'male' culture," one PR expert asserted, "doctors don't like nurses who see themselves as being equal to doctors and, worse, who can go about proving it."

Maureen McInaney, senior public information representative at the University of California San Francisco Medical Center, agrees: "Most hospital PR staff are not taught that promoting nursing is part of their brief, and too few institutions make it part of their brief. They conceive of hospitals as buildings with patients and doctors in them." McInaney explains, "Public information professionals are still more likely to seek out physician experts, often forgetting that nurses can respond to many of these inquiries."

Without institutional support and encouragement, communication specialists at medical centers and hospitals will be wary of promoting nursing even if they would like to. This is why, in the 1980s, the administration of Beth Israel Hospital in Boston gave its PR staff the resources and authority to promote nursing. "It took five years to sell primary nursing, which Beth Israel was developing and implementing, but eventually we did it," says Swartz-Lloyd, who directed the effort. According to Swartz-Lloyd, Mitchell Rabkin, MD, and Joyce Clifford, RN, then the hospital CEO and nurse in chief, respectively, not only encouraged the communication staff to go in a new direction but also shielded the staff from medical sniping. Time and again, through local and national print and television stories, Beth Israel proved that the nursing story is salable.

On the other hand, failure to promote nursing creates a self-reinforcing cycle. Nursing doesn't appear in the media when PR professionals don't send releases or pitch stories about nursing or educate journalists by talking with them about developments in nursing. So when a PR person approaches a journalist, as one Australian information specialist explained, the journalist discounts nursing as too "touchy-feely." If a PR staffer doesn't know how to counter that view of nursing, she or he may simply give up trying to pitch nursing stories. With no one initiating or pursuing the conversation, PR people don't get inquiries from journalists about nursing and thus conclude that nursing is not salable, and thus might discourage nurses who approach them with good stories.

Nurse executives and deans of nursing can provide the impetus to break that cycle.

Your Turn

Think of a story or two that you could pitch to journalists stemming from your work, institution, practice, research, or expertise. How does it relate to a timely, important concern or event? Try spinning the stories in various ways so that the same development can be connected to patient safety, health care financing, or treatment and care for specific groups.

CHAPTER 9

IN YOUR OWN VOICE: LETTERS TO THE EDITOR, OP-EDS, AND BLOGS

When we wrote the first edition of *From Silence to Voice*, opportunities for nurses to enter media discussions about health care were fairly limited. Nurses could write letters to the editor of newspapers and magazines. They could write opinion pieces known as op-eds to newspapers and other publications. They could write books. When we wrote the second edition of *From Silence to Voice*, the World Wide Web had made it easier for nurses to reach broader audiences with their concerns and opinions. Blog sites in particular were becoming popular.

Now, of course, the Internet, social media, personal digital devices, and instant connectivity mean that nurses can communicate with multitudes throughout the world essentially at any time and place. In a sense you could say that nurses no longer have an excuse to be absent from the health care discussions of our time. Technology has made it possible for nurses not only to communicate but also to communicate in great numbers.

There are many available vehicles. Nurses can use news media websites which more than ever welcome interaction with their readers and viewers in the form of comments, letters, blogs and even videos. Nurses can blog on any number of websites including their own. They can initiate and join larger conversations via Twitter, Facebook, Tumblr, YouTube, and many other platforms. They can illustrate their messages with art, photos, and videos. Nurses can share information on various issues with select groups or with the world at large. Today the issue is not so much how nurses gain access to public discourse but how willing they are to participate and what they are willing to say.

No matter which portal of entry you choose—blogs, op-eds, letters to the editor, posting on your Facebook page or creating a Facebook cause, writing a book or memoir—the rules for nurses are pretty much the same. You have to know your goal; target your specific audience; craft a credible, coherent argument; express your views or concerns with both sense and sensitivity; and pick the best vehicle or vehicles for making your point and telling your story. The web provides plenty of opportunities for sounding off with diatribes, attacks, and vulgarity. These kinds of communications do nothing to encourage support for nursing. The communication we are concerned with is the kind that enlightens and educates broader publics. There are useful structures for this purpose, among them letters to the editor and the personal or op-ed essay. In this chapter, we show how to construct letters, essays, and other messages and provide examples of various pieces written by nurses. The following guidelines apply to whatever vehicle you choose to express your opinions, concerns, or experiences.

Letters to the Editor

Media outlets have several forums for reader and viewer feedback. Most make it easy for you to post comments on issues that they cover. Social media platforms allow you to chime in with your thoughts in real time as you watch, say, a political debate on television. This kind of feedback can develop into an interesting discussion, but off-the-cuff comments may not be the most effective way for you to make your point. One reason is that although you need to register with websites in order to respond, the identities of those who write comments usually are not made public and thus the accountability bar is set pretty low. Letters to the editor are taken more seriously for two reasons—the writers are identified, and editors select only those letters for publication or posting that meet their standards. These are generally outlined on the publication's web page. The following guidelines from the *Milwaukee Journal Sentinel* are fairly typical:

1. Generally, we limit letters to two hundred words.
2. Name, street address, and daytime phone are required.
3. We cannot acknowledge receipt of submissions.
4. We don't publish poetry, anonymous, or open letters.
5. Each writer is limited to one published letter every two months.[1]

This is followed by a form on which a letter can be typed and submitted electronically. Note the suggested two-hundred-word limit. Editors are ready to condense letters submitted to them, but only up to a point. If you submit a letter that goes on and on, you are making it a better candidate for the delete button than for the letters page. News publications give preference to letters that address subjects that are of interest to readers in their area.

Usually a snail mail address also is given, but today that's pretty obsolete because the window of opportunity is tight. If an article that you want to respond to appears on December 2, it's best to write and transmit your letter that day. Indeed, you may see responses in the next day's newspaper or even alongside the original article online. The more days that pass, the lower your chances of getting published.

Note that all publications will want your name, address, telephone, and e-mail address. News publications do not run anonymous letters, and some call to verify that you are the writer. Under rare circumstances, the publication might withhold your name if you ask. But one of the reasons for writing letters to the editor is to make nurses and the work they do more visible.

When Elizabeth Gross Cohn read an op-ed in the *New York Times*, "Can Stop-and-Frisk Be Mended?"[2] she seized an opportunity to connect a controversial police procedure with health consequences. This is how her letter appeared in the Times.

Letter to the Editor

To the Editor:

As a nurse practitioner and a researcher working with the Harlem community, I know that men of color experience an increased prevalence of heart diseases, stroke, cancer and diabetes. Many causes contribute to these health disparities, but there is a growing body of research demonstrating that racial discrimination—perceived and actual—is a critical factor.

For example, the increased incidence of cardiovascular diseases has been recently linked to experiences with discrimination as published this year in *The American Heart Journal*, *The American Journal of Public Health* and *Current Hypertension Reports*.

I have grave concerns that stop-and-frisk may be undermining the health of the next generation of young men of color in our communities and across the country.

Elizabeth Gross Cohn
New York, June 19, 2012
The writer is an assistant professor,
Columbia University School of Nursing.[3]

Note that Cohn established her credentials and knowledge right off the bat by describing herself as a nurse practitioner and a researcher who works with the Harlem community. By describing her experience, she gives us a reason to pay attention to what she has to say on this issue. It is important to state your professional credentials in the body of your letter ("As a pediatric nurse") as well as with your signature ("RN"), and, if appropriate, your title ("Director of Nursing"). The reason for doubling or tripling up is that your nursing connection could disappear in the editing. Some publications identify physicians by putting MD after their names but do not list nursing degrees. The *New York*

Times no longer lists any degrees. As a case in point, RN and DNSc (doctor of nursing science) did not appear after Elizabeth Gross Cohn's name in the *Times*. The way to make sure that readers (and editors) can't miss the fact that you are a nurse is to say so in the letter and after your name. If you are a PhD and use only that as a credential, the nursing connection is likely to be lost. One other point: make sure your facts are accurate. News publications discard letters with obvious factual errors or exaggerations. Some publications fact-check letters before publishing them.

Nurses sometimes worry that they lack the expertise to challege the point of view of physicians and others who write about health care. But the things that nurses learn in their day-to-day work can be used to broaden the perspectives of others and provide editors, producers, and reporters with feedback on their coverage. The author of the following letter, Virginia Tyack, is not a nurse, but she once worked as a perfusionist trainee in a cardiac surgery OR. Because of that experience, she told us, she felt strongly about responding to an article in the *New Yorker* by the noted surgeon-journalist-writer Atul Gawande.

In his "Annals of Medicine" pieces for the *New Yorker*, Gawande explores innovative ways to improve medical practice and health care delivery. He often draws on his own experience and does not spare himself in discussing medical shortcomings. In a "Personal Best" column, Gawande explored how coaches can help athletes, muscians, teachers, and others improve their performance. He came off a little Lone Rangerish, however, when he suggested that personal coaches accompany surgeons in the operating room because: "Like most work, medical practice is largely unseen by anyone who might raise one's sight. I'd had no outside ears and eyes."[4] In her letter Tyack explained that there are other people in the operating room who could help surgeons do a better job.

October 24, 2012

Atul Gawande, in his article about using coaches to improve professional skills, shows an admirable desire to continue to hone his own skills as a surgeon ("Personal Best," October 3rd). But Gawande, like all surgeons, operates with other members of a surgical team, and his piece doesn't explore the shared experience of his team members, all of whom are vitally aware of the progress of a surgery. I once worked in a lowly position in an operating room. I was never consulted about how any aspect of a procedure, however minor, might be improved, until the hospital was faced with a malpractice lawsuit. Suddenly, it seemed, the surgeon, the hospital administrator, and the lawyers were interested in my intimate knowledge of that particular case and what I thought might have gone wrong. Perhaps another approach

Letter
to the
Editor

to improving patient outcomes might be routine "post-game" reviews with the entire surgical team. Good outcomes, after all, depend on the continuing development of everyone involved.

Virginia Tyack
Richmond, Virginia[5]

It can be quite a coup to get a letter published in major publications like the *New York Times* and the *New Yorker* magazine because they receive many letters from readers who want to be heard. The odds may be better with small and medium-sized news outlets that publish a higher percentage of the acceptable letters they receive. Smaller publications might also be willing to publish a longer letter that addresses a serious health care delivery problem and that cites statistics and research to make its point.

The New Hampshire nurse Kelly Clow wrote the following letter to the *Keene Sentinel* as an assignment in a course she was taking in the University of Massachusetts RN to BSN program. It refers to a law that went into effect in New Hampshire that would profoundly reduce the reimbursements that hospitals receive for caring for Medicaid patients. Indeed, a week after Clow's letter appeared, ten New Hampshire health care facilities filed suit claiming that the state had violated the Medicare Act by not fulfilling its legal obligations under the joint federal-state program. In her letter, Clow, a nurse at the Cheshire Medical Center, describes how budget cuts impact the ability of nurses to care for patients.

Letter
to the
Editor

Nurses Are Overworked

Tuesday, July 19, 2011

Patient safety is a priority for every nurse, for every patient, all the time.

As many hospitals across the state are faced with state budget cuts, some are cutting staff in effort to cut hospital costs ("Local Hospital Will Lose $6M" *The Sentinel*, June 23).

Cheshire Medical Center in Keene is going to lose Medicaid reimbursement totaling $6 million.

In the past two years, Cheshire Medical Center has already cut 100 positions. What do these cuts mean for patient safety? When the nursing staff available to provide care to patients is reduced, this could possibly put patients in danger. When there is a high patient-to-nurse ratio, there is an increased chance of adverse outcomes for patients, including, but not limited to, increased rates of medication errors, increased patient falls, increased chance of skin breakdown, increased patient and family complaints, increased infections and increased deaths.

An article published in the *New England Journal of Medicine* reports that the risk of death of a patient increases 2 to 6 percent when the registered nurse staff is below target levels.

This increased risk is too much for me to be comfortable with.

As a nurse, I have seen firsthand how staff reacts to an increased demand on their energy by having a larger personal patient census. Nurses are becoming burnt-out and many are leaving their jobs due to dissatisfaction.

A 2002 report titled "Hospital Nurse Staffing and Patient Mortality, Nurse Burnout, and Job Dissatisfaction" states "forty percent of hospital nurses have burnout levels that exceed the norms for health care workers, job dissatisfaction among hospital nurses is four times greater than the average for all US workers, and one in five hospital nurses report that they intend to leave their current jobs within a year."

Because nursing care is a 24-hour, around-the-clock, service there needs to be an adequate number of nursing staff employed to meet these needs. Cutting staff should not be seen as a way for hospitals to save money; this puts a patient's life at risk and leads to burnout for the nurses.

Kelly Clow, RN
Marlborough, NH[6]

For nurses, writing a letter to the editor is one of the simplest and most effective ways to do the following:

- Correct an error
- Increase nursing visibility
- Express an opposing point of view
- Affirm and encourage positive news coverage
- Educate journalists and the public about a particular issue
- Try to change the way a topic is perceived or covered

If you are trying to correct an error or a misconception about nursing, a direct but courteous approach works better than a harangue, according to Mark Jurkowitz, associate director of the Pew Research Center's Project for Excellence in Journalism and a former ombudsman for the *Boston Globe*. Maintain an even, reasonable tone in all contacts, oral or written, with the media. "No matter how angry you are, avoid conspiracy theories and vicious personal attacks," Jurkowitz advises. First call or email the reporter and bring the problem to his or her attention. If there is no resolution or the reporter can't be reached, the caller should try to get through to the editor of the section. A good way to build the bridge is to say you appreciate the reporter's effort and then calmly state your criticism. Give specific examples of what was underplayed, overplayed, or misreported and suggest what should be handled differently.

You don't have to be a specialist or a nursing professor to respond to coverage. You are an expert on your experience as a nurse, and your observations can

> You don't have to be a specialist or a nursing professor to respond to coverage. You are an expert on your experience as a nurse, and your observations can educate the public about nursing and health care.

educate the public about nursing and health care. If you've submitted a letter to the editor and it hasn't been published, you can submit it elsewhere, post it on a social media site, or use it in a blog. The letter form is a useful way to say a lot in a small amount of space. Writing letters to the editor provides practice in constructing clear, concise, and convincing arguments.

Blogs

"Blog" (both a noun and a verb) may be the most overused word in communication today as it is applied to just about anything that appears on the web. Wikipedia defines a blog (a condensation of web log) as "a discussion or informational site published on the World Wide Web and consisting of discrete entries ("posts") typically displayed in reverse chronological order (the most recent post appears first)."[7]

However, the form has been evolving and expanding. Once a blog was thought of as the work of an individual writing about a given subject. Some blogs are personal online diaries. More recently, according to Wikipedia, "multiauthor blogs" (MABs) have developed, with posts written by large numbers of authors and professionally edited. MABs from newspapers, other media outlets, universities, think tanks, interest groups, and similar institutions account for an increasing quantity of blog traffic. The rise of Twitter and other "microblogging" systems helps integrate MABs and single-author blogs into societal newstreams.[8]

Blogs have both expanded and blurred what is thought of as news media. An example is *The Huffington Post*, a content aggregator that describes itself as "The Internet Newspaper: News, Blogs, Video, Community."[9] *The Huffington Post* is known for the large number of blogs that it carries, some of which are targeted to readers in specific countries. Some blogs posted on this and other news sites are written by specialists in their fields and resemble the columns that appear in newspapers. The form, however, is elastic, and a "blog" can be almost anything—an opinion piece, a report, an announcement, an advertisement, and even a comedy routine.

In reality, blogs are a form of social networking in that visitors can leave comments, share with others, and message each other. Some blogs focus on particular subjects such as health, travel, and politics. Individuals blog to promote their work. Political activists and candidates blog to raise money and to get out the vote. Some blogs are promotional vehicles. Nursing and other organizational websites refer to their news releases as blogs. Some blogs are nothing more than pitches for products and services. Whatever blogs are, they are wildly popular. In 2011, there were over 156 million public blogs in existence.[10] You don't need much technical knowledge to start a blog or participate in the blogosphere. Today even countries have official blogsites.

Most of the nursing blogs we have seen are by nurses communicating with other nurses. Some of these are on organizational websites. Then there are the many individual blogs posted by nurses and student nurses on such blogsites as Wordpress and Tumblr as a way of connecting with their peers, venting their frustrations, asking for help, and instructing and inspiring each other. They tend to be an interesting mix of professional and personal subject matter. We have found a small percentage of these to be embarrassing, and even excruciating, to read in terms of the wildly inappropriate details that they reveal about the writer, sometimes even with photos and sometimes even under the writer's real name. It is puzzling that the writers of such blogs either don't realize or don't care that what they are posting can by seen by anyone and that it can come back to haunt them.

The kind of blogs that interest us most are ones that communicate with broader publics about the profession of nursing and the work of nurses even if they are targeted to other nurses. For example, journalists and members of the public would learn a lot about nursing were they to tune into one of our favorite blogs, ImpactedNurse.com. It is written, edited, and produced by Ian Miller, who describes himself as a registered nurse with nearly twenty-three years' experience working in the emergency department of a major teaching hospital in Canberra, Australia. The motto of his blog is "No fluff, no guff, no duff."[11]

Since 2002, Miller has been reporting on the latest clinical research. He offers nurses succinct clinical tutorials on such subjects as how to avoid air bubbles in IV lines and how to calculate pediatric fluid rates. He comments regularly on health care policy and delivery issues as they arise, like on a study that found Australian hospitals ill prepared to cope with a large-scale natural disaster or terrorist attack. He has a video on his website in which he cajols nurses to unearth their academic research and share it with other nurses. Successful blogs tend to exhibit a lot of personality, and that is certainly true of ImpactedNurse.com. Miller amuses readers with his own adventures and foibles like his struggle to fold up an ironing board. And his spoofs are priceless, like his report (complete with photos) that his ED brought in ultra-adorable puppies to carry around drugs in little backpacks after a study suggested that test subjects' performance and focus improved after viewing pictures of cute animals.

What stands out on ImpactedNurse.com is Miller's passion for learning and sharing, both of which go a long way toward establishing and maintaining a supportive community. One of his creative educational vehicles is the Thunder-box Paper series, named after the Aussie term for an outhouse. The reason is that the series consists of one-page overviews of a clinical subject (e.g. "Normal blood electrolyte/glucose values") that are meant to be stuck on the toilet door and read and memorized while one is doing one's business there.

We don't know how many lay people look at this or other nursing blogs, but we can't help but think that blog communities have the capacity to positively influence how nurses think about their work and how nurses might communicate about that work with others. Stories by nurses can be very potent, like this sensitive (but definitely not saccharine) piece by Ian Miller reflecting on the dehumanizing effects of healthcare protocols.

Blog

The Re-Identification of Our Patients

Suspend, for just a moment, our professional obligation to maintain patient confidentiality. To de-identify and to cohort. Suspend all our preconceptions of the sanctity of this. Just for a moment.

Imagine that it became hospital policy to use every patient's name, and a short bio, and a picture of them (perhaps with their family) at every case presentation, teaching session and every review of an adverse outcome. Especially every review of an adverse outcome.

Imagine if patients were routinely asked to write a a few paragraphs about themselves that would be read out to the operating team by the surgeon prior the first incision.

Imagine if the family of confused, elderly or demented patients were encouraged to fill a small informing scrap book (provided by the hospital) and all hospital staff from the treating consultant to the attending cleaner were expected to familiarise themselves with it.

Imagine that it became policy for a senior representative of the hospital executive to be present with every family during times of difficult discussions, decisions and deaths.

Imagine if there was a large wall or an open room in the main foyer of every hospital that allowed families (and staff) to commemorate and celebrate the life of a family member who had died that month, in any way they chose.

Imagine if we re-identified our patients instead of de-identifying them.

What would that be like?[12]

A number of nurses who blog identify themselves with only a pseudonym. One of the blogs we check in on is *Not Nurse Ratched*, by an anonymous nurse-writer whose picture nonetheless is posted and who says of herself: "I'm a former medical editor, current ER nurse, Apple geek, writer, photographer, ranter, and inveterate smartass."[13] Not Nurse Ratched frequently writes about her experience as a nurse, but notes under the heading of "HIPAA": "Any patient mentions are scrambled like an egg. If you think you recognize yourself or anyone who actually exists, it's purely accidental." To further protect herself from retribution, she adds an "Institutional disclaimer: This blog is my own. I write as myself and not as a representative of any institution." Not Nurse Ratched is wide ranging in her subject matter. We think that any member of the lay public who happens upon this blog, or a number of others, will get a serious and unvarnished view of nursing.

Op-Eds

Despite the popularity of blog sites, the op-ed sections of printed and online newspapers and newsmagazines remain powerful forums. If you have enough material for a 750-word essay, by all means write an op-ed. An op-ed is essentially a short essay that addresses a timely issue with a strong point of view. The term op-ed is newspaper jargon. It stems from the traditional placement of opinion columns on a page *op*posite the *edi*torial page. There's no reason that a letter to the editor or a blog couldn't be shaped into an op-ed.

Some women's and consumer magazines run op-ed type essays from outside contributors, although they probably refer to them as blogs. The kind of pieces they accept can range from opinion columns to slice-of-life features. Business websites provide another market for the op-ed contributor, as do many magazines that serve specific "communities" such as college alumni or members of religious denominations. Some publications reserve slots for longer unsolicited analytical pieces. Sunday week-in-review and analysis sections of newspapers may accept pieces that are up to fifteen hundred words. Public policy outlets may also accept longer submissions. These are just a few of the outlets that nurses can use to reach broader audiences.

What Are Op-Eds About?

- An op-ed can propose a solution to a pressing problem.
- An op-ed can present an unaddressed aspect of an issue or give a unusual twist to the discussion.
- An op-ed can expand on news coverage.
- An op-ed can present a personal experience that relates to a public issue.

Even with stiff competition for access, the op-ed remains a forum of choice. For nurses, time dedicated to learning how to compose op-eds will be well invested. Expect to rewrite your essay many times. It takes skill to deliver a snappy op-ed. That skill develops from practice. Don't be discouraged when your submission is rejected. Submit it somewhere else. Above all, try, and try again.

An op-ed should address a timely issue, one that has been in the news but has not yet been talked to death. It must confidently express an opinion. Unlike a news article, an op-ed is not designed to present only the "facts" or to take an "on the one hand, on the other hand" tone. An op-ed demands an assertively articulated point of view.

The Nuts and Bolts of Op-Ed Writing

An op-ed is only 750–800 words long, $2\frac{1}{2}$ to 3 double-spaced, typewritten pages. The standard form consists of four parts: (1) lead, (2) focus, (3) elaboration, and (4) kicker.

1. The opening paragraph, or lead, sets the scene and tone for the reader. It may state the main point or direct the reader toward the point. The lead could be in the form of (a) an anecdote or scene-setter, (b) a summary of what has happened before, or (c) a direct statement calling for a specific action.

2. The second paragraph usually contains the focus of the piece (if it isn't already in the lead). The focal paragraph is known in journalistic jargon as the "nut graf" (meaning the core paragraph, or "graf" for short) or "billboard" (meaning the paragraph that "advertises" to the reader what the article is about). Every op-ed, indeed every type of article, must have a nut graf. If you start submitting articles for publication, sooner or later an editor will ask you about your nut graf, maybe in just those words.

3. The rest of the article elaborates on the focus and moves from point to point in an interesting manner using some or all of the following: (a) factual statements, (b) statistics, (c) examples, (d) quotations, (e) anecdotes, (f) explanations.

4. The kicker, or the last paragraph, wraps up the op-ed and ties it with a bow. The kicker could be (a) a different, dynamic, or snappy restatement of the point; (b) a direct call to action; (c) a quotation; (d) an anecdote; or (e) a warning.

The op-ed must be concise. Most op-eds run no longer than 750 or 800 words, and some may be only 400 to 600 words. Submissions that vastly exceed the standard length run the risk of rejection on that basis alone.

The first and second paragraphs of an op-ed must offer an engaging or novel point of view. An editor sifting through submissions may not read much beyond the first two paragraphs before hitting the "reject" button.

Some editors may be so intrigued by a strong point of view that they will go beyond the normal editing and offer to help cut or reshape the piece. This is rare, though. Longer commentaries—those between one thousand and fifteen hundred words—should be directed only to sites that accept that length.

An op-ed—even a humorous one—must address something that people do or should care about. Health care certainly offers enough facets to keep op-ed writers busy for years. The best time to get published is when the news media are paying attention to an issue—not before it has been raised or after it has crested. Precisely because of the broad nature of health care, however, the op-ed writer must resist the temptation to address several points in one essay. While an op-ed can be about any number of things, the successful op-ed is about only one. The secret to op-ed writing is to organize the article around one point and stick to that point. The strength of an op-ed is that it can give a new perspective to an issue. This is what nurse practitioner Joyce Penrose brought to her op-ed for the *Pittsburgh Post-Gazette* about meeting the need for primary care.

Providing Primary Care for the Poor: Nurse Practitioners and Physician Assistants Stand Ready to Meet the Challenge, Again

Op-Ed

October 11, 2012

BY JOYCE PENROSE

A sentence in the article "Can Medicaid Solve Our Ills?" in the Sept. 9 *Post-Gazette* caught my eye. Quoting Dr. Alan Yeasted, reporter Bill Toland wrote, "There is somewhat of a shortage of PCPs (primary care physicians) and a bigger one looming in the future." This will especially be true in Pennsylvania if the governor expands Medicaid coverage under the provisions of the Affordable Care Act.

I couldn't help but remember similar concerns expressed in the 1960s when primary care physicians also were in short supply, a shortage sure to be exacerbated with the passage of Medicare and Medicaid.

What's different, though, is the changing face of primary-care delivery, which now includes the extensive use of nurse practitioners and physician assistants. Indeed, it was the legislation that created Medicare and Medicaid in 1965 that spurred the development of these professions.

The prospect of providing access for the elderly poor to primary care, from which they had been excluded, mainly due to cost, raised thorny questions. How could we possibly care for so many who were so sick? For there was no doubt that the elderly poor, having gone without primary care for most of their lives, were sick and needed help.

The '60s was a time of ferment in America, with civil rights, women's rights, the antiwar movement and other struggles challenging long-accepted norms. One norm that changed was the role of nurses.

At the time, nurses, virtually all of them women, were educated in hospitals and largely worked in hospitals. Their functions diverged sharply from those of physicians, and many state nursing laws prohibited nurses from performing "acts of medical diagnosis."

Fast forward to 2012 when we encounter nurse practitioners in retail clinics, physician offices, emergency departments, family planning programs and in many other settings.

This change took almost 50 years. The first programs to educate nurse practitioners and physician assistants were founded in 1965 by visionaries who saw that nurses could handle health promotion and disease prevention and that military corpsmen could build on their service-related experience to extend the reach of physicians. The University of Colorado hosted the first nurse practitioner program, which focused on the care of children. Duke University in North Carolina created the first physician assistant program.

The need for additional primary-care providers and the effectiveness of nurse practitioners in filling that role has resulted in a tremendous growth of nurse practitioners in Pennsylvania. According to the Pennsylvania Coalition of Nurse Practitioners, more than 7,000 currently practice in the commonwealth.

These nurses hold degrees at the master's level. In the near future, nurse practitioners will be prepared at the doctoral level, earning Doctor of Nursing Practice degrees. This reflects the growing responsibility shouldered by nurse practitioners in providing primary care to a diverse population.

Furthermore, nurse practitioners are more likely to work in rural and remote areas than are other primary-care providers. When, in 1965, caring for the large influx of poor and sick strained the resources of organized health care delivery, the country responded by developing community health centers. Care provided in these centers is judged to be among the most cost-efficient provided in our health system. New models of care delivery, utilizing teams of physicians, nurse practitioners and other health care professionals, are needed as we face new challenges.

Almost 50 years after the first nurse practitioners graduated from the University of Colorado, their importance to the provision of primary care was recognized by the Institute of Medicine in its 2010 publication "The Future of Nursing: Leading Change, Advancing Health." Nurse practitioners have been studied since their field was created, and their ability to deliver high-quality, cost-effective health care has been demonstrated repeatedly. They, and their physician assistant colleagues, stand ready to again help alleviate a looming shortage in primary care.

Joyce Penrose is a family nurse practitioner and adjunct associate professor in the School of Nursing at the University of Pittsburgh (jep87@pitt.edu). She spent the first seven years of her career caring for the rural poor at a community health center in central Virginia.

Op-Eds Using Nursing Research

Nursing research that adds new dimensions to issues or events that are reported in the news is an excellent way for nurses to help the public understand that they are, in fact, scientists whose work can contribute to solving critical problems. Letters to the editor and opinion pieces, whether published by conventional newspapers or through Internet publications, are an excellent way for nurses to be recognized as newsmakers and sources for comment on the news.

Over the past thirty years, several factors have made it essential for physicians to communicate with the public. Over time, insurers and government were no longer willing to write blank checks for health care services, and demands for reform of the system were increasing. If doctors were going to influence the funding and delivery of health care, they had to be willing to take their case to the public. At the same time, competition was growing for research funds, and patients were seeking more information from their doctors. In the United States, medical organizations did a turnabout. They dropped their bans against advertising, encouraged physicians to raise their public profiles, and taught them how to use the media effectively.

Today, the impetus to communicate with the public about health care is even stronger. "Funding agencies are eager to see that research results are disseminated to appropriate scientific, professional, and lay audiences," says Ross Koppel, a medical sociologist at the University of Pennsylvania's Department of Sociology and Center for Clinical Epidemiology and Biostatistics. "They require a dissemination plan that typically involves presentations to professional meetings, publication in refereed journals, releases to popular venues like newspapers or magazines if appropriate, and, if possible, book-length manuscripts for wider audiences. To reach wide audiences," Koppel told us, "funders today want researchers to be able to talk about their work in ways that nonspecialists and laypeople can understand."

For many years, the widely quoted bioethicist Arthur L. Caplan has been urging doctors to learn how to express themselves so that they can gain public support. He has even taught his students at the Center for Bioethics at the University of Pennsylvania how to write for popular audiences. We heard Caplan tell nurse executives attending a University of Pennsylvania conference that they must talk to the media both to inform the public about current health care issues and to influence the democratic process of decision making. He urged nurses to "take tough positions, advocate your views, and don't be wishy-washy."

Medical journal editors have paved the way for nurse researchers willing to follow this advice. They have convinced journalists that dry, seemingly incomprehensible study reports can be fascinating and worthy of media and public attention. They have made research findings reader friendly for reporters, who, in turn, have learned how to translate that research into understandable, everyday language.

Using their own voice, nurse researchers can do the same. This is precisely what nurse researchers Kathleen McPhaul and Jane Lipscomb and Matthew London did when, in 2010, a physician at Johns Hopkins Hospital was killed by an irate family member in his office. Longtime researchers into workplace violence and workplace violence prevention, McPhaul and Lipscomb were very aware that too many people—including politicians, policy makers, health care administrators, and even journalists—consider workplace violence inevitable, the result of a few bad apples and unamenable to system change. The two researchers at the University of Maryland School of Nursing had written many scholarly papers on the subject. Patricia Fanning, at the communications department at the university's Baltimore campus where the two work, had also encouraged them to respond to any coverage of workplace violence in the news. When this story hit the papers, McPhaul and Lipscomb took advantage of the opening and with Fanning's help wrote the following op-ed and submitted to the *Baltimore Sun*, which published it on September 22, 2010.

Op-Ed

The Public Should Care that Healthcare Workers Face Dangerous Working Conditions

Even though much of the public was stunned to learn of the shooting of a physician by a patient's family member at The Johns Hopkins Hospital last Thursday, we shouldn't be! Health care workers experience four times the risk of assault on the job when compared to all other types of workers; for those working in psychiatric units and the emergency department, the risk is considerably higher. Fortunately, most of the assaults do not involve handguns and near fatal injuries as was the case here, but many of them are life altering, career- ending injuries. Most of the discussion following last week's events focused on metal detectors, but metal detectors don't prevent the violence toward staff by patients who use their hands, which is far more common. What does prevent this type of violence is a strong violence policy, referring competent patients to the judicial system (i.e., pressing charges), being immediately responsive to staff concerns about safety and providing adequate staffing levels, video surveillance, personal alarms, more training, or limiting access to hospitals and clinics. Johns Hopkins officials stated that customer service will suffer if they put metal detectors at their 80 entrances, but we would ask them why they need 80 entrances and to weigh the benefits of that number of separate entrances verses the costs of limiting some of these points of access.

Judging from the momentum of the patient safety movement, the public seems increasingly aware that hospitals can be dangerous places for patients. But what the public does not appreciate is that hospitals are also dangerous places for employees and that those working conditions, in turn endanger patients. Workplace violence is an invisible but deadly epidemic for healthcare workers all over the world. Depending on the type of patient and the type of unit, estimates range from 30% to 100% of hospital staff experience verbal and physical violence each year. In the case of any other epidemic (salmonella, H1N1) these statistics would generate alarm. But violence toward healthcare workers remains largely invisible to the public; remaining the purview of a few active unions, nursing associations, and researchers.

Patient and staff safety are linked. If your nurse, doctor, or patient care technician is not safe, your loved one is not safe either. As such, the public must recognize and demand improved working conditions and safety of healthcare workers. Health care organizations must demonstrate that staff safety is as high a priority as patient safety and that they will work with clinicians to improve security while not compromising the quality of care for which institutions such as Johns Hopkins are world renowned.

What the public fails to realize is that the dangerous jobs of the past such as Baltimore's famed steelmaking, shipbuilding and construction trades were made safer over time by strong workplace regulations and strict enforcement. With manufacturing on the decline, the "new economy" is the service sector where different but dangerous working conditions exist. In the past, the Maryland Occupational Safety and Health Administration (MOSH) led the country making construction and shipbuilding jobs safer. It's time to regulate workplace safety in our hospitals in order to reduce the daily risk of violence faced by the healthcare workforce. Other states have done so including California, Washington State, New York and New Jersey. Regulations that protect health care workers from violence on the job will not turn hospitals into fortresses. Instead regulations in these others states require clear policies, a thorough risk assessment, adequate staffing and security resources, employee training, and ongoing recordkeeping and monitoring. Is it too much to ask for us to join voices and support a MOSH regulation to keep health care workers, patients and visitors safe from this workplace violence?

Kathleen M. McPhaul, PhD, MPH, RN
Jane Lipscomb, PhD, RN, FAAN
Matthew London, MS[14]

When they wrote their commentary, their goal, Lipscomb says, was to make sure people understood that something can be done about workplace violence. Being a target of violence is not, as many administrators seem to contend, a part of the job description of any person who works in a health care facility, whether at the very top or bottom of the hierarchy. The authors wanted health care workers and the public to understand that there are specific strategies and programs that can be put into place to curtail health care violence. Their column extended the discussion about the particular incident to health care workplace violence in general. Their op-ed prompted more coverage and discussion of the issue on radio, TV, and in newspapers.

Conveying Real-life Experiences and Describing What Nurses Do

Snapshots of physician practice are a staple of op-ed pages. Many physicians contribute stories about their moral dilemmas, relationships with patients, and successful, and unsuccessful, interventions. These narratives position physicians as the primary actors in weighing and resolving the ethical dilemmas that confront our advanced technological society. If nurses are to convince the public that they too are storehouses of human insight and health care expertise, they must dramatize this fact with compelling narratives.

Since we wrote the second edition of *From Silence to Voice*, a new nursing voice has appeared in the pages of U.S. newspapers and on various websites. Because of her talent as a writer and her persistence as a patient advocate, Theresa Brown has become a regular commentator on health care issues for the *New York Times* health pages and also for its *Well* blog.

Brown's journey from bedside nurse to columnist is an interesting one. She earned a PhD in English at the University of Chicago and was a lecturer in the English department of Tufts University in Boston until 1997. After having three children, Brown decided to become a nurse. Originally she had contemplated becoming a nurse midwife. "I was talking to a friend who is a nurse and who is also named Theresa and I described my experience of having a midwife when I had my twins and I told her how cool it was. She said, 'Well, you could do that.'"

That conversation helped her decide to go to nursing school. While raising her children, she took one of the science courses each semester that was required for nursing school. Then she entered an accelerated program at the University of Pennsylvania. When her husband got a new job in Pittsburgh, she transferred to the program at the University of Pittsburgh.

Brown changed her mind about midwifery when she realized how difficult it would be to combine that field with raising small children. She also made a switch because, in nursing school, she discovered bedside nursing. "Before I went to nursing school," Brown told us, "I didn't know much about what hospital nurses do and how important they are. Once I learned more I knew I wanted to be a bedside nurse."

When Brown graduated, she got a job as an oncology nurse at the University of Pittsburgh Medical Center (UPMC). In the spring of 2008, she had a disturbing experience when a patient she was caring for with lung cancer bled out and died very quickly. She decided to write about the experience and then tried to get her article published. "I sent it to the *New York Times* health science section and they accepted it. Because they had a backlog of stories, it took a long time for them to publish it and it didn't come out until September 2008."

The article captured the attention of an editor at Harper Studio book publishers, who approached Brown, asking her to write about nursing. Brown didn't hesitate. She quickly signed a contract to write a book about her first year in nursing. *Critical Care: A New Nurse Faces Death, Life, and Everything in Between* was published in 2010.[15]

Brown's literary agent, who also represented Tara Parker-Pope, the editor of the Times' *Well* blog, knew that Parker-Pope was looking for a nurse to write for the blog. She put the two together and Brown was asked to do a monthly column for the *Well* blog based on her experiences as a practicing bedside nurse. "Tara helped me figure out what kind of stories were appropriate for *Well*, what kind had staying power and were interesting," Brown explained.

Initially Brown worked for free and then she contracted with the *Times* for payment. At this writing, she has a contract with the *Times* to produce a monthly column that appears either on an op-ed page or in the *Opinionator* blog on Sundays.

Many doctors, among them Atul Gawande, Jerome Groopman, and Richard Selzer, have used their experience in practice to write books and articles. With a few exceptions—Echo Heron, Peggy Anderson, and Cortney Davis—nurses have not done the same. Brown is the only bedside nurse writing today who uses her own experiences with patient care to write about nursing and health care issues for a major publication and perhaps the only nurse in recent history to do so on an ongoing basis. Although hospitals have not only tolerated but actually advertised their physician writers—who chronicle serious problems within their systems as well as their heroic triumphs—hospital administration has not been encouraging to nurses. Brown says she has always been very careful to respect patient confidentiality while working at UPMC and worked out various parameters for her writing with the hospital. In 2011, however, she was told that many restrictions would be placed on her writing, so many that it would effectively be impossible for her to continue working at UPMC and also pursue her writing. She decided that she would not stop writing and left that job. She has since found another and continues to write, although she does not identify the hospital where she is employed.

The fact that UPMC imposed so many restrictions on Brown's work illustrates a double standard at hospitals when it comes to allowing practicing professionals to explain their work and express their concerns. Brown has written scores of commentaries over the past few years. We have chosen this one about nurse-physician relationships because it illustrates not only how nurses can use their experiences to write op-eds but also how such op-eds can stimulate lively debates about health care issues.

Op-Ed

Physician, Heel Thyself

BY THERESA BROWN, PITTSBURGH

May 7, 2011

It was morning rounds in the hospital and the entire medical team stood in the patient's room. A test result was late, and the patient, a friendly, middle-aged man, jokingly asked his doctor whom he should yell at.

Turning and pointing at the patient's nurse, the doctor replied, "If you want to scream at anyone, scream at her."

This vignette is not a scene from the medical drama "House," nor did it take place 30 years ago, when nurses were considered subservient to doctors. Rather, it happened just a few months ago, at my hospital, to me.

As we walked out of the patient's room I asked the doctor if I could quote him in an article. "Sure," he answered. "It's a time-honored tradition—blame the nurse whenever anything goes wrong."

I felt stunned and insulted. But my own feelings are one thing; more important is the problem such attitudes pose to patient health. They reinforce the stereotype of nurses as little more than candy stripers, creating a hostile and even dangerous environment in a setting where close cooperation can make the difference between life and death. And while many hospitals have anti-bullying policies on the books, too few see it as a serious issue.

Today nurses are highly trained professionals, and in the best situations we form a team with the hospital's doctors. If doctors are generals, nurses are a combination of infantry and aides-de-camp.

After all, patients are admitted to hospitals because they need round-the-clock nursing care. We administer medications, prep patients for tests, interpret medical jargon for family members and double-check treatment decisions with the patient's primary team. Nurses are also the hospital's front line: we sound the alert if a patient takes a serious turn for the worse.

But while most doctors clearly respect their colleagues on the nursing staff, every nurse knows at least one, if not many, who don't.

Indeed, every nurse has a story like mine, and most of us have several. A nurse I know, attempting to clarify an order, was told, "When you have 'M.D.' after your name, then you can talk to me." A doctor dismissed another's complaint by simply saying, "I'm important."

When a doctor thoughtlessly dresses down a nurse in front of patients or their families, it's not just a personal affront, it's an incredible distraction, taking our minds away from our patients, focusing them instead on how powerless we are.

That said, the most damaging bullying is not flagrant and does not fit the stereotype of a surgeon having a tantrum in the operating room. It is passive, like not answering pages or phone calls, and tends toward the subtle: condescension rather than outright abuse, and aggressive or sarcastic remarks rather than straightforward insults.

And because doctors are at the top of the food chain, the bad behavior of even a few of them can set a corrosive tone for the whole organization. Nurses in turn bully other nurses, attending physicians bully doctors-in-training, and experienced nurses sometimes bully the newest doctors.

Such an uncomfortable workplace can have a chilling effect on communication among staff. A 2004 survey by the Institute for Safe Medication Practices found that workplace bullying posed a critical problem for patient safety: rather than bring their questions about medication orders to a difficult doctor, almost half the health care personnel surveyed said they would rather keep silent. Furthermore, 7 percent of the respondents said that in the past year they had been involved in a medication error in which intimidation was at least partly responsible.

The result, not surprisingly, is a rise in avoidable medical errors, the cause of perhaps 200,000 deaths a year.

Concerned about the role of bullying in medical errors, the Joint Commission, the primary accrediting body for American health care organizations, has warned of a distressing decline in trust among hospital employees and, with it, a decline in the quality of medical outcomes.

What can be done to counter hospital bullying? For one thing, hospitals should adopt standards of professional behavior and apply them uniformly, from the housekeepers to nurses to the president of the hospital. And nurses and other employees need to know they can report incidents confidentially.

Offending parties, whether doctors or nurses, would be required to undergo civility training, and particularly intransigent doctors might even have their hospital privileges—that is, their right to admit patients—revoked.

But to be truly effective, such change can't be simply imposed bureaucratically. It has to start at the top. Because hospitals tend to be extremely hierarchical, even well-meaning doctors tend to respond much better to suggestions and criticisms from people they consider their equals or superiors. I've noticed that doctors otherwise prone to bullying will tend to become models of civility when other doctors are around.

In other words, alongside uniform, well-enforced rules, doctors themselves need to set a new tone in the hospital corridors, policing their colleagues and letting new doctors know what kind of behavior is expected of them.

This shouldn't be hard: most doctors are kind, well-intentioned professionals, and I rarely have a problem talking openly with them. But unless we can change the overall tone of the workplace, doctors like the one who insulted me in front of my patient will continue to act with impunity.

I wish I could say otherwise, but after being publicly slapped down, I will think twice before speaking up around him again. Whether that was his intention, or whether he was just being thoughtlessly callous, it's definitely not in my patients' best interest.[16]

This op-ed provoked a lot of commentary, particularly in the physician community. Internist Kevin Pho, who writes for *USA Today* and has his own website, KevinMD (which claims that he is "social media's leading physician voice"), attacked Brown both on his website and on the blog of the *Atlantic* magazine. Ignoring the fact that Brown had previously written about nurse bullies,[17] Pho argued that Brown was unfairly picking on doctors. He also insisted that her goal was not to raise consciousness about a serious issue—bullying in the health care workplace—that could affect patient safety but simply to use the pages of a major magazine to get back at a doctor.[18] Many nurses and other health care workers, however, concurred with Brown's argument, and their comments and letters were widely published and circulated. In fact, about a year after Brown's op-ed appeared, physician patient-safety expert Lucian Leape and colleagues published a two-part series of articles in *Academic Medicine* discussing the problem of lack of respect in the health care workplace and citing the particularly thorny issue of physician behavior toward nurses.[19]

Try and Try Again

In writing letters, op-eds, and longer articles, remember that you can't succeed without trying. There are many publications that are looking for intelligent, fresh points of view.

Nurses who are frequently published in letters pages or op-ed sections rarely have all or even most of their work accepted. "I've had many letters to the editor published in major newspapers like the *New York Times* or *Philadelphia Inquirer*," says Claire Fagin, dean emerita of the University of Pennsylvania School of Nursing. "I've succeeded because I've written so many. When I see something I like, I write to compliment the reporter. When I see something that concerns me, I go to the computer and express my views. Because people see me in print, they think that my scorecard is better than it is. For all the pieces I've had published, I've had many more rejected. In fact, I could publish a volume called *The Unpublished Letters and Articles of Claire Fagin*. My advice is just keep writing."

Today, if your letters or op-eds are rejected, you can use social media to publish them.

Our advice is, if you come across something that concerns you in the papers, on the radio or TV, in the movies, or in any of the mass media, do something about it. Write a letter, make a phone call, send an e-mail, start a blog. If you don't like what you hear or see, don't keep it to yourself. If you like it, praise it (the media need as many pats on the head for the good things they do as slaps on the wrist for the bad). If you're an oncology nurse and you see something erroneous written about pediatric nursing, don't wait for a pediatric nurse to write a letter to the editor; do it yourself. If you see something disturbing written about health policy, don't hesitate to respond because you're "just a nurse," not a PhD in health policy. You have more real experience with health than most of the highly paid consultants who tell administrators—or even national health systems in many countries—how to organize their services. Speak up, speak out, make a difference.

Social Media

In the section on blogs above, we discussed one small area of social media, which nurses can use to convey information about their work to a variety of publics. Social media, however, constitute myriad ways to help the public understand nursing work.

When people talk about social media, they are referring to a large and changing number of Internet, web, and mobile-based tools for sharing information. Because social media is a moving target, it is beyond the scope of this book to outline how, precisely, nurses can use these platforms. We have, however, consulted with experts who understand both the promise and problems of participating in this technological universe and who offer advice on how to navigate its sometimes overwhelming aspects.

Robert Fraser, a nurse and author of *The Nurse's Social Media Advantage: How Making Connections and Sharing Ideas Can Enhance Your Nursing Practice*, describes social media as "an evolution of communication technology that has changed how we can share, publish, and communicate ideas."[20] He told us that nurses need to explore the range of tools available to them "to advance work we're interested in and issues we care about."

Megen Duffy, a nurse, blogger, and self-described techie, has outlined the most popular social media platforms and how to use them in her "iNurse" columns for the *American Journal of Nursing*. She encourages nurses who have not already done so to become adept at using these media. In one of her articles, Duffy outlined the benefits: "Social media sites have a huge potential for improving our practice by increasing our networking sources and improving access to current information, particularly in areas of nursing we might not encounter daily (for example, I follow an infusion nurse on Twitter who regularly adds to my knowledge of IV skills). They can also add to our quality of life by introducing us to other nurses in our field, sometimes validating our experiences and feelings (for example, when I was a new nurse

I received many tips from Twitter nurses about how to manage my time in the real world)."[21]

Christina Young, a social media consultant, told us that many people are intimidated by what they consider to be a complicated social media landscape, but from a technological point of view, social media platforms are no more complicated than sending an email to a friend. "What you're doing, when you hit publish rather than send, is the technical equivalent of sending a message to an open audience," she said.

Fraser says that trying to determine which social media tools are most effective "is where the challenge emerges and where people sometimes get lost." He likens social media to a hammer—"How you use it depends on your goals. For example, if you had a best practice you wanted to share, using digital tools you can share that in different ways. You can share it as the research is being developed. Throughout the process of development you can, in fact, not only help others improve the work they're doing but learn from the experience they have working in similar fields. Social media tools offer a much quicker way of getting out information than has been previously available."

Fraser offers these recommendations:

1. "Know the tools. When you hear about a new social network or digital tool, you should find out what it is actually accomplishing. You might not need it today, but it may be useful down the road if you have a project that it can help promote. For nurses just venturing into digital technology, using simple profiles like LinkedIn, are the easiest way to begin. On these platforms, people can find you based on your expertise, knowledge, and experience. From there may want to test and use other on-line tools, like research networks such as Mendeley.com that allow you to share research articles and connect to people studying similar areas. Or you can create a blog to share your experience in school, on a research project, or in professional development."

2. "Test and experiment. As nurses, we're scientists and clinicians who understand scientific method. Because there isn't a perfect way to use Twitter or Facebook, or others, we need to experiment for our purposes. Here's just one idea. Try to use Twitter once a week to check for news and updates for people you follow. If you're trying to promote an organization, then use it once a day to share a piece of information about your work or information in the field. It's useful to take a bit of time to look at what your followers or people around you are saying. By doing this, you can, over time, be effective. But only if the technology meets your goal and purpose. If it doesn't, then consider modifying it or using something else. At the end of all this, if it isn't being useful don't use it. Remember the hammer analogy.

These tools are like a hammer, you may not need it and everything may not be a nail."

Setting Boundaries

The fact that social media can reach an open audience is, for nurses, the source of both their promise and their potential problems. The promise of social media is that nurses can go beyond their personal network to discuss issues of concern and share ideas, research, problems, and solutions. People working in health care can use Facebook or another platform to alert others and campaign for action on a critical issue like safe staffing. They can post a clever video on You-Tube illustrating how quickly infections move through hospitals because health care workers persist in wearing ties, jewelry, and lab coats.[22] Hyperlinks allow people to broadcast ideas, events, and information to other outlets instantly. Ideas can go viral and reach not merely hundreds of people but tens of thousands, even millions.

The downside, as Young explains, is that you're also communicating with an "unseen audience that people using social media cannot control." A staff nurse may write something on Facebook venting about her unit being short-staffed on a particular evening. She may think she's just sounding off to her network of close "friends." But those "friends" have "friends" that may include the family of a patient on that unit. And the Facebook post in question may also come to the attention of her employer, who may have a personnel policy (see examples of what is lawful and unlawful cited below) that attempts to restrict social media use by hospital employees.

Young also reminds us that many businesses now use Internet monitors to track what is being said about them (and by whom) on various social media platforms. "Through devices like Google alerts, companies (and these include health care employers) have people constantly monitoring what is being said—good, bad, or indifferent—about them," Young explains. "Any smart company has someone monitoring social media all the time. If anyone thinks they can write about their company and somehow be flying under the radar, that's naive."

"Boundary setting is an important part of using digital tools that some people worry about a lot and some people don't worry about enough," Robert Fraser told us. "People need to understand that digital tools blur the boundary between what is public and private. It's important for nurses to realize that on social networks anything that is being saved or posted may potentially become public. Just as emails get forwarded beyond intended recipients, privacy policies on social networks such as Facebook may change from time to time. That's why people need to speak professionally, maintain professional standards, and heed their legal obligations. Consider the following example. You put something on Facebook telling all your friends that you hate your manager. You may not even mention where you work or discuss her by name. But you forgot that your profile says where you work or live. Or maybe you have posted about your institution before mentioning the hospital's or even the manager's name. When someone puts these pieces of information together, you end up sharing more information than you have may have realized and certainly intended. This may mean that, at a minimum, you are perceived as unprofessional. Even worse, depending on what other information you share, you may be perceived of as having violated professional or organizational policies or standards."

Megen Duffy observes that "younger nurses may be more susceptible to courting social media disasters than older nurses simply because they're more used to sharing intimate details of their lives online. Nurses who have been on Facebook their entire high school and college careers may be more likely to see it as a place for private conversation and not as a public forum, while for older nurses social media may be a totally new arena." She lists the things that are "likely to get you fired, cost you your license, or both." These include posting obvious identifiers of patients (including photos), posting information about a celebrity patient, making fun of a patient you've identified, posting how dangerous or unsafe your facility is, and publicly harassing or bullying co-workers.[23]

Does setting boundaries mean you can't use the social media to talk about your work at all?

"No, that is not true," Robert Fraser says. "Setting boundaries doesn't mean we can't talk about work. It does mean that we need to have a more professional dialogue. Just as our textbooks talk about patients in ways that don't violate confidentiality, with these tools we have to do the same. My general rule is that if I wouldn't be comfortable publishing what I am saying or doing in a professional publication with my picture next to it then I won't save it. It's too easy to press send, save or post."

So how exactly can nurses use social media to talk about their work without violating patient privacy under HIPAA (the Health Insurance Portability and Accountability Act)?

"Say you had a patient whom you took care of yesterday and you felt she was a total bitch," Fraser says. "You really didn't like her. You could in fact talk about that situation on Facebook in a very professional way. You don't give away specific details that violate legal obligations and you don't create an unprofessional image and dialogue. You might say something like, "some patients can be challenging. They may be anxious or frightened about their treatments and we, as nurses need to honor their concerns."

Even assuming that nurses stick to professional discourse, there are managers and health care facilities that are attempting to prohibit nurses from using social media in various ways. Megen Duffy advises nurses to "read your institution's policies about social media. Closely. . . . You may be prohibited from using Facebook or Twitter at work, but even if these networks are barred from work computers, tweets or status updates from your company-owned smartphone are still time-stamped. You may work for one of the more draconian hospitals that ban employees from social media altogether. In my experience, banning blogging and Facebook simply drives nurses underground into anonymity, which does nothing to promote professionalism—and dramatically increases the chances that these nurses, falsely lulled into a sense of security by supposed anonymity, will violate HIPPA."[24]

According to Robert Fraser, "Many managers take a very old school approach to any kind of communication outside of the institution. They feel that if we talk about anything that goes wrong it will be bad for our image or that of the institution for which we work. Today, there is a greater transparency in health care and this can be very positive. It can lead to much needed discussions of things like the challenges of dealing with a high caseload, or staffing models that are introduced in the case of cutbacks."

Such a discussion occurred in May, 2012, when NPR (National Public Radio) in the United States put a "call-out" to nurses on Facebook. It was prompted, according to the producer Patti Neighmond, by a survey by NPR, the Robert Wood Johnson Foundation, and the Harvard School of Public Health that found 34 percent of patients hospitalized for at least one night in the past year said "nurses weren't available when needed or didn't respond quickly to requests for help." NPR wanted to know what was going on from nurses themselves.

NPR reported that it received hundreds of responses: "piles of stories about nurses feeling overworked, getting no breaks, no lunches and barely enough time to go to the bathroom. Even worse, many nurses say breaks and lunchtimes are figured into their salaries and deducted, whether they take them or not." Most of the nurses who agreed to be interviewed would do so only anonymously. But their stories were stunning. As a result of the nurses stories, which would not have been available without social media, NPR interviewed Linda Aiken, a noted expert on nurse staffing, who put her finger on the problem: "There's not an actual nursing shortage," Aiken said. "There's a shortage of nursing care in hospitals and other health care facilities."[25]

Nurses can also use a website titled Help a Reporter Out (HARO).[26] Reporters sign on to HARO and place queries seeking information and people sign on as sources to provide information. This is a great way for nurses to reach out to journalists.

If your goal is communication between a few close friends and co-workers and no one else, then social media platforms may not be the best tool to use. If your objective is to inform fellow employees about conditions in your workplace because you want to change them through collective action or legislation, then by all means use social media for that kind of outreach. Several Facebook-based campaigns for education and action to promote nurse-patient staffing legislation have greatly benefitted from the web's quicker and easier way of gathering endorsements, fundraising, and collecting contact information.

Any attempted muzzling of nurses as advocates for public policies that benefit patients and themselves is not healthy for health care institutions or our larger society. But it reflects a broader trend in which more corporations are now actively promoting their own views on legislative/political matters or economic policy questions, while tolerating less workplace dissent from employees whose preferred form of civic engagement differs from their own.

As reported in 2012 by the general counsel of the National Labor Relations Board (NLRB), many employers are now "drafting new and/or revising existing policies and rules covering such topics as the use of social media and other electronic technologies, confidentiality, privacy, protection of employer information, intellectual property, and contact with the media and government agencies."[27]

This NLRB document goes on to provide summaries of recent unfair labor practice cases in which the Labor Board concluded that "at least some of the provisions in [these] employer policies and rules were overbroad and thus unlawful under the National Labor Relations Act." This useful report also includes a model "social media policy" that did manage to pass NLRB muster, by properly balancing workers' rights and legitimate employer concerns.

When confronted with management directives regarding social media use by employees in your workplace, you should first get a copy in writing. Then, compare its provisions to the NLRB-approved version referenced above because it may include improper and legally unenforceable restrictions.

If you are represented by a union, management will, in many cases, be obliged to bargain with employees about any proposed personnel policy changes related to social media use, before they are implemented. Anytime management unilaterally introduces new rules about social media use—whether in a unionized workplace or nonunion one—those affected should scrutinize such rules closely and seek reliable advice about their legality.

As noted earlier, private sector management most often interferes, either knowingly or unwittingly, with workplace speech and communication that involves "concerted activity" legally protected under section 7 of the NLRA. For example, some employers who have "merit pay" systems have been known to discourage coworkers from sharing data, among themselves, about individual compensation. As noted by the NLRB, they claim that this is "personal information about another employee." Fortunately, under federal labor law, management can't use this "privacy" excuse as a basis for prohibiting workers from discussing any terms or conditions of their employment, whether they do so one on one, in groups, or via social media tools like Facebook.

Likewise, some employers have tried to curb employee "comment on any legal matters, including pending litigation or disputes." This free speech limitation is unlawful because "it specifically restricts employees from discussing the protected subject of claims against the employer." That is to say, if a worker has filed a discrimination complaint or any other kind of job-related legal claim (over an occupational hazard or injury, improper overtime pay, or denial of pension or health benefits), both the complaining party and his or her coworkers have the legal right to discuss such "disputes" because they are related to wages, hours, or working conditions. (Employees also have the right to take legal action over such matters without being subject to employer retaliation.)

Our final advice about what you do or say, with or without the megaphone of the social media, is simple: use common sense, keep it civil, and don't back down just because your manager says, "You can't." It may be necessary for you and other nurses to politely, but firmly, assert your legal rights in order to care for patients safely and ensure fair treatment of yourselves. By contacting the nearest regional office of the NLRB, you can obtain the simple paperwork needed to file a formal "unfair labor practice" charge against an employer, guilty of social media policy transgressions (which may include unlawful discipline based on overly restrictive rules). The NLRB agent on duty can assist you in this process (whether or not you have a personal attorney or union representative aiding you as well).

> Our final advice about what you do or say, with or without the megaphone of the social media, is simple: use common sense, keep it civil, and don't back down just because your manager says, "You can't."

Combined with traditional media, social media now give nurses an unprecedented opportunity to use their own voices to make their work, concerns, and policy suggestions heard. As we have seen above and throughout this volume, some nurses have taken advantage of this opportunity to challenge traditional images of nursing and to present important opinions and ideas that would otherwise be absent from the broader debate about health care. We encourage many more nurses to jump into the debate.

CHAPTER 10

GETTING IT RIGHT

In this chapter we present several examples in which hospitals, nursing organizations, educational institutions, and individual nurses have acted strategically to present nursing as knowledge work. In these examples, nursing is also integrated into broader institutional promotions rather than excluded from them.

In 2004, as the Hospital of the University of Pennsylvania (HUP) sought Magnet accreditation, its chief nursing officer (CNO) Victoria Rich and its nursing governance council decided to take a critical look at how nurses were presented within the institution. Rich asked Suzanne Gordon to analyze the nursing department's public communications, and Gordon suggested a number of changes. Rich called in the public relations firm that then worked with the hospital to discuss the negative effect of some of the traditional images of nurses that were being promoted in the broader University of Pennsylvania Health System, which includes HUP as well as Pennsylvania and Penn Presbyterian Hospitals. The company immediately set about redesigning the hospital recruitment material.

The results of this redesign were a complete departure from the status quo. In brochures and ads there were no more posed pictures of nurses smiling inanely at the camera. Instead, photos of nurses depicted them in action. Headlines and text emphasized the knowledge and skill of nurses at the institution and created an overall effect of intelligence and competence. Anyone looking at these images could immediately ascertain that these nurses were using their brains, not just their hearts.

In one photo, a nurse reaches into an isolette on a neonatal ICU as she cares for a tiny baby tethered to a tangle of tubes and lines. The ad copy reads, "OUR NURSES ARE AN ARTFUL BLEND OF SCIENCE AND CARING." In another image, a nurse whose face broadcasts intelligence is engaged in a high-tech treatment. The text reads, "OUR NURSES ARE RESPECTED FOR THEIR EXPERTISE." In yet another, physicians and nurses are shown working in the background as a male OR nurse in the foreground reaches toward an array of surgical instruments. The text reads, "OUR NURSES ARE RELENTLESS IN THE PURSUIT OF EXCELLENCE." The captions on other images make similar points such as one that reads, "OUR NURSES ARE AS MULTIFACETED AS THEIR SKILLS."

Every image and word was carefully chosen to suggest knowledge, skill, cutting-edge treatment, and dynamism. Yet these presentations never undermine the idea that nursing is about attention to human beings and not just their diseases. Rather than science and emotion being set up in opposition, the two elements are consistently integrated to create an image of a Penn nurse who is at the front lines not only of high tech treatment but also of attention, compassion, and concern.

The hospital has since moved to another ad agency and changed its campaign design but not the underlying message. The look of the new campaign is crisp, clean, ultra-modern. Photos and text are accompanied by structural images of hexagons, arrows, and cubes in which key words appear. In one ad, a nurse with an OR mask draped under his chin looks at the camera as if to affirm the ad copy, which states, "You turn game changing into life saving." What is remarkable is that these ads appeared not only in nursing newsletters and journals but were also placed in major publications and were plastered on the doors of elevators in the hospitals that are part of the University of Pennsylvania Health/Penn Medicine system. In this way the internal and external messages meshed and nursing became more visible throughout the hospital system.

Just a Nurse

Changing its recruitment material was not the only way that the nursing department at Penn challenged nursing's virtue script. In 2007 CNO Rich asked Gordon and her colleague Earl Dotter, a photographer who is widely known for his images of workers, to spend a week at the Hospital of the University of Pennsylvania interviewing nurses and photographing them in action. The result was an exhibit of 110 museum-quality images of HUP nurses. Each of the photographs shows a nurse doing her or his actual work and is accompanied by interview text that explains what the nurse was thinking at that particular time. The collection—titled *Just A Nurse*—was displayed for three weeks in the hospital atrium before, during, and after Nurses Week. The exhibit began with Gordon's poem "Just a Nurse" and was divided into six sections, each presenting images of activities that nurses perform. The first section outlined the history and meaning of Nurses Week and contained the following text:

> Hospitals all over the United States and the world celebrate Nurses Week. With the best intentions, however, many focus more on nurses' hearts than on their brains. HUP has chosen to deviate from that path. In this exhibit, what becomes apparent is not only how kind and attentive nurses are but how knowledgeable, immensely skilled, technologically proficient, and medically astute are the nurses who work in this institution. We see, in these photographs, nurses who are constantly vigilant—on the lookout for the most subtle, almost imperceptible changes in a patient's status or in the care environment. They use their mastery with their colleagues in an intricately choreographed exercise in teamwork and then, when alone with a patient or family members, mobilize their skill of involvement. Learning and teaching is central to their mission. Plus they are up to date on the latest in science and technology. A rainbow of diversity, all of the men and women pictured here show what it means to be "just a nurse."

Other sections of the exhibit were titled "Vigilance," "Learning and Teaching," "Science and Technology," "Teamwork," and "The Skill of Involvement." Here is an excerpt from the "Science and Technology" section:

> Nurses have always based their practice not only on the latest scientific and technical knowledge but on cumulative wisdom. Think, for example, of a Daughter of Charity in 18th century France. On completion of her preparation, she left Paris for the provinces equipped with "three boxes of lancets and ligatures plus a case of surgical instruments. . . . " Nurses conduct research—on their own and in collaboration with medical researchers—that is transforming hospital care as well as care in the home and community. In fact, many experimental medical research studies are run by nurses. And let's not forget the ICU, which was developed to deliver intensive nursing care.

The following text appeared in the "Learning and Teaching" section:

> A lot of people believe that nurses were "born to care." In fact, nothing could be further from the truth. Nurses aren't born; they're educated, both in school and on the job.
> A new patient analgesia pump comes on the market. Nurses have to *learn* how to use it safely. Patients in the hospital—and leaving it—are on complex medication regimens. Nurses have to *learn* how to safely administer them as well as how

to educate patients about how to safely manage their own care once they've left the hospital. Nurses teach one another and they also teach doctors in training as well as veteran physicians.

"The Skill of Involvement" was described in the following excerpt:

Nurses are known for their compassion, their caring, their ability to be with and there for human beings in need. Because of this some people think of nurses as angels of mercy, or saints, or human beings with otherworldly gifts . . . Yet the things we most closely associate with nursing are, in fact, hard-won skills. Nurses' caring and compassion, for example, constitute what the nursing theorist Patricia Benner calls "the skill of involvement." In a world that values independence and invulnerability, the ability to tolerate human dependence and to accept the inevitability of mortality are hard-won skills indeed.

Nurses don't just *feel* when to move in close because a patient needs them, or when to back off because a patient wants some space. When they have mastered the skill of involvement, nurses are able to make these critical decisions on a daily, sometimes minute-by-minute basis. That's what it means not simply to be a nurse but also to think like a nurse.

"Vigilance" was described in the following manner:

Look at their eyes, the expression on their faces, the cock of their heads as they listen—nurses are constantly on the alert. Anticipating. They know that a patient's condition can change in a matter of seconds. A need can arise. A piece of information can emerge in a seemingly banal conversation. A stray comment is decoded. The key to a medical and nursing mystery suddenly appears—and is quickly grasped.

In their educated glance nurses combine another crucial skill, the ability to protect patients from danger without making them feel endangered. To see like a nurse is to be constantly prepared to prevent crises and take advantage of an opportunity for growth and healing that emerges, quicksilver-like at the most unpredictable moments.

During the three weeks that the exhibit was displayed in the main hospital's atrium, over seventy thousand people viewed it, The exhibit received coverage on local TV stations and in the *Philadelphia Inquirer*.

At the same time as nurses were being presented to the public in photos and ads, a significant change was occurring in how they presented themselves to patients and families and colleagues in their daily work. CNO Rich and her leadership team felt that the normal presentation of nurses did not create a professional image and was confusing to both patients and other staff as to the roles of those going into and out of patients' rooms. So Rich launched a campaign to replace this quasi-uniform with more professional-looking attire, as she described in her story, "Real Nurses Don't Wear Wings." It appeared in *When Chicken Soup Isn't Enough*. A condensed excerpt appears in the text box below.

While nurses at all three Penn hospitals changed their uniforms to navy blue, nurses in the OR still remained in their hospital-provided green surgical scrubs. As they watched the transformation, the nurses no longer wanted to wear the same green that everyone else in the OR wore, Rich said. They wanted to be distinguished as nurses. They asked the nursing administration to purchase three new machines that would dispense navy blue scrubs in small, medium, and large for OR nurses. Although this change cost the hospital money, Rich stated that she and other hospital executives readily agreed to support this.

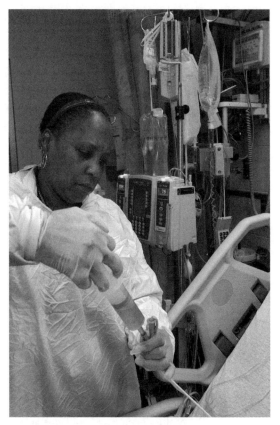

"You've got to have eyes in the back of your head. You continuously look at the monitors, the patients, and the chart concurrently. That's why they're in the ICU," says Jewell Howard, RN. (Photo by Earl Dotter.)

Real Nurses Don't Wear Wings

By Victoria L. Rich

Since bedside nurses abandoned the white cap and starched white uniforms, nurses' image in the workplace has gone from rigidly circumscribed to pretty much anything goes. . . . I knew that the people I saw in these outfits were nurses. But few others—particularly patients and physicians—shared that critical knowledge since many other categories of workers wore similar outfits. Unfortunately, I'd been unable to do much to change it until I was presented with a perfect storm of events in 2004.

Our hospital system as a whole was dealing with the issue of creating a more respectful workplace. One of our major concerns was nurse/physician collaboration. . . . The Dean of the Medical School, Dr. Arthur Rubinstein, was also concerned about these issues and the University of Pennsylvania Medical School had also set up a respectful workplace committee on which I sat. As we talked in our executive group, it became clear that no one knew with whom they were working. People didn't know who was a doctor, a nurse, a nurse's aide, a respiratory therapist. People rarely said, "Hello, I'm Doctor so and so, or I'm nurse so and so." Name tags were almost always turned front to back. In fact, lots of people didn't even wear name tags. And uniforms were no longer identifiers of a professional or occupational group.

Well, I thought, I can't control the physicians in this organization, but we, as RNs, can control who we are and how we present ourselves. . . . We needed to be easily identifiable as nurses . . . Even though, we, as nurses, often complain that we don't get enough respect, that patients don't know who we are, that doctors don't ask us about our concerns, when I broached the idea of a uniform change to HUP nurses, they were quite resistant. They felt they had a right to express their individuality at work by wearing—obviously within limits—pretty much whatever kind of uniform they wanted to wear.

How could I convince them that if we really believe that we are the most important person to the patient we have to not only talk the talk and walk the walk, but wear the garb that conveys our hard-earned professional stature? After all, we, like the police and firefighters, are critical to patient safety and rescue. They are identifiable. Why aren't we? We had many meetings on this subject at HUP. I discussed the issue with the nursing staff as well as the nursing shared governance committee that included thirty-five leaders chosen by each unit in the hospital. We conducted an on-line survey about the issue. We finally got nurses to agree that they should indeed all wear a unique one-color uniform. The nurses themselves decided on navy blue scrubs. We also decided to embroider on them the symbol for the HUP nursing model of excellence and professional practice. Because people still wanted to maintain a sense of individuality, nurses decided not only to put "RN" on the uniform but also to identify the unit they worked on—for example, the cardiothoracic unit, neurosurgery, oncology.

Then we had to deal with the issue of cost. How much would this cost nurses who had already purchased a stock of uniforms? I asked. I was absolutely determined that this important issue would not get in the way of success in this effort. So I went to our CEO—who along with many of the physicians—was very committed to the idea that nurses should be easily identified. (Some of the physicians suggested that we go back to whites with caps. "No way is that ever going to happen," I said, putting an end to that idea).

To the CEO and COO, I proposed that we purchase two sets of the scrub uniforms for every nurse. However, we had to get our CEO and COO not only to agree to this financial outlay but to help us deal with apparel in other hospital departments. For example, in the peri-operative area, the surgeons had just given all the peri-operative surgical techs and instrument staff navy blue scrubs. If nurses were to be identified by their navy blue, then respiratory and surgical techs or transport workers couldn't wear them too. The CEO and COO agreed. They would do what it took to make sure that only RNs at HUP would wear navy blue. Their willingness to make such an agreement allowed me to go back to our nurses with a powerful message: look how much this organization is prepared to invest to underscore the importance of nursing at HUP.

Over the next months. . . we invited uniform manufacturers into the hospital to put on fashion shows, so nurses themselves could decide which material and style of uniform they preferred. All registered nurses, including me and the nursing leadership team, wore navy blue scrubs when rounding on the units.

After two years of work, RNs in our organization have really embraced this change. About ten times a year I'll receive an email from a HUP nurse telling me that she—or he—has had a family member admitted to another hospital. Invariably they tell me that it's impossible to figure out who is—and who is not—a nurse. . . . Not only has HUP changed but, at our sister institution, Presbyterian Hospital, all RNs are navy blue. Moreover, RNs at all of our 125 ambulatory practices now wear navy blue. We have also gotten many letters from patients telling us how much they appreciate being able to easily identify the nurses and we've also received very positive comments from physicians.

Perhaps the most compelling evidence of how important this change has been occurred in the fall of 2008, when we had a fire on the 12th and 14th floors at HUP. In the midst of the smoke, blaring alarms and chaos, we had to safely evacuate 75 patients. The process went very smoothly. When we debriefed about what had happened, everyone identified a key factor that helped determine a successful outcome: Because all the nurses were in navy blue, critical players in this evacuation were easy to spot. In a true disaster, everyone ended up safe in large part because everyone knew who was a registered nurse.

Maimonides Medical Center

Maimonides Medical Center, with 705 inpatient beds, is in one of the most diverse sections of Brooklyn, New York. For the institution's 2011 centennial celebration, Maimonides produced videos for its webpage and other materials describing the series of innovations for which the hospital is known. One video focused on a century of education at the institution segued into another video devoted to nursing at Maimonides and seamlessly integrated the discipline into the larger hospital narrative.

This video is an apt template for anyone wanting to highlight the practice of direct care nurses. It introduces a cardiothoracic intensive care nurse, Rook Rampersaud, who has worked at the hospital for twelve years. Not surprisingly, what we noticed first was the fact that Rook actually has a last name. As she talks to us about nursing, the camera follows her while she cares for a critically ill patient, who has just had open-heart surgery. We watch her manipulate complicated devices, deliver multiple medications, and make sure the patient is turned and constantly monitored. While explaining her work to the viewer, Rampersaud addresses the virtue lens through which many members of the public view nursing. "Nurses are often thought of as angels," she says. This ignores, she explains, that many nurses have a college-level education and a science background. Nurses, she says, have a range of critical thinking skills that they apply "to take care of both people and their illnesses."

In this video she is shown doing exactly that. In caring for her patient who has just been extubated, she constantly talks with him, explaining what she is doing. While we

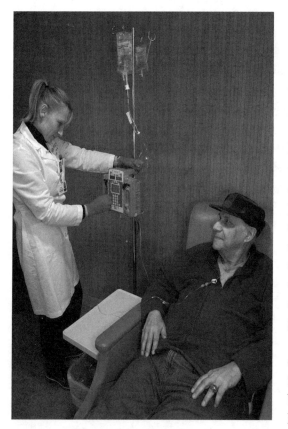

Iryna Durnyeva, RN, NP. (Photo by Earl Dotter.)

see her monitoring multiple machines, delivering medication, giving her patient chest physical therapy, and teaching him lung expansion and coughing techniques, we also learn why she is doing these things. At the same time that she is caring for this patient, she is readying the room for her next admission. She is also teaching a newly graduated nurse. She shares with the new recruit the anxiety that she felt as a new nurse and what it means to move from novice to expert in nursing. By the time she was off orientation, she says, she had the tools she needed to "admit her patient, know when there was a problem, and know when to call for help." She then describes for us the preceptor program that teaches both student and new nurses.

Tom Smith, the chief nursing officer at Maimonides, explained that the nursing department worked closely with the hospital's communications department to depict nursing accurately in the centennial promotions. The professional introduction of Nurse Rampersaud in the video was quite deliberately thought out. As Smith explained:

> At Maimonides, we felt it was very important to include the nurses' full name and credentials and title. We also wanted to highlight her knowledge and skill. She is on top of everything, every detail of the care which this patient required, and was also seen mentoring a new nurse in the ICU. We wanted to show the depth and breadth of nursing practice, which involves caring for a human being as well as managing the environment in which care is being delivered. This means managing technology and equipment, medication delivery, relationships with other disciplines, and care of the patients' family members. Nursing isn't hearts and flowers, it's bringing knowledge and skills to a relationship. We did this video not to talk to nurses but to help the public understand what nurses do at Maimonides.

New York's Hospital for Special Surgery

The Hospital for Special Surgery (HSS) in New York City boasts that it has done more knee and hip replacements than any other hospital in the world. If it followed the typical template, its advertising and website would have focused solely on its surgeons. That has not been the hospital's approach. Virtually every mention of doctors in the hospital's full-page ads in the *New York Times* has been paired with a statement about its nurses.

A typical ad in 2011 incorporated this heading: "Best Hospital. Best Doctors. Best Nurses." Text under it read: "You'll find many of our doctors in *New York* magazine's 'Best Doctors' issue, year after year, after year. And our nurses have been awarded the nation's highest nursing award not once, but twice. . . .

HSS has a leading infection prevention program partnering with doctors, nurses, and operating room staff to continually improve processes for patient safety."[1]

HSS went further in December 2011, when it achieved Magnet status for the third time. It used the award to run a full-page *Times* ad focusing exclusively on its nurses. Although a photo at the center of the page featured the standard image of a nurse holding the hand of a patient, it specifically pointed out that nurses are one of the primary reasons the hospital has been able to attain excellence. It boasted that since the hospital had been rated number one in orthopedics by the *US News & World Report*'s "Best Hospitals" issue, "it's no wonder that we attract some of the best qualified nurses in the country. 92% of our nurses are educated at the baccalaureate level, a significant percentage as compared to other hospitals in our peer group. And after they join us, we teach them to be even better."

The ad went on to describe nurses' roles at the hospital:

> HSS nurses receive specialty training in musculoskeletal medicine and surgery, operating room nursing, and autoimmune diseases.
>
> Our nurses participate in clinical decision making, contributing to better patient care and higher patient satisfaction.
>
> Educational programs for patients initiated and run by our nurses have helped speed up recovery and reduce the length of stay for HSS patients dramatically. . .
>
> By educating our patients and family members before treatment, our nurses, along with the interdisciplinary team, make them active participants in their own recovery. . . . Nurses work collaboratively with physical therapists, case managers, nutritionists, and physician assistants to develop an individual assessment of functional status, psychosocial needs, and medical history. . . .
>
> And, even after patients leave the Hospital, our nurses are still checking on them. Each patient receives a post discharge phone call from their nurse to make sure recovery is going smoothly.
>
> Hospital for Special Surgery nurses have partnered with doctors and operating room staff to create a leading infection prevention program. And nurses make a major contribution to our ranking in the 99th percentile for 'likelihood to recommend the hospital to others' when compared against hospitals in our peer group.[2]

The ad copy repeated HSS's slogan: "Best hospital. Best doctors." Then it added, "And absolutely, unequivocally, the best nurses."

What's perplexing is not that HSS features nurses in its advertising and marketing, but that so many other hospitals do not. You'd think it would be a no-brainer: if you want to recruit nurses, and patients who value nursing, you should make them visible in a way that moves beyond the typical smiling face and angel of mercy image.

Emphasizing interdisciplinary care is smart in terms of quality of care, patient satisfaction, and hospital reputation, according to an article by an editor at Press Ganey Associates, a large hospital consulting firm, that was posted on HSS's website.[3]

The article, published in late 2011, stated that HSS's challenge has been to balance a surge in surgical volume with quality of service. The most strategic approach to meeting that challenge, according to the article, was "an interdisciplinary approach toward communication and coordination of care." Nurses, the article continues, were in the vanguard in developing the hospital's "Patient Experience Strategic Plan." The program they came up with included a nurse-staffed call center; a clinical nurse liaison specialist to communicate with families; hourly postoperative rounding by nurses and others to stay on top of pain management, among other things; nursing councils, to "foster open dialogue about care and service issues"; creation of a clinical nurse specialist position, "to enhance nursing staff orientation"; a nursing career ladder and point-of-care education; and discharge phone calls by nurses. These initiatives, the article asserted, raised patient satisfaction scores, "reflected in the fact that 91% of patients discharged from HSS would recommend this hospital to their friends and family."[4]

Because federal reimbursement is increasingly based on clinical quality and patient satisfaction, health care in the United States is "moving from a system that encourages the most intensive and technologically advanced treatments for patients to one based on the value of delivered services," according to Press Ganey's 2011 Pulse Report "Perspectives on American Health Care."[5] In terms of patient satisfaction, "nurse communication always is the key to higher . . . scores," the report states.

If nursing is so central to hospitals' financial health, hospitals have interesting options. They can demand that nurses go into patients' rooms every hour to tell them that "I am here to give you very good care," and discipline nurses if they do not smile in hallways or when they are on the phone, or they can involve nurses more directly in care and service programs. In any event, nursing should become a much more visible part of hospital marketing.

The *Pulse* at the University of Toronto Faculty of Nursing

When Sioban Nelson became the dean of the faculty of nursing at the University of Toronto in 2005, this premier nursing school in Canada did not have a premier-level communication strategy. The school occasionally published a magazine that went out mainly to its alumni and it had a monthly newsletter that announced events. "It was like a church newsletter," Nelson recalls. "The people who wrote it had no professional writing experience and no broader strategy for positioning nurses as the kind of thought leaders that one would look toward in a first-class research-intensive university program."

Nelson decided to change that. She wanted a publication that could reach a larger professional community comprised not only of alumni and students but also nursing regulators, working nurses, members of professional nursing associations and unions, and people in other health professions. Nelson wanted something that would explore how nursing both fit into and contributed to changes in health care.

Her mission was given a huge boost when the school received a ten-million-dollar gift from Toronto financier Lawrence Bloomberg who also wanted to expand the school's profile in the larger health care community. To do this, Bloomberg and Nelson met with Roger Martin, dean of the university's Rotman Business School, which produces a popular magazine simply called *Rotman*. In a meeting with these two high-level businesspeople, Nelson learned about Rotman Business School's promotional strategy.

"The school," Nelson explains, "never pays for advertising. It gets media coverage because it has positioned itself as a go-to institution on issues that are critical to the business community. Its prize-winning magazine has helped the school establish and maintain this reputation by covering timely and substantive topics important to the community. Key to this effort is the dean's involvement indicated by, among other things, the lead article he writes for every issue of the magazine."

Nelson decided to emulate the business school's strategy to position her faculty as intellectual leaders on health care issues: "As I began to think about this, I realized that what is missing in nursing is big picture, analytical thinking on critical health care issues. Many university nursing magazines focus almost exclusively on internal issues—what the faculty is doing. They are a lot like our newsletter was, a kind of social or research calendar that describes what people inside the school are up to. This misses a larger consideration of broader health care issues. In nursing there is a great deal of talk about critical thinking but there isn't a lot of analysis. We lack a big picture."

In 2008, the school launched *Pulse,* a magazine concerned with the health of Canadians and with global health. The magazine highlights the work of U of T nursing faculty, students, and alumni, but in addition covers issues stemming from and of concern to others in the larger nursing community such as regulators, professional associations, and the faculty's hospital and clinic partners.

"By looking at critical health issues," Nelson remarked, "we can tell the story of what our faculty are doing in a way that showcases the role of a research-intensive university in health care. The magazine allows me to do what a dean is supposed to do, which is to tell everyone how wonderful we are. But we do it in a way that illuminates the critical role and contributions nurses make to the health care system." Like the business school dean, Nelson writes a lead article that encapsulates the central topic of each issue of the magazine.

Pulse has produced a number of themed issues. "In one on cardiac care, we described a range of clinical initiatives in which our partners were involved," she said. "We also looked at new roles for APRNs [advanced practice registered nurses], and used personal stories of alumnae who have had cardiac illnesses. Another issue was about community care and engagement. This gave us an opportunity to talk about interesting work nurses are doing in community outreach, in homeless shelters, and palliative care."

One issue of the magazine was on knowledge translation and described how scientific findings can affect practice. Another was on partnership and looked at how research-intensive universities can cooperate with the community.

Nelson has departed from the traditional academic nursing school recipe by insisting that not every illustration or photograph be of a nurse or nursing. She has also banned traditional virtue script images. "Illustrators always want to come back with an image of nurses but often in ways I don't like, like caps and hearts and hands. So I have banned all that," she says. "But we might play off of a traditional image and do a surreal cap as an illustration. When we talked about knowledge translation, we had an image, not of a nurse, but of a man with a light going off in his head.

"I think of this as a grown-up nursing magazine," Nelson concludes. "So many other nursing magazines or newsletters rely on

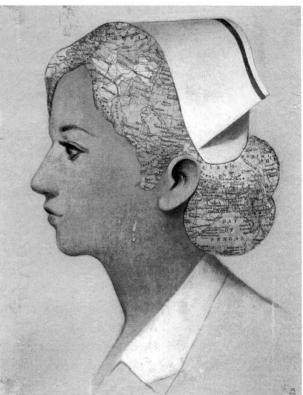

Pulse magazine illustration, courtesy of the Lawrence S. Bloomberg Faculty of Nursing, University of Toronto.

the virtue script and whatever endorphin button nurses have that makes them feel loved. It's what's known as affect bias. We aren't doing that anymore." The magazine, Nelson says, has not suffered by banishing virtue script text and images. "It's interesting how much people like the *Pulse*. I get tons of feedback from older and younger alumnae. Everyone really likes it."

Swiss Nurses Association

When it comes to both internal and external communication, one of the most innovative and active nursing associations in the world is the Swiss Nurses Association (ASI). Both a union and a professional association, ASI has developed creative promotional campaigns to challenge traditional understanding of nursing practice.

In 2001, the association began to transform the traditional image of nurses in Switzerland by introducing a dramatic new symbol: Power Nurse. A female action hero, the Power Nurse, as described by Pierre-Andre Wagner, an RN and the association's legal counsel, "darts through the air, her red hair flying. She wears a tight green shirt, a blue miniskirt, red boots and carries a thermometer. She looks like Superman's twin sister. She is the Power Nurse."[6] That year the Power Nurse became a symbol of the emancipation of nurses in Switzerland as nurses challenged the Swiss parliament to legally redefine nursing as an autonomous profession instead of as assistive personnel to physicians.

"The association knew that it needed the support of the public if it was to succeed," ASI's Wagner explains. "To the disbelief of many longtime members of the association, we hired a high-profile public relations firm to design a campaign that would convince the public that nursing was able to stand on its own. The firm submitted a number of ideas to us and one of them was the Power Nurse. This superwoman-like image was a hit. It directly countered the passive docile image of the nurse—the one who acted only when a doctor told her what to think and do."

When the association unveiled its campaign it had to deal with some disgruntled members. "Many nurses loved her—many hated her. Many hated us—their association—for doing this to them," Wagner says. "They were shocked, but what shocked them was exactly what filled others with enthusiasm. The diversity of our profession was made obvious by the multiplicity of the reactions to the Power Nurse: the conservative faction was appalled by her immodesty. The postfeminist faction lambasted the use of allegedly sexist imagery. The vast majority just loved it. Thousands of nurses who occasionally wear tight shirts,

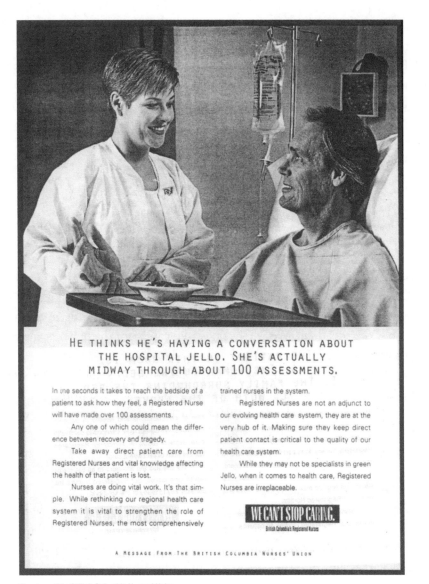

HE THINKS HE'S HAVING A CONVERSATION ABOUT
THE HOSPITAL JELLO. SHE'S ACTUALLY
MIDWAY THROUGH ABOUT 100 ASSESSMENTS.

In the seconds it takes to reach the bedside of a patient to ask how they feel, a Registered Nurse will have made over 100 assessments.

Any one of which could mean the difference between recovery and tragedy.

Take away direct patient care from Registered Nurses and vital knowledge affecting the health of that patient is lost.

Nurses are doing vital work. It's that simple. While rethinking our regional health care system it is vital to strengthen the role of Registered Nurses, the most comprehensively trained nurses in the system.

Registered Nurses are not an adjunct to our evolving health care system, they are at the very hub of it. Making sure they keep direct patient contact is critical to the quality of our health care system.

While they may not be specialists in green Jello, when it comes to health care, Registered Nurses are irreplaceable.

WE CAN'T STOP CARING.
British Columbia's Registered Nurses

A MESSAGE FROM THE BRITISH COLUMBIA NURSES' UNION

Courtesy of the British Columbia Nurses' Union.

miniskirts, and boots—not to work of course—and thousands of nurses who don't, understood that the Power Nurse was not meant to represent *a nurse*. She was a tongue-in-cheek way of symbolizing what we cherish about our profession: its modernity, its self-consciousness and self-assurance.

"The media loved her. For quite a long time, the Swiss nurses, as well as their association, had been pretty much media averse, content to work in the shadow of front-page politics—to do good and shut up. As for public opinion, it had been content to admire nurses almost above any other profession, without having to bother to understand what exactly they were admiring them for.

"Even though the legislation [to redefine nursing] passed the Chamber, it did not pass the Senate," Wagner told us. "But the heated discussion it generated gave politicians a new appreciation of nursing, which has helped us a great deal. They knew they had *to* talk to nurses not just *at* them. For the nurses of Switzerland, the world will never be the same again. With the Power Nurse, they have crossed a line and there will be no way back."[7]

Alison Whittaker and the Play "Vital Signs"

Alison Whittaker has been a nurse at the University of California at San Francisco Medical Center for more than ten years. According to Whittaker, "Being a nurse is about knowledge and knowing your patient, listening to them and being able to assess them. We are the ones advocating for the patients and managing patient safety."

Whittaker went into nursing as a second career. As soon as she started working, she recognized its drama and value. "When I started working at UCSF, I was so excited by all the diversity and all the different characters I worked with," she says. "Suddenly I was working with all these people of different ethnicities and races." Whittaker felt compelled to translate her daily experiences for the stage.

She took classes in theater to learn playwriting and acting. She then wrote a one-woman play that she performs. In it she dispenses high doses of humor to introduce the audience to the realities of patient care. As she acts out the role of the nurse, she demonstrates the kind of expertise that nurses develop on the job. Whittaker also slips into the personas of other health care characters—patient care aides, unit clerks, housekeepers, and other nurses—the village members it takes to care for the sick. Among her characters are "difficult" and "easy" patients and a gay/transsexual/cross dressing patient-care aide who just got a breast implant.

The success of her play is instructive: a public raised on TV medical shows has a high threshhold for graphic imagery and is more than ready to listen to a no-holds-barred view of the realities of nursing work. Whittaker's audiences don't flinch when she begins her play with the following monologue:

"If I asked you to smile and stick your tongue out, you would. If I asked you to follow my finger, you would. If I told you to take off your pants and show me your genitalia, you wouldn't argue with me. You'd take off your pants and show me your genitalia. Believe it or not, if I told you to bend over and spread your buttocks and show me your anus, you'd willingly bend over, spread your buttocks and show me your anus.

"I could stick a suppository in you or give you an enema. If neither a suppository nor an enema worked for you, I'd glove up, lube up my finger, gently slide it up your anus and disimpact you. I'd do what it takes. I'd get it out. I could put a tube up your penis, all the way to your bladder; you'd thank me. I do these things, these extremely intimate things to stangers, people I've just met, people like you. It's my job. I'm a nurse."

As she wrote her play, Whittaker was careful to not violate patient confidentiality regulations nor the trust of her co-workers. "I disguised every patient," she says. "I changed details, changed the diagnoses. I made many of them composites from different settings in which I work. I also checked with all of the people with whom I work to make sure they were okay with the play. They were."

After due diligence, "Vital Signs" was ready for showtime in 2011.

Whittaker first performed her play at the Women's Festival at the Shotwell Theater in San Francisco. Audiences received it so well that the theater gave her a two weekend run. She then auditioned the play at the Marsh theatre in San Francisco's Mission district. She brought in an audience by printing up postcards about the play and delivering them to nurses, aides, and doctors at UCSF. She also asked her friends and those in nursing networks to tell people about the play. This produced the kinds of audiences that convinced the Marsh to do the show again in 2012.

Her second run that summer was extended into early fall. Originally, the play was supposed to be performed only on Saturday and Sunday, but packed houses led the theater to add Friday night performances. (Whittaker has also performed the play at the Boulder and San Francisco Fringe Festivals.)

Whittaker has learned how to promote her play to prospective audiences. For her second run at the Marsh, she handed out postcards at five San Francisco hospitals, plus UCSF. She created a website for the show, and the Marsh also promoted it.[8] She worked both the traditional and social media to publicize her play. The result: a cover story in the lifestyle section of the *Independent Journal of Marin*, positive reviews in the the *San Francisco Chronicle and Examiner*, the *San Francisco Theater Blog*, the *San Francisco Weekly*, and *Beyond Chron*.

Although Whittaker depicts a variety of characters in her play, one group is missing. Physicians. This was not accidental. "I feel like there is so much about doctors but there's nothing about nurses and nurses' aides," she explains.

"I work on the night shift. It's kind of the joke on the night shift—where are the doctors? Patients are constantly saying, 'I need to talk to the doctor,' and we're thinking, 'well good luck.' I am certainly not anti-doctor and I work with some great doctors. In fact, the first night of my run a female neurosurgeon came to the show and gave me a standing ovation."

CHAPTER 11

APPEARING ON TELEVISION AND RADIO

One fall morning, Cindy Dalton, a nurse who works in a Montreal community health center, was about to make her television debut. As she waited in the greenroom near the set of the program *Montreal Today*, she reflected on the fact that the sum total of her media experience consisted of being interviewed for five minutes on the radio. Now she was about to appear on a major television show to talk about the nursing crisis in Quebec. She was to have a fellow guest: Suzanne Gordon. Dalton told Gordon that she was nervous. Gordon suggested that she rehearse. Gordon pointed out that the segment on nursing would be only six minutes long. "Deducting the time spent on questions from the host, we'll each have about two and a half minutes," she said. She suggested that Dalton prepare an anecdote so that she could use that time to convey the importance of what nurses do.

Dalton thought for a moment. "I work as a community health nurse in the area of family health," she began. "I begin working with families during pregnancy and continue until the kids are six years of age. The other day a pregnant Chinese woman had trouble getting her needs across when she visited the obstetrician. Doctors don't have much time these days, so it's important to ask them the right questions. I worked with her to prioritize her questions and make a list."

Since it was close to airtime, Gordon interrupted. "The problem with this anecdote is that it doesn't focus on you, the nurse," she said. "It focuses on the physician, on the busy man or woman who has no time. You want to highlight the importance of nursing. Is there another anecdote you could use?"

Dalton considered the question. Then she described her home-care work with a multiple sclerosis patient who could no longer walk on his own. The man spent his days sitting on the sofa while his wife cared for their two children, a two-and-a-half-year-old and an infant. Although he was unsteady using a walker, the patient refused to use a wheelchair or modify his home to accommodate his condition. He was depressed because the only thing he could manage was to go to the bathroom. He was so afraid he would drop his infant that he wouldn't even hold the baby. As she began explaining how she helped this patient, Dalton suddenly stopped.

Gordon asked her why.

Dalton looked frozen. "I can't use that anecdote. It's private," she said. "The patient might listen to the show. Telling his story would be a breach of patient confidentiality."

"Just change the details," Gordon said. "Make him a woman; change the ages of the children."

"But if I do that, I'm lying," Dalton protested. "Then I'm going to have trouble being truthful while I'm on the air." Dalton said she was also concerned that if she pared her story to a few sentences, people would not "hear the nursing." Gordon assured her that she would feel more comfortable with a little practice and that if she talked about her nursing work, listeners would not miss the point.

As the two approached the set, Gordon coached Dalton to "take advantage of whatever opening the host gives you to bring up your anecdote."

When the cameras rolled, the host Leslie Roberts said to Dalton, "Tell me a bit about your work if you can. You've been a nurse for twelve years. Is it getting worse? Do you see the crisis, or is it being blown up by the media?"

"Definitely nurses are more challenged in the present health care system," Dalton said. "Every time there's a challenge you have to adjust to it, and today the challenges are coming more quickly, and the period of adjustment is shortened."

The host had been asking for a general description of nurses' problems. But Dalton astutely took advantage of the opening he gave her to bring the audience into the world of daily nursing practice.

"I can give you an example of the kind of work I do," she continued. "At the moment I'm working at a CLSC [community health center] with families with young children. But I also work with people who have chronic illnesses. When I went to visit one family in their home recently, I found they had a newborn baby and the wife had multiple sclerosis. It was a challenge for me to work with her because she was very depressed. The husband was taking on more and more work with the newborn baby. For the first time in her life, the wife couldn't walk, but she was reluctant to use a wheelchair. I knew she could fall, and if she fell, it would cost more health care dollars because she would need more services." Dalton then explained that she helped to rearrange the house so the wife could navigate in her wheelchair, taught her how to safely hold her baby, and helped the family alleviate her depression.

When Dalton had finished relating her anecdote, Roberts interviewed Gordon about the problems nurses face in the United States. Turning back to Dalton, Roberts asked if Canadians should solve their health care crisis by becoming more like Americans.

Although Dalton is not a health policy expert, she did not hesitate to voice her opinion. "No," Dalton answered. "The solution is to strengthen the present health care system. My own personal opinion is that under privatization there would be people who need services and couldn't afford them or would not get good services."

Roberts argued that Canada already has a two-tiered health care system, with some people getting better care than others. Dalton agreed that while "there are some services you can pay for and get quicker, we still have universal health care and we should maintain it. It's very important."

Then she bridged to more discussion of nursing.

"Nursing is also very important," she explained. "When you go to the emergency room, the first person you see is a nurse. When you're going to have an operation, the person who prepares you before surgery is a nurse. What's the first thing that happens when you open your eyes? Who are you going to see at your bedside? Who will make sure that you recover with no complications? A nurse. When you're going to ring your call bell at night for help because you're in pain, or you're worried about being sent home the next day, who's going to come to your room and make sure you know how to take your medications safely at home? A nurse."

After the show Dalton was exhilarated. "As I started to talk about nursing, I became more and more energized," she said. "At first I was preoccupied by the set, the lights, the people walking around making strange signals to one another. Because the host kept nodding his head, I was worried that I was taking too much time and that he wasn't interested in what I had to say. I was too focused on his agenda. I was letting the setting paralyze me.

"Then I remembered why I was here. I was here for a purpose—for nursing. I realized I had to focus on my agenda. Once I got comfortable, the ideas started coming to me. At the end, I felt I could do this again. If I did, I would be much better."

With preparation, a sense of purpose, and the conviction that nurses have a right to speak for themselves and their profession, most nurses will find that it

> ## Basic Rules for Appearing on Radio and Television
>
> - Prepare, prepare, prepare
> - Create three "bumper stickers"
> - Be credible
> - Be enthusiastic
> - Speak with conviction

isn't all that hard to speak on television or radio, in front of a live audience, or to a journalist who is interviewing them for a story.

How to Feel in Control

As with patient care, the best way to feel you're in charge is to get as much information as possible in advance.

If a reporter or producer calls you to arrange an appearance on a radio or TV program, ask the name of the show and of the host who will be interviewing you. Producers rather than the on-air reporters or talk show hosts usually make the initial contact.

Find out if the show is on health care or public policy. Is it an entertainment show? Is it a show that encourages conversational dueling? This will tell you what kind of audience it attracts and how to prepare.

Ask how much time you will be allowed to talk. We've been on radio and television news programs where we've had less than two minutes to present our case.

There are different kinds of television and radio programs. Some are fast-paced entertainment shows that rely on glib retorts. Some try to generate controversy for controversy's sake. Others are more interested in drawing out solid information on a particular problem. You can find out about these shows by asking the host, a friend, or an organizational PR person or by tuning in yourself. It's a good idea to observe the format of the show, particularly if you don't have a great deal of on-air experience.

You'll need to know if a show is live or taped and if it is done in a studio or if, in the case of radio, the interviewer will call you at home or work. Most radio interviews are done outside the studio. Some shows are taped in advance and aired later. You will want to know if the show has call-ins. Callers' comments limit your on-air time. In addition, you'll have to respond to differing perspectives and to a wide and unpredictable variety of questions.

Ask the producer or interviewer if there is a particular slant to his or her thinking on the subject that will be addressed. Ask if you will be the only guest or one of several. Ask how many and who they are. Get a sense of their expertise or point of view. If you know you will be debating someone with an opposing point of view, consider what they are likely to say. Find out how long you will be on the air. You need to know whether you will have two minutes or half an hour in which to make your points.

Many shows do a preinterview to screen potential guests. This is useful to both you and the show's producers and reporters. Your responses to questions and your stage manner will help them decide if they want you on the program. This preinterview will give you an idea of the slant so that you can prepare your comments for the show.

Your attractiveness as a guest will depend on your ability to get your points across vividly and succinctly. The syndicated newspaper columnist Ellen Goodman once told us that when she is unenthusiastic about being on a show, she tells the preinterviewer that the subject has many facets and then she proceeds to elaborate on all of them. Interviewers quickly terminate the call.

It's important to know how a show plans to use nurses—for their clinical or health care expertise or for entertainment value. When a television show ostensibly focuses on the "health care team," producers tend to position the show around a physician or physicians and use nurses as props for the physician-centered narrative.

Several years ago, for example, Sally Jesse Raphael, a daytime television host, planned a show on the care of her son, who had been in an automobile accident and was hospitalized for a month. A group of nurses were invited to the program. To thank the doctors and nurses who had cared for her son, Raphael presented video clips of his hospital stay and asked the experts to talk about his treatment.

The "experts" were all MDs. Dressed in suits and ties, they sat with Raphael on the show's main set. The young man's nurses, on the other hand, had been invited en masse. Dressed uniformly in scrubs, they sat in the audience, where they dutifully applauded or laughed on cue. None was asked to speak about either the medical or nursing issues that were involved in the complex case.

A similar dynamic is at work in the media conferences that hospitals stage to keep the press updated on high-profile cases. For example, when the Cleveland

Clinic arranged a media conference in 2008 to report on the procedures it used for its first surgical face transplant and to demonstrate the success of the surgery by introducing the patient who received it, the physicians involved were on a dais and the nurses and other staff were seated like an audience in rows of chairs on the floor.

With the current popularity of emergency department "reality" shows, viewers do get a chance to see real nurses in action doing their real work as a camera crew follows them around. But when producers interpret the work, or when hospital public relations people structure media events, there is usually a division of duties between the physicians and nurses. As we saw in the extensive coverage of Congresswoman Gabrielle Giffords's injuries and recovery, physicians were cast as the knowledge workers and nurses as the emotion workers. Questions about the patient's status and treatment in this case and many others that we have observed were addressed by physicians even when nursing care was involved. When public relations people refer reporters to nurses, it is almost always for the "human interest" angle, which means for emotion-laden anecdotes about the patient's feelings and those dealing with intimate interactions between the patient and the nurse.

When working with the media and with media relations specialists at their institutions, nurses and nursing administrators need to hash out in advance what is significant about nursing work and what needs to be shown. Nurses must use their leverage to avoid reinforcing images that aren't going to help them or the public. The media needs you and your cooperation as much as you need media attention. It's a two-way street.

In response to Sally Jesse Raphael's request, the hospital PR and nursing departments should have insisted that at least one nurse be on the panel to talk about nursing care. That should have been a condition for nursing's participation. If Raphael refused, the nurses could have refused to appear. Even more hardball, nurses had the power to embarrass a daytime woman's show host whose son was saved by nursing yet wouldn't allow his nurses to appear on a panel of experts. This would have been a good story to leak to the news media. Using nursing's leverage in this way may sound risky. Nurses may be concerned that they will alienate the media—or their institutions—if they do so. Hospitals that want free publicity may pressure nurses to cooperate with media requests that demean nurses. But why should nurses agree to reinforce inaccurate stereotypes? The very process of negotiating these matters might teach reporters and PR staff to show more respect toward individual nurses and their profession. For decades, doctors have negotiated the rules of engagement with television. What is being sought is not propaganda for nurses but an accurate and complete picture of what nurses do.

Your Turn

Imagine that your hospital PR department informs you that a TV crew will be in your hospital filming a documentary on your emergency department. You're a nurse manager in the ED. How will you prepare yourself and the nurses in the department to talk to the journalists? What do you want the nurses to highlight? How will you help them to avoid traditional stereotypes? How will you alert them to possible pitfalls? What will you do if you see a doctor-centered, nurse-as-cheerleader narrative emerging?

Being Interviewed at Work or at Home

Some shows will ask you to come to their studio. Others will interview you at your workplace or home. Communication satellites make it possible for radio or television programs originating across the country or the globe to set up a telephone conversation or live appearance that sound and look as though everyone is in the same room.

In the case of radio, if an interviewer calls for a comment and you are in the middle of something or just feel unprepared, ask him or her to call back in a few moments so that you can pull your thoughts together. Sometimes interviewers will be on deadline and will want you immediately. Buy a little time to think by asking a few questions about the show.

If you don't feel ready, you don't have to agree to the interview. But remember, you're the health care expert. The program is seeking your expertise. Try to compose yourself and speak from your heart about what you know. Most of the time people sound and look much better on radio and television and on web broadcasts than they think they do.

If you have advance notice of an interview that will take place at your home or workplace, give yourself a little breathing space. If you've just seen ten patients or had your management skills tested to the limit, and you are stressed and harried, don't go directly to the phone. Try to take a fifteen-minute or even a five-minute breather. Take some deep, relaxing yoga breaths and collect your thoughts.

Do the same if you will be receiving a call at home. If it's an early morning show (you'd be surprised by how many are) set your alarm to wake you at least a half hour before you're supposed to be called. Have a cup of coffee or tea. Put on your clothes. It's amazing how talking on the radio in your bathrobe at six in the morning can undermine your professionalism even though no one can see you. Some people like to stand up to give radio interviews because it makes them feel more dynamic and authoritative.

It is not unusual for television programs to bring their cameras to you, in which case you will want to be prepared to receive them. If you are going to a radio or TV station for an appearance, give yourself plenty of time to get there. It's better to arrive fifteen minutes early than exactly on time but frazzled. Air times are locked in stone. If you're five or ten minutes late, you may miss the opportunity to be on at all.

Appearance

How you appear and behave on radio and television affects the way the audience receives your message. Whether you're a staff nurse or a researcher, you want to appear knowledgeable and credible. Your dress and body language will help or hinder this effort.

Look professional. Women should never appear in midthigh skirts that hike even higher when they sit or low-slung pants and skimpy tops that bare their midriff and even more. Wear neat, tailored clothes. Don't be bland, but don't be jarring. You should have some color in your attire, but bright reds and oranges go neon on the screen. Whites tend to fade out. Keep away from checks, herringbone tweeds, small stripes, and other small patterns that tend to wiggle on TV. Avoid flowered, sweet, or cute clothing. Depending on the type of show, men should wear suits, sports jackets and ties, or smart-casual clothing. Stretched or holey T-shirts don't lend themselves to credibility.

Since television's bright lights tend to wash out even the rosiest complexion, it helps to wear some makeup. Foundation, rouge, and powder will do. Men may also want to apply some powder, particularly to a shiny scalp, and perhaps foundation too. Some national shows have staff who will apply your makeup. Assume, however, that you won't be made up there and apply your own cosmetics before you go to the studio. If you are going to appear on television a lot, you might want to invest in a lesson from a makeup artist.

Avoid excessive jewelry, particularly the clanking variety. You don't want necklaces or bracelets to jangle against sensitive microphones or strike desks or chairs. Dangling earrings are a distraction. So are long, Barbra Streisand–type nails. The grunge look or an elaborately teased hairdo also compromises a credible presentation.

When you are seated, try to look alert but relaxed and comfortable. Don't slump. Sit up straight and lean forward slightly. This is an attentive posture. If you are asked to stand for the interview—a format at some stations—stand up straight, try to look relaxed, and let your hands hang easily at your sides. Make eye contact with the host.

Don't worry about the camera. It will follow you; you don't have to follow it. Try not to be distracted by camerapeople and producers who are signaling one another or the show's host. These people are not signaling because you've made a mistake. They are communicating with the host or each other about timing and production details. If the host looks at people in the studio while you are talking, or reviews notes, or seems to be listening in an earpiece to what someone is saying, he or she knows the camera is on you and is counting on you to continue talking.

Always assume that your microphone is on and recording even if the show goes to commercial breaks or seems to be over. Don't say anything during these breaks and begin talking normally only when your mike has been removed.

With today's automated sets, you might find yourself in a booth or a newsroom with a remotely operated camera aimed at you. You might even find yourself talking just to a computer screen. If you go to a studio to be interviewed for a program based in another city, your "face-to-face" with the host will be via his or her image on a monitor or his or her voice in your earpiece. This can be unnerving. Keep in mind that on television it will look like you are actually having a conversation with the interviewer. Your job is to regard the robotic camera (which may advance and back away eerily) as though it were a human being and talk directly to it. You will get an indication of when the show has gone to a commercial and you can relax for a moment. But when the discussion is going on, don't assume that you are not on camera because someone else is talking. A camera may be taking reaction shots of you. The famous "split-screen" and the supposedly turned-off microphone has undone more than one politician. This is such an artificial environment that you may feel as though they have put you in isolation and forgotten about you. But you are very much part of the program. If you have something to say, and no one has given you a chance, politely, but assertively, interject.

When you are asked a question, don't look toward the ceiling as if waiting for the angels to send you an answer. Keep your eyes on the host (or robot camera). Some people blink rapidly when they are working their way through an answer. If you have this tendency, consciously override it so that you have a steady look. If you're responding to another guest on the show, look at him or her (or at the robot camera as though it were that guest). Make hand gestures, but don't let them get out of control. You want viewers to listen to what you say, not get caught up with your mannerisms.

When someone else is talking, look interested. Don't scratch your head, scowl, roll your eyes, or snicker if you think what the person said is absurd. The camera might pan toward you at any time and catch your reaction. When someone is asking you a question or making a statement, resist grunting or uttering affirmative "uh-huh" sounds. Similarly, don't automatically nod your head. Affirmative nods and sounds are intended to show the other person that you are taking in what he or she is saying, but they can be a distraction and may give the impression that you agree with what the person is saying even if it is outrageous or contradicts your argument. Just looking attentive is sufficient. This is also the correct demeanor for participating in a panel discussion or engaging in questions and answers from a lecture podium.

State Your Qualifications and Set Ground Rules

Before you go on air, establish how you will be identified and how the host and other guests will address you. This is essential. Tell the producer exactly how you want to be identified.

Give the correct spelling of your name and title for the identifier that will flash on the screen when you are talking. Make sure *RN* or *nurse* is included in the identification. If you have another title, such as *professor*, your nursing identification may disappear unless you insist that it be present. Identifications in radio and TV land (and even in most mainstream publications) are short, so get in the essentials, and accept that no one is interested in the fact that you are the Florence Nightingale/Lavinia Dock/Lillian Wald Professor of Physiological and Anatomical Nursing at the University of Such and Such School of Nursing. What they need to know is that you are an expert on a certain subject and a professor at the University of Such and Such School of Nursing.

Make sure you establish ground rules for oral introductions. Ask to be introduced with your specialty and perhaps the number of years you have been a nurse, as in "Joanne Clarke is with us today. She's been a psychiatric nurse for twenty years and works with adolescents." If you are a staff nurse, provide additional details too. For example, you might want to be introduced as "Tom Smith, who has been a medical-surgical nurse at General Hospital for ten years. Nurse Smith works extensively with elderly patients."

If you're a PhD nurse, beware of being called "Dr." over and over again. The audience will probably think you are a physician. If you use your *Dr.* title, be sure to preface statements with "As a nurse . . ."

If you are not a PhD and you are going to be on air with MDs or PhDs, insist on being addressed as Mrs., Miss, Ms., or Mr. (last name) or Nurse (last name). Unless you intervene, hosts will call doctors "Dr.," professors "Professor," and you Joan or Jim. Even if you have to intervene while on the air, do not allow yourself to be called by your first name while others are being addressed with titles that convey expertise.

Tone of Voice and Interview Etiquette

Tone of voice is important, especially on radio. Maintain an even, measured tone even if you are provoked. Don't get riled by what a caller, another guest, or the host has said. Maintain your composure just as you would with a difficult patient. Combat their comments with a powerful argument, not by raising your voice, making personal attacks, mocking, or being sarcastic.

To be polite and still make your point, you can say, "That was interesting, but let's think about this aspect of the issue," and move on to your message.

Regard negative and insulting comments as opportunities to make your points. For example, if a host says, "It's surprising to me that nurses know so much about diseases and medications," pick up on the host's language and respond, "You know, what's surprising is that you're surprised." Then describe what nurses know. For example, "I've been an oncology nurse for ten years. I am very familiar with toxic chemotherapy drugs and how to administer them so that patients don't develop fatal complications."

If you're talking about the consequences of a shortage of nurses or understaffing on hospital floors, a host might concur in a way that subtly demeans nurses. "So what we're missing in health care," he might offer, "is the TLC nurses bring."

To this, you can reply, "Nurses definitely bring a great deal of caring and compassion to their patients and to their patients' families. But the real problem with a shortage of nurses is that there won't be anyone in hospitals to rescue patients from complications that could lead to death. That's what nursing is, a matter of life and death."

If you're on a show where the host or the guests are constantly interrupting and shrieking at one another, your challenge will be to resist retreating into frustrated silence or joining in the shouting match. Try an amused tone to interject, "Well, if I could just get a word in edgewise," or, "If one of you would just let someone finish a sentence." When someone interrupts, you can say firmly, "I've given you the courtesy of letting you respond. I'd appreciate the same courtesy."

The most important thing is to be interested, enthusiastic, and cooperative rather than withholding and monosyllabic. When Dick Cavett had a conversation show years ago, we watched him interview the famous Russian ballet dancer Rudolf Nureyev, who appeared wearing a snakeskin suit and matching platform boots. Cavett asked the dancer an intelligent question, to which Nureyev responded, "Yes." Then Cavett asked another excellent question, to which the dancer responded, "No." Another perceptive comment received a terse yes, followed by yes, yes, and no. After the first few minutes, it must have been agonizingly clear to Cavett that he was living the interviewer's worst nightmare: he had to fill up airtime with a talk show guest who refused to talk.

If you're nervous or suspicious, don't pull a Nureyev. The way to deal with this is to be prepared, and then talk your way out of your anxiety.

Be Prepared

You must know in advance which points you want to make. Years ago Christopher Lydon (the former host of *The Connection* on National Public Radio) told Bernice Buresh before interviewing her on television that she should think of her points as "bumper stickers." This is a useful image. Bumper stickers represent the essence of your message and are easy to remember. You can embed your bumper sticker into an anecdote, example, or rejoinder. But the main point must be short and clear. Realistically, you may not have time to make more than three points and may only get a chance to make one, but you can make it count.

Hang In There!

The advice to be prepared with bumper stickers has come in handy on more than one occasion but no more so than on an early morning television news show in Milwaukee that Bernice Buresh appeared on several years ago. In preparation, she talked with the producer the day before and asked how much time she would be given. The producer said three minutes.

Buresh started out the next morning at 5:30 A.M. and drove through blowing snow to get to the station in advance of the 6:20 A.M. segment. At the

station entrance, she rang the buzzer repeatedly until someone from security came and let her in. An assistant greeted her and briskly led her into the
newsroom, sat her on a stool, stuck an earpiece in her ear, clipped a small
microphone onto her sweater, and disappeared.

After a while, Buresh motioned over a news writer she spotted across
the room and asked when she would be on and how much time she would
have. The news writer relayed the question to the hosts, who were visible on
a monitor but situated in a studio elsewhere in the building. Buresh heard
the voice of one of them in her earpiece. "Oh, Bernice," she said. "We're so
sorry. We're only going to have about a minute and a half because we need
to talk more about the snowstorm." Buresh politely protested that she had
been offered three minutes and had made the trip downtown on that basis.
"Well, maybe we can stretch it to two," the host said.

Buresh, seated on the stool in front of a robot camera, looked at the piece
of paper on which she had written five bumper stickers, and she crossed out
two. She quickly rehearsed in her mind how she would present the remaining three.

The two women hosts, who had a format in which they chatted with
each other, spent a lot of time discussing a new survey about whether
cats or dogs are more popular as family pets. Then abruptly one of the
hosts segued to a thirty-second intro on the nursing shortage, which cited
Milwaukee hospital vacancy stats, introduced Buresh as a journalist, former
Milwaukeean, and coauthor of a public-communication book for nurses, and
then noted, while footage of hospital nurses at work appeared on the screen,
that applicants were being turned away from nursing schools because there
weren't enough slots available.

In a thirty-second answer directed to the camera in front of her, Buresh
documented the extent of the nursing shortage, made sure to name the university that had set up her appearance ("as I told students yesterday during
my lecture at the University of Wisconsin–Whitewater"), and emphasized
the serious consequences of the nursing shortage (the closing of ICUs,
emergency room diversions).

One of the hosts asked a twelve-second question on what could be done
about the nursing shortage.

Buresh replied that money wasted in the U.S. health care system needed
to be shifted into resources for nursing because of the critical importance of
nursing. She said that nurses were leaving clinical settings because of poor
working conditions and that the nursing shortage would not be remedied unless nurses could have long-term, satisfying careers so that working nurses

would want to stay on the job and the best and brightest candidates would want to enter the profession and stay for the long run. Her answer took fifty seconds, the later part of which was overlaid with more footage of nurses at a Milwaukee hospital.

The instant Buresh was finished, her camera shut off. One host turned excitedly to the other and said she was dying to hear the answer to the important question posed earlier—were dogs or cats more popular?

After learning that the answer was cats, and after getting a pro forma thank you for her appearance, Buresh morosely made her way out of the station into the dark early morning thinking the whole thing had been a waste of time.

It wasn't. A lot of people saw the segment and remembered it even though it was only two minutes and two seconds long in its entirety. When she reviewed the tape later, Buresh saw that the segment was informative about nursing and had used positive images of nurses doing their work. The program had got her name and identification right, and, amazingly, she looked relaxed and cheerful on camera, in contrast to how she had felt.

Earlier we talked about preparing three anecdotes on nursing. For television and radio, these anecdotes must be reduced to a few sentences that can be delivered quickly in a conversational style to make a point. Write down your points, and the statistics or facts that will bolster them, and take them with you to the studio. Review the points before you go on air.

Remember to translate jargon into ordinary language. It's *critical care unit*, not *CCU*; *cancer*, not *CA*; *heart attack*, not *MI* or *myocardial infarction*.

Your Turn

Think of three bumper stickers you'd use to describe your work or make your point. For example:

- Nursing is a matter of life and death, not TLC.
- Nurses are the ones who see patients first in the emergency department, and nurses decide how sick they are, how urgently they need to be treated, and who needs to treat them.

Bridging

Bridging is a technique for getting to your bumper stickers. It means using a question or comment as a bridge to make your point.

That's what Cindy Dalton did on *Montreal Today*. She briefly answered the host's question then seized the opportunity to describe the challenges nurses face in their daily practice. Later, when the discussion turned to health care policy, she directed the conversation to the nursing component.

A bridge is merely a transitional statement, such as the following:

- "You know that's an interesting issue, but so is this . . . "
- "Let me tell you about . . . "
- "While we're talking about what's important to patients, consider this . . . "
- "The real issue is . . . "
- "Here's another factor that hasn't been mentioned . . . "

Questions from interviewers come in various forms, some of which may surprise you. Here are a few common types and possible ways to respond.

The Flattering or Gift Question

An interviewer might say, "Oh, nurses are wonderful people. They do such important work." Or, "It's just terrible what's happening to nursing."

These "nonquestions" can derail you because it's hard to know how to respond. Treat them as an invitation to take the conversation in the direction you'd like to go. "Thank you," "Yes, that's true," or "I'm glad you feel that way" are reasonable prefaces to a follow-up such as "Nurses hope the public will transform private gratitude into public support for nursing. Those listeners who share your views about nursing may want to call their political representative to support increased funding for nursing education, staffing, or research. In fact, there's now a bill in the state [or provincial] legislature that would allocate more money to nursing. We need public support for it . . . "

The Open-Ended Question

"What's it like to be a nurse?" Taken too literally, this type of question can have you chasing all over the landscape. Regard it as an invitation to tell an anecdote that contains one of your bumper stickers. "Well, one of the things we do in hospitals is prevent major complications like bedsores that can cause the patient terrible suffering and sometimes even lead to death and can cost between four thousand and seventy thousand dollars to heal."[1]

The Double-Bind Question

By confronting you with two untenable options, these questions are a classic catch-22.

An example: "Did you become a nurse because you didn't have what it takes to get into medical school, or because you're just too nice to be a doctor?"

Without repeating the question, one answer would be "I became a nurse because I wanted to apply my intelligence to caring for the sick and vulnerable. I work on a surgical unit where, among other things, I make sure that patients don't develop pneumonias, blood clots, or wound infections after their operations . . . "

The Erroneous-Assumption Question

Like the double-bind question, this query throws negative material at you. The challenge is to quickly dispense with the negative and turn to the positive.

A Canadian radio interviewer once interrupted a guest who was describing the burdens being placed on nurses with "So if nurses don't get enough respect, why don't they just all move up the food chain and become doctors?"

To which the guest responded, "In my view, nurses are already at the top of the food chain. Think about it; if all the nurses became doctors, who would provide twenty-four-hour care of the sick?"

Never be afraid to challenge erroneous assumptions or misinterpretations of nursing. You are being interviewed because you are the expert, and therefore it is your role to correct mistaken ideas about nursing. Be prepared to do so.

Several years ago, nurses being interviewed by the journalist Bill Moyers for a documentary series, *Healing and the Mind*, seemed taken aback when Moyers misidentified their work.

In the documentary, Moyers observed nurses working with fragile premature infants and their teenage parents at Parkland Memorial Hospital in Dallas and then talked with the nurses about what they were doing. Clearly impressed, Moyers nonetheless demonstrated at the end of the segment how even the most intelligent and sensitive people can be confused about nursing. "You're *more* than nurses, you're *more* than technicians," he exclaimed. Then placing their work in the context of innovations in medicine, Moyers declared, "That's what *medicine's* about today."

Your Turn

Practice doing an interview with a friend or colleague and then critique it, paying attention to the following:

- Are you speaking in ordinary language?
- Are you describing your work briefly and concretely?
- Are you conveying your enthusiasm?
- Are you expressing a strong point of view?

Moyers's response was startling. But imagine the effect the nurses might have had on millions of viewers if they had been ready for a predictable misinterpretation. They could have politely, but firmly, responded, "No, Bill, what you have just seen is the very essence of *nursing.*"

The Absent-Party Question

The interviewer may use a comment made by a general or specific absent party to inject controversy or discredit your arguments.

An interviewer might say, for example, "Many people are now saying that nurses have become too vociferous in their demands." To which you might respond, "Most people tell us quite the contrary. They are glad that nurses are standing up for patient care."

A variation of the form might be "I have a friend who teaches chemistry at a prestigious university and he says that nursing students are the dumbest ones in his class."

This technique is insidious because you know neither the person nor what he really said. Yet the absent party is set up as an authoritative commentator. To this statement, you might reply that you had not heard the comment and then describe the rigors of nursing education—"Sorry I haven't heard that one. But in nursing school we learn pharmacology, anatomy, and pathophysiology, not to mention family health and how to communicate with patients and families."

The Loaded-Preface Question

An interviewer might pack a lot of information—some of it inaccurate or provocative—into a question. He or she might say, "I know your organization

Interview Tips

- Find out in advance what the interview will be about.
- Find out how much time you will have.
- Prepare three "bumper stickers."
- Don't be a captive of the question. Bridge from the interviewer's question to the points you want to make.
- Use anecdotes, personal stories, statistics, sparkling language.
- Avoid jargon, technical terms, and alphabet soup (i.e., initialisms and acronyms).
- Tell the truth; don't exaggerate to win an argument.
- Don't repeat a negative question or offensive words.
- Know in advance what you will not divulge. Whether it is personal or has to do with your institution or profession, know how far you are willing to go and go no further.
- Assume everything is on the record. Don't comment if you don't want your comment to be aired.
- If you don't know something, say so. Then talk about what you do know.
- Be cooperative and communicative.
- Enjoy your experience on air.

doesn't represent many people and has not established a track record in this area. What is its mission in this campaign?"

Take a mental breath and use the question to describe the importance of your organization and its key role in the current issue. "Our organization represents seventy thousand RNs. We've just done a study that documents how violence in the workplace harms patients and exacerbates the nursing shortage."

The Irrelevant or Non Sequitur Question

Depending on the tone of the show, an interviewer may incorporate a statement that has no bearing on the subject, such as "My mother-in-law just loves the nurses on *ER*."

Use this bland statement to make a point: "Yes, nurses who work in emergency rooms are great. In fact, they do a lot more than is shown on that show . . ."

The Direct-Accusation Question

How about getting hit with this? "You're complaining about violence against nurses. What about all those nurses who kill their patients?"

You might reply by saying, "There aren't many nurses in that category, but workplace statistics indicate that more must be done to protect *nurses* from violence." Whatever else, do not repeat the phrase "nurses who kill their patients."

The Inconsistency Question

This type of question suggests that you are unable to make up your mind and thus can't be trusted.

An interviewer might say, "Nurses complain that they have to do too much non-nursing work, but now they're saying they don't want more nursing assistants to help them."

Nurses and other caregivers are often criticized when they "break frame" by doing something that seems out of synch with their conventional image such as asking for something for themselves or going on strike. Journalists may imply that nurses are being selfish or hiding behind patient care to get something for themselves, as in the question "Are you really trying to protect your patients, or are you just trying to protect your job?"

A picket line interview during a strike might produce the following: "Why are you abandoning your patients? Isn't your job to be at the bedside no matter what?"

Because nurses don't want to be perceived as selfish and uncaring, they tend to spend time trying to prove how unselfish and caring they are. A better tack might be to state forthrightly, "We certainly do want to protect our jobs. That's because our job is to save your life."

Or you could say, "A hospital's job is to care for patients and to support and sustain the people—professional nurses and other staff—who provide that care twenty-four hours a day. Because hospitals have cut too many nursing jobs, staff nurses are frequently asked to work two back-to-back, ten-hour shifts. The nurse may be exhausted and have no time to go the bathroom or take a lunch break. Studies now show that these conditions lead to errors that can harm patients."

To which the response might be "Nurses are doing too many non-nursing activities like transporting patients, answering phones, or cleaning up. We want nursing assistants to help with that, not to give patients baths or medications or monitor their vital signs."

The Question You Don't Know How to Answer

Sometimes interviewers will ask you questions you simply can't answer. If you're an oncology nurse, an interviewer could come from left field and ask you a question about the treatment of diabetics or the latest proposal for health care reform. If you know about diabetes or have an opinion about the latest health care reform proposal, voice it. If you don't, don't take a stab at it. Simply say, "That's an interesting question, but it's not my field. You might want to talk to a nurse who specializes in diabetes," or, "You can get a lot of good information on health care reform by talking to people at the American Nurses Association." Then, use the question to bridge into what you do know about.

Call-in Shows and Nurse-Run Shows

Thanks to the myriad call-in shows that are on television and radio, you can use the electronic media to make your point even if you are never invited to appear on a show. If you are at home, at work, or driving in the car and you hear people discussing health care, listen carefully. If you're thinking, "I have something to say about that topic," punch in the number and express your point of view. People who call in to shows are generally not asked to give their last names. So if you're worried about retaliation, this is a perfect forum. Some shows take

Beware of repeating negative statements. While it's a normal response for people to repeat the negative to refute it, you may inadvertently give it more weight than it deserves. If an interviewer asks you about "nurses who kill their patients," and you say, "Nurses don't kill their patients," the listener has just heard the words "nurses . . . kill . . . patients" twice.

When people are under stress they might even introduce a negative suggestion themselves, as Richard Nixon did in 1973 in the statement that became emblematic of his unraveling presidency: "People have got to know whether or not their president is a crook. Well, I'm not a crook."

If people make allegations, simply refute them. Don't raise new ones yourself.

e-mailed questions and comments as well, and the host reads them on the air. If you can't get through or don't want to make a call, your view may still be aired.

We've been on a number of shows where nurses have called in spontaneously. Some have recounted heart-wrenching experiences. Some have talked about the work they do with patients. Others have discussed their research. Most have significantly advanced the discussion.

The show doesn't have to be on nursing to allow you, as a nurse, to contribute. It can be about health care reform, legislation, a political candidate's stand on issues, women and gender, or education—whatever topic provokes and inspires you to interject your experience and expertise. If you are listening and feel that something should be added, you're just the one to do it.

CHAPTER 12

OPPORTUNITIES AND CHALLENGES AHEAD

As we conclude this edition of *From Silence to Voice*, nurses and others in health care who have long been denied the respect and resources they need have an unprecedented opportunity to make their work better understood and their voices heard.

Three interconnected challenges create this opportunity for nurses. One is escalating health care costs. The second is patient safety. The third is the new focus on interprofessional education and practice.

In most health care institutions, nurses are at the forefront of patient safety. Keeping patients safe reduces health care costs. Every preventable medical error and injury adds unnecessary costs—extra hospital/nursing home/rehab days, extra medications, extra lines and tubes, and extra sheets and meals, not to mention extra pain and suffering. Every time nurses or other caregivers get sick because of the patient load they bear, from lack of sleep or a surfeit of stress, patients become less safe, and nurses turn into patients themselves, thus adding more to health care costs.

We are learning just how the traditional image of the nice nurse who sacrifices for her or his patient actually compromises patient safety. We now know that tired caregivers who are "always there when someone needs them" not only make more errors but also are physiologically incapable of providing the empathy patients want. We know more about how assertive nurses prevent problems. As we explained in the introduction, many physician patient safety advocates even argue publicly that nurses should express their concerns and that doctors and health care administrators should listen to them. As they campaign for patient safety, these physicians are helping the public to understand nurses' roles in protecting patients.

Many nurses are using their voices to explain to the public what they do to provide high-quality patient care. But too many nurses and their organizations seem trapped in the confines of the saccharinized care narrative we have described in previous chapters. Many seem to be unaware that there is a contradiction between asserting that they should have a leading role in modern health care and simultaneously promoting nursing for the "feminine" virtues that have limited nurses' leadership for centuries.

We see these limitations at work when patients express surprise that nurses "know so much" and compliment the "smart nurse" by exclaiming, "Why, you could be a doctor!" The fact that consultants think they can make money by reengineering nurses' facial expressions into a permanent smile is testament to how little the decision makers in our society grasp why nurses are at the bedside or in health care institutions. That nurses should be asked to "always be there" for patients, or be honored for their unpaid labor and the extra mile they go (rather than for the miles they routinely run day after day), suggests that many do not understand that nurses' need for respite is closely linked to patient care outcomes.

Today, as most nurses correctly believe, too many members of too many publics do not fully understand the connection between nursing and quality patient care. Instead of nursing realizing its potential, nursing remains under constant threat as hospitals and other health care institutions consider ways to replace higher-paid, more educated professionals with cheaper, lower-skilled staff. Because of society's failure to understand the importance of nursing work—and its lifesaving and cost-saving potential—health care facilities in industrialized societies often try to turn nurses into assembly line workers who don't have the necessary time to practice up to their scope.

Not only is the basic direct care nurse being asked to do more and more with less and less; so are nurse practitioners, other advanced practice nurses, home-care and school nurses, nurse managers, and even nurse executives. Nurse practitioners (NPs) who act as primary care providers were once lauded for the time they spent with patients. Now many are limited to the same ten- to fifteen-minute slots as primary care physicians. Similarly, acute care NPs in hospitals spend too much of their time in front of computers ordering medications and thus have less time to spend with patients. Many nurse managers supervise two or three units instead of one and sometimes have over a hundred staff members reporting to them. Chief nursing officers may be managing not one but several hospitals. All are under pressure to cut costs, work longer hours, spend more time documenting than delivering care, and accept constant insecurity and instability.

Many nurses have welcomed the recent report, *The Future of Nursing: Leading Change, Advancing Health*, by the Robert Wood Johnson Foundation and the prestigious U.S. Institute of Medicine, because it seems to portend great things for the profession.[1] Nurses, the report says, should be viewed as equal partners with physicians, should practice to their scope, and should help redesign and lead health care systems as well as guide people toward better health and health outcomes. The report emphasizes the roles that advanced practice nurses could play in the health care system.

The Future of Nursing also identifies barriers that "need to be overcome to ensure that nurses are well-positioned to lead change and advance health." It notes that nurses do not have sole power to make necessary changes. It states that "many diverse parties"—government officials, insurers, health care researchers, licensing bodies, educational institutions, philanthropic organizations, and so on—must work together with nursing to "ensure that the health care system provides seamless, affordable, quality care that is accessible to all and leads to improved health." In other words, nurses need to secure the cooperation and commitment of others to fulfill their potential and improve health care. How is that possible if members of these influential publics misunderstand nursing? To succeed in this enterprise, nurses must communicate what they really do in practice and make a credible case for why they should lead this movement and where they will lead it.

Communication will be critical if the global economy continues to slow. Economic bad news is usually detrimental to the nursing profession and to the patients who depend on nurses for their lives and health. In the coming years, we may experience the same kind of pressures to cut nursing staffs as those at play in the 1990s. Indeed, as we were finishing this book, we received a glimpse of this in a webinar notification by HealthLeaders Media on how hospitals could cut nursing labor costs. The announcement read, "With the economy in a very slow recovery, cost-sensitive financial leaders are moving beyond 'low-hanging fruit,' digging into labor budgets to find savings. Nurse labor is one area that is sure to attract scrutiny. Healthcare leaders must understand how to optimize nursing staff, when to offer overtime, and how to build and use a flexible in-house nurse pool."[2]

> By expanding their care narrative to include the many ways nurses put their caring into concrete action, we will see just why nurses should lead and how they can help us enhance our health and well-being.

Higher professional status for nurses does not guarantee that the pressures on the profession will disappear or that nurses will be able to deal with them effectively (one has only to look at the industrialization of medicine to see how little protection status offers when facing the marketization of health care). Improvement will come about only if influential segments of the public understand the concrete benefits of nursing work and the need for more resources for patient care.

We believe that the widespread interest in improving health care while controlling costs gives nurses unprecedented opportunities to communicate with receptive publics about nurses' roles in patient safety and cost-effective care. By expanding their care narrative to include the many ways nurses put their caring into concrete action, we will see just why nurses should lead and how they can help us enhance our health and well-being.

In more than two decades of writing about nursing, we have been struck by how receptive people are to stories about the real work of nurses when nurses describe how they save lives, prevent pain and suffering, and also save money. Nurses may fear that if they tell these stories, they will lose patients' trust or even alarm patients by revealing the dangers inherent in today's high-tech health care system. Nothing could be further from the truth. As documented in studies by Dominick Frosch and others, patients are well aware of these dangers, which is why they want to participate in decisions about their treatment and care.[3] To know that a nurse understands these dangers and is there to prevent problems is far more reassuring than frightening.

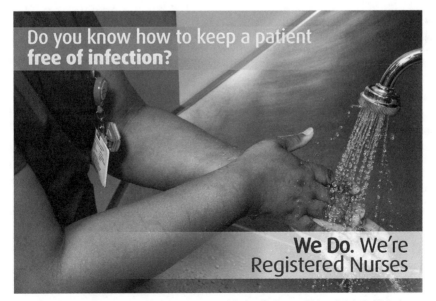

An example of an effective advertisement for how nurses prevent infection. (By Suzanne Gordon; photo by Earl Dotter.)

Nurses often tell us that they do not feel authorized to tell their stories to the public because they are "just a nurse." Suzanne Gordon wondered what would happen if the phrase *just a nurse* were "spun" to illuminate the richness and importance of nursing. She conceived of the script that follows as a promotion for nurses. Many nurses regard "Just a Nurse" as a poem and have posted it in their workplace. We encourage nurses, wherever they work and in whatever capacity they practice, to show what it means to be "just a nurse."[4]

Just a Nurse

by Suzanne Gordon

I'm "just a nurse"; I just make the difference between life and death.

I'm "just a nurse"; I just have the educated eyes that prevent medical errors, injuries, and other catastrophes.

I'm "just a nurse"; I just make the difference between healing and coping, and despair.

I'm "just a nurse"; I just make the difference between pain and comfort.

I'm "just a nurse"; I'm just a nurse researcher who helps nurses and doctors give better, safer, and more effective care.

I'm "just a nurse"; I'm just a school nurse who makes sure children stay healthy so they can learn in school.

I'm "just a nurse"; I just work in a major teaching hospital managing and monitoring patients who are involved in cutting-edge experimental research.

I'm "just a nurse"; I just educate patients and families about how to maintain their health.

I'm "just a nurse"; I'm just a geriatric nurse practitioner who makes a difference between an elderly person's staying in his own home or going to a nursing home.

I'm "just a nurse"; I just make the difference between dying in agony and dying in comfort and with dignity.

I'm "just a nurse"; I'm just the real bottom line in health care.

Wouldn't you like to be "just a nurse" too?

HOW WE CAME TO WRITE THIS BOOK

Our inquiry into nursing and public communication began in 1989 when we served as news media consultants to the Nurses of America (NOA) project, a national public relations campaign to rectify the nursing shortage by attracting high-quality candidates into the field. As journalists all our professional lives, we have written about social and political actions in the United States, including the civil rights, women's, antiwar, gay rights, labor, and community organizing movements. We have also covered mainstream electoral politics. We have seen how marginalized groups managed to bring their agendas to the forefront of public attention and win important legal and social victories. So when NOA asked us to help, we were delighted to accept.

The NOA project was funded by almost a million dollars from the Pew Charitable Trusts and administered by a council of representatives from major nursing organizations. It sponsored activities designed to analyze public attitudes toward nurses and to project a positive image of contemporary nursing. The project undertook studies, monitored the media, distributed press materials, and "media trained" nurses so that they would be more skilled in talking to reporters, appearing on television, and developing "media events" to stimulate coverage of nursing.

We were particularly interested in press coverage of nursing. We wanted to know whether and to what degree journalists used nurses and nursing organizations as sources of information on health and health care. We devised a study to examine the representation of nurses in the health coverage of three major newspapers. Before the explosion of Internet media this was a particularly important line of inquiry because a profession's public status and credibility are enhanced through having its expertise acknowledged in the journalistic media. Today, the forms of media may have changed but not the media's importance in our culture.

We were quite sure that nursing—the largest health care profession by far—would be shown to be vastly underrepresented in news coverage. But we didn't expect nursing to be virtually missing from health reportage. This is what the study "Who Counts in News Coverage of Health Care?" documented.[1]

We found that practically everyone had more of a public voice on health and health care than nurses. When we analyzed the sources of 908 direct quotations by "occupation," we found that physicians were by far the most frequently quoted occupational group. They accounted for nearly one-third of the quotations. But nurses were not a close second, third, or even fourth. After physicians, eleven other groups were quoted more frequently than nurses. These included sources from government, business, nonprofit organizations, education, public relations, and medical organizations, as well as patients, family members, and an assortment of professional and nonprofessional health care workers. Nurses were at the bottom of the list, accounting for only ten, or 1.1 percent, of the quotations. No matter how we analyzed public visibility, nurses were either in or tied for last place.

This discovery had far-reaching implications. If there was little trace of nursing in the serious coverage of health and health care, then how could anyone, including those in a position to supply nursing with needed resources, understand and recognize its value? When medicine is consistently depicted as the center of the health care universe, physicians get credit for every contribution to health care, even in those instances when it should go to nursing or another profession.

Concerned about what might be a systematic journalistic bias against nursing, we were determined to acquaint our fellow journalists, particularly those who specialize in health and medical reporting, with this serious omission in their reporting. Armed with the study, we and small groups of nurses met with journalists to discuss the fact that they seemed to be ignoring nurses as sources of health care information and nursing issues as news. We made sure our study was widely circulated. It was distributed to journalists at conferences and its findings appeared in the journalism trade press.

Many journalists acknowledged that they knew nothing about nursing. To help them get a better grasp of the field, we prepared a media packet that contained information on nursing and on newsworthy nursing projects, as well as biographies of nurses. These materials linked nursing with contemporary health care issues, suggested potential stories, and gave reporters the names of expert nurses to talk to.

Later on, with the support of major nursing organizations, we created a nursing source directory for journalists so that they would have the names of nurses (instead of only physicians) whom they could call for information on health care. This project was suggested and partially funded by the Ms. Foundation for Communication and Education.

In general, reporters and editors welcomed this material. Some readily acknowledged that they had not paid much attention to nursing. Many said they were interested in doing stories that included nurses. When groups of nurses provided them with materials on current health care issues, many in fact did stories that included nurses as primary spokespersons. In most cases, when nurses sought meetings with editorial boards to discuss health coverage, they received positive responses and discussed how coverage could be improved.

At this point, approaches to increasing the visibility of nursing seemed straightforward enough. The news media constituted the major conduit. Nurses had to work on educating journalists about nursing so that they would be more receptive to covering the profession. Nurses and nursing organizations had to be much more active in presenting journalists with newsworthy material. All this could be accomplished if more nurses developed public communication skills. Indeed we would write a public-communication book for nurses that would help them develop these skills.

We anticipated that the NOA project would provide the foundation for a cooperative communication program by nursing organizations, and there was some discussion of such a plan. We also expected nurses who had been media trained to take an active role in media outreach. We ourselves wrote articles about nursing and thought that more journalists would routinely cover nursing.

But these expectations did not come to fruition at the time. Rather, nursing was thrust onto the public stage in connection with the health care upheaval of the mid-1990s. Many nurses became alarmed when hospital restructuring experiments endangered their patients, and some courageous nurses did speak up. Still, journalists covering this story had a difficult time finding nurses who would talk with them about these events or even about routine nursing practice so that they could understand the changes that were going on.

Journalists still complain that they are frustrated in their attempts to find nurses who will do even the basics of communication—return phone calls or answer simple questions about their work. These complaints are echoed by public relations specialists in nursing organizations, nursing schools, and hospitals and medical centers. They tell us they might interest a journalist in an idea for a story only to discover that they can't find nurses willing to talk to reporters, even about noncontroversial subjects.

These experiences made us realize that we had underestimated the significance of cultural issues in the relationship between nursing and the public world. Whereas we once thought that nursing could become significantly more visible by using more or less generic public relations techniques, we now believed that communication considerations specific to nursing must be addressed.

Our metaphors also changed over time. Initially we thought in terms of the *invisibility* and *visibility* of nursing. We began, however, to feel that the operative terms were *silence* and *voice*. That is why we called this book *From Silence to Voice* and why we began to focus, in the second edition, on moving beyond a "virtue script" that idealizes nursing toward messages that accurately depict nursing and its importance in health care.

The "scripting" of nursing is central to this third edition of *From Silence to Voice*. It continues to be a constant concern—one that has become sharper as new players encourage nurses to remain cloaked in a virtue script that we believe to be a threat not only to nursing but also to patient care.

NOTES

Introduction

1. Jeffrey M. Jones, "Record 64% Rate Honesty, Ethics of Members of Congress Low; Ratings of Nurses, Pharmacists, and Medical Doctors Most Positive," Gallup report, December 12, 2011, http://www.gallup.com/poll/151460/Record-Rate-Honesty-Ethics-Members-Congress-Low.aspx (accessed May 7, 2012).

2. American Nurses Association, news release, December 13, 2011, http://www.nursingworld.org/FunctionalMenuCategories/MediaResources/PressReleases/2011-PR/Nurses-Keep-Top-Spot-in-Poll.pdf (accessed May 7, 2012).

3. Barron H. Lerner, "A Life-Changing Case for Doctors in Training," *New York Times*, August 14, 2011, http://www.nytimes.com/2009/03/03/health/03zion.html (accessed May 7, 2012).

4. "ACGME Duty Hours Standards Fact Sheet," Accreditation Council for Graduate Medical Education, http://www.acgme.org/acWebsite/newsRoom/newsRm_dutyHours.asp (accessed May 7, 2012).

5. Darshak Sanghavi, "The Phantom Menace of Sleep-Deprived Doctors," *New York Times Magazine*, August 5, 2011, http://www.nytimes.com/2011/08/07/magazine/the-phantom-menace-of-sleep-deprived-doctors.html?_r=1&pagewanted=all (accessed May 7, 2012).

6. Ibid.

7. Alison M. Trinkoff and Jeanne Geiger-Brown, "Sleep-Deprived Nurses: Sleep and Schedule Challenges in Nursing," in *First, Do Less Harm: Confronting the Inconvenient Problems of Patient Safety*, ed. Suzanne Gordon and Ross Koppel (Ithaca, N.Y.: Cornell University Press, 2012), 168–179.

8. Paul Starr, *The Social Transformation of American Medicine* (New York: Basic Books, 1982). See the introduction, "The Social Origins of Professional Sovereignty," 3–29.

9. Sioban Nelson and Suzanne Gordon, "The Rhetoric of Rupture: Nursing as a Practice with a History?" *Nursing Outlook* 52, no. 5 (September 2004): 255–261.

10. George Lakoff, *Don't Think of an Elephant: Know Your Values and Frame the Debate* (White River Junction, Vt.: Chelsea Green, 2004), xv.

11. Daniel Kahneman, *Thinking, Fast and Slow* (New York: Farrar, Straus and Giroux, 2011), 119.

12. Erving Goffman, *The Presentation of Self in Everyday Life* (New York: Anchor Doubleday Books, 1959).

13. Institute of Medicine, *The Future of Nursing: Leading Change, Advancing Health* (Washington, D.C.: National Academies Press, 2011).

14. Sioban Nelson and Suzanne Gordon, *The Complexities of Care: Nursing Reconsidered* (Ithaca, N.Y.: Cornell University Press, 2006), 13–29.

15. *The American Heritage Dictionary of the English Language*, 4th ed. (Boston: Houghton Mifflin 2000), 838.

16. Suzanne Gordon, ed., *When Chicken Soup Isn't Enough: Stories of Nurses Standing Up for Themselves, Their Patients, and Their Profession* (Ithaca, N.Y.: Cornell University Press, 2010).

1. Ending the Silence

1. Bernice Buresh, Suzanne Gordon, and Nica Bell, "Who Counts in News Coverage of Health Care?" *Nursing Outlook* 39, no. 5 (1991): 204–208.

2. *The Woodhull Study on Nursing and the Media: Health Care's Invisible Partner*, Indianapolis, Center Nursing Press, Sigma Theta Tau International Honor Society of Nursing, 1998, http://www.nursingsociety.org/Media/Documents/Forms/DispForm.aspx?ID=1 (accessed October 20, 2012).

3. Alex Berenson, "Long-Term Care Hospitals Face Little Scrutiny," *New York Times*, February 10, 2010, http://www.nytimes.com/2010/02/10/health/policy/10care.html?pagewanted=all (accessed February 12, 2010).

4. US Department of Health and Human Services Centers for Medicare & Medicaid Services, "Statement of Deficiencies and Plan of Correction" 2007–2009 reports for Select Specialty Hospital of Kansas City, http://documents.nytimes.com/health-inspection-reports-from-5-hospitals#p=1 (accessed October 20, 2012).

5. http://www.massgeneral.org/ (accessed June 5, 2012).

6. http://www.mghpcs.org/Nursing/index.asp (accessed June 5, 2012).

7. http://healthcare.partners.org/streaming/mgH/Nursing/NursingWeek20110502/index.html (accessed June 5, 2012).

8. http://www.emoryhealthcare.org/index.html (accessed June 5, 2012).

9. http://www.emoryhealthcare.org/about-us/index.html (accessed June 5, 2012).

10. http://www.mc.vanderbilt.edu/ (accessed June 5, 2012).

11. http://stanfordhospital.org/ (accessed June 5, 2012).

12. Geralyn Martinez, "Flying to New Heights," *Stanford Nurse*, Spring 2012, 16–17.

13. Theresa Mallick-Searle, Martha Berrier, et al., "Peering through the Mask of Pain," *Stanford Nurse*, Spring 2012, 5–7.

14. February 29, 2012, http://www.bannerhealth.com/NR/rdonlyres/FDB12264-ADA3–47D1-B29B-46061A9FF49F/60044/SimulationSystemNewletter22012.pdf (accessed June 7, 2012).

15. http://www.bannerhealth.com/_Health+Professionals/For+Nurses/Nursing+Research.htm (accessed June 7, 2012).

16. http://www.med.nyu.edu/ (accessed March 14, 2012).

17. http://research.med.nyu.edu/about-us/research-publications/doctor-radio (accessed June 7, 2012).

18. http://www.med.nyu.edu/about-us (accessed June 7, 2012).

19. Office of Communications and Public Affairs, Advertising and Branding, New York Langone Medical Center, 2009–2011, http://communications.med.nyu.edu/advertising-branding/advertising/nyulmc-any-given-moment (accessed March 14, 2012).

20. Julie Fairman and Joan Lynaugh, *Critical Care Nursing: A History* (Philadelphia: University of Pennsylvania Press, 1998).

21. New York Langone Medical Center, http://communications.med.nyu.edu/advertising-branding/advertising/nyulmc-any-given-moment (accessed March 20, 2012).

2. The Daisy Dilemma

1. Nurses Week Greeting Cards, Nurse Gifts, Nurse Day, http://www.nursesweek.org/ (accessed November 12, 2012).

2. Richard G. Shuster, "A Nurse Is More," May 10, 1999, http://www.appleseeds.org/nurse-is-more.htm (accessed March 26, 2012).

3. "Salute to Nurses," advertising supplement, *Boston Globe*, May 6, 2012, 5.

4. Ibid., 6.

5. Ibid., May 8, 2011, 1.

6. Ibid., May 6, 2012, 1.

7. Ibid., May 8, 2011, 5.

8. "National Nurses Week," special advertising supplement, *Virginian-Pilot*, May 9, 2012, 11, http://www.bluetoad.com/publication/index.php?i=110953&m=&l=&p=3&pre=&ver=flex (accessed June 26, 2012).

9. "A Special Supplement," *Portsmouth Daily Times*, May 6, 2012, http://matchbin-assets.s3.amazonaws.com/public/sites/504/assets/6B5Y_05_02_2012_1335991503.pdf (accessed June 20, 2012).

10. "Salute to Nurses," advertising supplement *Boston Globe*, May 6, 2012, 1.

11. J. Adams Barnes, Secretary, Foundation for the Elimination of Diseases Attacking the Immune System, Form 1023 Application for Recognition of Exemption, US Department of the Treasury Internal Revenue Service, April 3, 2000.

12. Statements from Mark and Bonnie Barnes, unless otherwise noted, are from an interview by Bernice Buresh on June 20, 2012.

13. DAISY Foundation home page, http://daisyfoundation.org/ (accessed October 30, 2012).

14. Washington Office of Secretary of State, Charitable Solicitations Program Charity Profile Report for 2010, http://www.sos.wa.gov/charities/search_detail.aspx?charity_id=27386 (accessed June 17, 2012).

15. DAISY Foundation home page, http://daisyfoundation.org/ (accessed October 30, 2012).

16. Ibid. (accessed June 30, 2012).

17. Ibid. (accessed June 30, 2012).

18. Kathy Douglas, "Staffing Unleashed: Through the Eyes of Gratitude," *Nursing Economics* 30, no. 1 (2012): 42–44, 49.

19. DAISY Foundation home page, http://daisyfoundation.org/ (accessed June 27, 2012).

20. Ibid.

21. NCSBN (National Council of State Boards of Nursing), "A Nurse's Guide to Professional Boundaries" brochure, https://www.ncsbn.org/2551.htm (accessed June 1, 2012).

22. Cinnabon Cinnamon Roll Facts, http://www.livestrong.com/article/251148-cinnabon-cinnamon-roll-nutrition-facts/ (accessed June 2, 2012).

23. K. Han, A.M. Trinkoff, C.L. Storr, and J. Geiger-Brown, "Job Stress and Work Schedules in Relation to Nurse Obesity," *Journal of Nursing Administration* 41, no. 11 (Nov. 2011): 488–495.

24. David A. Kessler, *The End of Overeating: Taking Control of the Insatiable American Appetite*, Rodale, 2009, 32.

25. Ibid., 77.

26. Erving Goffman, *The Presentation of Self in Everyday Life* (Anchor Books, 1959).

27. Cindy Lefton and Rick Breugger, "Literature Review on Meaningful Recognition in Nursing," Psychological Association Associates and DAISY Foundation, 2009. Copies available by request from the DAISY Foundation.

28. AACN (American Association of Critical-Care Nurses) Standards for Establishing and Sustaining Healthy Work Environments, Executive Summary, 2005, http://www.aacn.org/WD/HWE/Docs/ExecSum.pdf (accessed May 4, 2010).

29. On Nursing Excellence, http://www.onnursingexcellence.com/about.html (accessed November 7, 2012).

30. Karen Schmidt, *Region*, "Script Not Included," May 1, 2012 http://www.onnursingexcellence.com/downloads/CRP_fea_film_NEW.pdf (accessed October 31, 2012).

31. On Nursing Excellence, http://www.onnursingexcellence.com/index.html (accessed October 31, 2012).

32. http://www.youtube.com/watch?v=D4G3DXY_VKI&feature=player_detailpage (accessed October 31, 2012).

33. Institute for Staffing Excellence and Innovation, http://www.staffingexcellence.org (accessed November 7, 2012).

34. The DAISY Foundation, http://daisyfoundation.org (accessed June 2, 2012).

35. Johnson & Johnson, Campaign for Nursing's Future, http://campaignfornursing.com/portraitofthanks/ (accessed March 16, 2012).

36. Karen Donelan, Peter I. Buerhaus, et al., "Awareness and Perceptions of the Johnson & Johnson's Campaign for Nursing's Future: Views from Nursing Students, RNs, and CNOs," *Nursing Economics* 23, no. 4 (2005): 153.

37. Johnson & Johnson, Campaign for Nursing's Future, *Progress Report* 1, 6.

38. Ibid., 3.

39. Alison P. Smith, "J&J's Campaign for Nursing's Future: The Gift That Keeps on Giving," *Nursing Economics* 23, no. 4 (2005): 200.

40. http://www.discovernursing.com/gang/ (accessed March 22, 2012).

41. Alison M. Trinkoff and Jeanne Geiger-Brown, "Sleep-Deprived Nurses: Sleep and Schedule Challenges in Nursing." In *First, Do Less Harm: Confronting the Inconvenient Problems of Patient Safety*, ed. Ross Koppel and Suzanne Gordon (Ithaca, N.Y.: Cornell University Press, 2012), 168–179.

42. Mark John Somers, Linda Finch, and Dee Birnbaum, "Marketing Nursing as a Profession: Integrated Marketing Strategies to Address the Nursing Shortage," *Health Marketing Quarterly* 27 (2010): 299.

43. Ibid., 302.

44. Ibid., 299.

45. Ibid., 298.

46. Melissa E. Wayne Rudy, "New Grad Still Seeking Job," http://content.healthaffairs.org/content/28/4/w657.abstract/reply#healthaff_el_17390 (accessed March 23, 2012).

47. Allnurses.com, "New Grad RNs: Do You Hate Nursing Already?" http://allnurses.com/florida-nurses/new-grad-rns-471519.html (accessed March 23, 2012).

48. Peter L. Buerhaus et al., "The Recent Surge in Nurse Employment: Causes and Implications" *Health Affairs* 28, no. 4 (2009).

49. Samantha King, *Pink Ribbons, Inc.: Breast Cancer and the Politics of Philanthropy* (Minneapolis: University of Minnesota Press, 2006), 9.

50. P. Rajan Varadaragan and Anil Menon, "Cause-Related Marketing: A Coalignment of Marketing Strategy and Corporate Philanthropy," *Journal of Marketing* 52, no. 3 (1988).

51. Barry Meier, "Hip Implant U.S. Rejected Was Sold Overseas," *New York Times*, February 14, 2012, http://www.nytimes.com/2012/02/15/business/hip-implant-the-fda-rejected-was-marketed-abroad.html (accessed March 23, 2012).

52. Food and Drug Administration, "FDA Drug Safety Communication: Modified Dosing Recommendations to Improve the Safe Use of Erythropoiesis-Stimulating Agents (ESAs) in Chronic Kidney Disease," http://www.fda.gov/Drugs/DrugSafety/ucm259639.htm, 6/24/11.

53. Michael Diamond and Bob Bielk, "Woes for Johnson & Johnson," *USA Today*, November 20, 2011.

54. Jerome P. Kassirer, *On the Take: How Medicine's Complicity with Big Business Can Endanger Your Health* (New York: Oxford University Press, 2005), xvii.

55. The Institute of Medicine, "The Future of Nursing: Leading Change, Advancing Health" (report brief, National Academies, Washington, D.C., October 5, 2010), 2–3.

3. From Virtue to the Voice of Agency

1. Isabel Marcus, "Dark Numbers: Domestic Violence, Law, and Public Policy in Russia, Poland, Romania, and Hungary" (unpublished manuscript).

2. Suzanne Gordon and Sioban Nelson, "Moving beyond the Virtue Script in Nursing," in *Complexities of Care: Nursing Reconsidered*, ed. Sioban Nelson and Suzanne Gordon (Ithaca: Cornell University Press, 2006), 16.

3. Sioban Nelson, *Say Little, Do Much* (Philadelphia: University of Philadelphia Press, 2001), 123.

4. Susan M. Reverby, *Ordered to Care: The Dilemma of American Nursing, 1850–1945* (Cambridge, U.K.: Cambridge University Press, 1987), 4.

5. Kathy Douglas, "Staffing Unleashed: Through the Eyes of Gratitude," *Nursing Economics* 30, no. 1 -(2012): 42.

6. Sara Ruddick, *Maternal Thinking: Toward a Politics of Peace* (Boston: Beacon Press, 1989); Laurel Thatcher Ulrich, *A Midwife's Tale: The Life of Martha Ballard, Based on Her Diary, 1785–1812* (New York: Vintage, 1990); Patricia Benner, Christine A. Tanner, and Catherine A. Chesla, *Expertise in Nursing Practice* (New York: Springer, 1996).

7. St. Mary's Hospital website, http://www.stmarysmadison.com/pages/default.aspx (accessed May 6, 2012).

8. "Salute to Nurses," advertising supplement, *Boston Globe*, May 6, 2012, 5.

9. Wikipedia, "The Shannon-Weaver model," http://en.wikipedia.org/wiki/Shannon%E2%80%93Weaver_model (accessed March 12, 2012).

10. Amartya Sen, *Development as Freedom* (New York: Anchor Books, 2000), 19.

11. Ibid., 189–192.

12. Florence Nightingale, *Notes on Nursing: What It Is and Is Not* (New York: Dover, 1969), 133–134.

13. Patricia Benner, *From Novice to Expert* (Reading, Mass.: Addison-Wesley, 1984).

14. *New York Times*, February 8, 2012, A11.

15. *New York Times*, May 23, 2012, A5.

16. http://www.hcahpsonline.org/home.aspx (accessed June 30, 2012).

17. Theresa Brown, "Hospitals Aren't Hotels," *New York Times*, March 14, 2012, http://www.nytimes.com/2012/03/15/opinion/hospitals-must-first-hurt-to-heal.html?_r=1 (accessed June 30, 2012).

4. Presenting Yourself as a Nurse

1. Daniel Kahneman, *Thinking, Fast and Slow* (New York: Farrar, Straus and Giroux, 2011).

2. Erving Goffman, *The Presentation of Self in Everyday Life* (Garden City, N.Y.: Doubleday Anchor Books, 1959), 17, 30.

3. Mallory Stark, "Creating a Positive Professional Image: Q&A with Laura Morgan Roberts," *Harvard Business School Working Knowledge* (2007), http://www.scribd.com/doc/96820337/Creating-VeImage (accessed October 25, 2012).

4. American Association of Colleges of Nursing, CNL White Paper, 2007, http://www.aacn.nche.edu/publications/white-papers/cnl (accessed June 16, 2012).

5. Suzanne Gordon and Elizabeth M. Grady, "What's in a Name?" *American Journal of Nursing* (August 1995): 31–33.

6. Dominick L. Frosch et al., "Authoritarian Physicians and Patients' Fear of Being Labeled 'Difficult' among Key Obstacles to Shared Decision Making," *Health Affairs* 31, no. 5 (2012): 1030–1038.

7. Ibid.

8. Crystal Lindaman, "Talking to Physicians about Pain Control," *American Journal of Nursing* (January 1995): 2–3.

9. Arthur Kleinman, *The Illness Narratives: Suffering, Healing, and the Human Condition* (New York: Basic Books, 1988).

10. Linda H. Aiken, S. P. Clarke, D. M. Sloane, and Julie Sochalski, et al., "Hospital Nurse Staffing and Patient Mortality, Nurse Burnout, and Job Dissatisfaction," *Journal of the American Medical Association* 288, no. 16 (2002): 1987–1993; J. Needleman and P. Buerhaus, "Nurse Staffing and Patient Safety: Current Knowledge and Implications for Action," *International Journal for Quality Health Care* 15, no. 4 (2003): 275–277.

11. Erving Goffman, *Asylums: Essays on the Social Situation of Mental Patients and Other Inmates* (New York: Doubleday Anchor Books, 1961).

12. American Nurses Association, "Workplace Violence," *Nursing World*, http://nursingworld.org/MainMenuCategories/Policy-Advocacy/State/Legislative-Agenda-Reports/State-WorkplaceViolence (accessed October 25, 2012).

13. National Institute for Occupational Safety and Health (NIOSH), *Violence: Occupational Hazards in Hospitals* (publication 2002–101, Department of Health and Human Services, Center for Disease Control and Prevention, Cincinnati, 2002), http:www.cdc.gov/niosh/2002–101.html (accessed September 8, 2005).

14. American Nurses Association Center for Ethics and Human Rights, "Code of Ethics for Nurses—with Interpretive Statements," 2001, provision 4.2, http://www.nursingworld.org/ethics/code/protected_nwcoe303.htm#4.2 (accessed September 8, 2005).

15. John Seabrook, "The White Dress," *New Yorker* (March 18, 2002): 122–127.

16. Nancy M. Albert et al. "Impact of Nurses' Uniforms on Patient and Family Perceptions of Nurse Professionalism," *Applied Nursing Research* 21 (2008): 181–190.

17. Hajo Adam and Adam D. Galinsky, "Enclothed Cognition," *Journal of Experimental Social Psychology* 48, no. 4 (2012): 918–925.

18. Sandra Blakeslee, "Mind Games: Sometimes a White Coat Isn't Just a White Coat," *New York Times*, April 2, 2012, http://www.nytimes.com/2012/04/03/science/clothes-and-self-perception.html (accessed June 17, 2012).

19. Celia Davies, *Gender and the Professional Predicament in Nursing* (Buckingham, U.K.: Open University Press, 1995), 120.

5. Tell the World What You Do

1. International Council of Nurses, "The ICN Code of Ethics for Nurses, Revised 2012," 3 (available at www.icn.ch).

2. NCVSBN (National Council of States Boards of Nursing), "A Nurse's Guide to the Use of Social Media" (white paper, August 2011), https://www.ncsbn.org/ (accessed March 2, 2012).

3. Theresa Brown, *Critical Care: A New Nurse Faces Death, Life, and Everything in Between* (New York: HarperCollins, 2010), xii–xiii.

4. Barry Morley, "The World Is Loud but Nurses Remain Silent," *Australian Nursing Journal* (Australian Nursing Federation), July 2005.

6. Creating Anecdotes and Arguments

1. Claude M. Steele, *Whistling Vivaldi: And Other Clues to How Stereotypes Affect Us* (New York: W.W. Norton, 2010), 12–13.

2. Ibid., 166, 216, 176.

3. Suzanne Gordon, *Nursing against the Odds: How Hospital Cost-Cutting, Media Stereotypes, and Medical Hubris Undermine Nurses and Patient Care* (Ithaca, N.Y.: Cornell University Press, 2005), 360–362.

4. Jo Stecher, "The Overlooked Symptoms," in *When Chicken Soup Isn't Enough: Stories of Nurses Standing Up for Themselves, Their Patients, and Their Profession*, ed. Suzanne Gordon (Ithaca, N.Y.: Cornell University Press), 67–68.

5. Institute of Medicine, *Keeping Patients Safe: Transforming the Work Environment of Nurses*, ed. Ann Page (Washington, D.C.: National Academy Press, 2004); Institute of Medicine, *Nursing Staff in Hospitals and Nursing Homes: Is It Adequate?* ed. Gooloo S. Wunderlich, Frank Sloan, and Carolyne K. Davis (Washington, D.C.: National Academy Press, 1996), 560.

6. Institute of Medicine, *To Err Is Human: Building a Safer Health System*, ed. Linda T. Kohn, Janet M. Corrigan, and Molla S. Donaldson (Washington, D.C.: National Academy Press, 1999).

7. Courtney H. Lyder et al., "Quality of Care for Hospitalized Medicare Patients at Risk for Pressure Ulcers," *Archives of Internal Medicine* 161 (2001): 1549–1554; Susan Skewes, "Skin Care Rituals That Do More Harm Than Good," *American Journal of Nursing* 96, no. 10 (1996): 33–35.

8. John A. Heit, W.M. O'Fallon, T.M. Petterson, C.M. Lohse et al., "Relative Impact of Risk Factors for Deep Vein Thrombosis and Pulmonary Embolism: A Population-Based Study," *Archives of Internal Medicine* 162, no. 11 (2002): 1245–1248.

9. Institute of Medicine, *To Err Is Human*.

10. Sanjay Saint, R.H. Savel, and M.A. Matthay, "Enhancing the Safety of Critically Ill Patients by Reducing Urinary and Central Venous Catheter-Related Infections," *American Journal of Respiratory Critical Care Medicine*, 165, no. 11 (2002): 1475–1479.

11. Sanjay Saint, "Prevention of Nosocomial Urinary Tract Infections," in *Making Health Care Safer: A Critical Analysis of Patient Safety Practices*, Evidence Report/Technology Assessment 43, Agency for Healthcare Research and Quality, 2001, http://www.ahrq.gov/clinic/ptsafety/chap15a.htm (accessed May 28, 2005).

12. Sanjay Saint, R.H. Savel, and M.A. Matthay, "Enhancing the Safety of Critically Ill Patients by Reducing Urinary and Central Venous Catheter-Related Infections," *American Journal of Respiratory Critical Care Medicine*, 165, no. 11 (2002): 1475–1479.

13. Anne E. Rogers, W. T. Hwang, L. D. Scott, Linda H. Aiken, et al., "The Working Hours of Hospital Staff Nurses and Patient Safety," *Health Affairs* 23, no. 4 (2004): 202–212.

14. Suzanne Gordon and Bernice Buresh, "Finding the 'I' in the 'We,'" *American Journal of Nursing* 96, no. 1 (1996): 21–22.

15. Institute of Medicine, *Keeping Patients Safe*.

16. Milt Freudenheim, "As Nurses Take On Primary Care, Physicians Are Sounding Alarms," *New York Times*, September 30,1997, A1, D4.

7. How the News Media Work

1. Lois Monteiro, "Nightingale and Her Correspondence: Portrait of the Era," in *Florence Nightingale and Her Era: A Collection of New Scholarship*, ed. Vern L. Bullough, Bonnie Bullough, and Marietta P. Stanton (New York: Garland, 1990).

2. "Press Widely Criticized, but Trusted More Than Other Information Sources," Pew Research Center for the People and the Press, September 22, 2011, http://www.people-press.org/2011/09/22/press-widely-criticized-but-trusted-more-than-other-institutions/?src=prc-headline (accessed July 2, 2012).

3. John Hohenberg, *The Professional Journalist: A Guide to the Practices and Principles of the News Media* (New York: Holt, Rinehart & Winston, 1978), 44.

4. Marc Lacey and David M. Herszenhorn, "In Attack's Wake, Political Repercussions," *New York Times*, January 8, 2011, http://www.nytimes.com/2011/01/09/us/politics/09giffords.html?pagewanted=all (accessed April 23, 2012).

5. Jennifer Medina, "Surgeon and Sudden Celebrity, and Trying to Balance the Roles," *New York Times*, January 12, 2011, http://www.nytimes.com/2011/01/13/us/13rhee.html (accessed April 23, 2012).

6. Jennifer Medina, "Doctor Cautions That Rehabilitation Process for Giffords Is Likely to Be a Long One," *New York Times*, January 20, 2011, http://www.nytimes.com/2011/01/21/us/21giffords.html (accessed April 23, 2012).

7. James C. McKinley Jr., "Giffords Arrives at Rehabilitation Facility in Houston," *New York Times*, January 21, 2011, http://www.nytimes.com/2011/01/22/us/22giffords.html (accessed April 23, 2012).

8. "The Court and Medical Care," *New York Times*, June 29, 2012, A20.

9. Andrew Pollack, "In Reversal, F.D.A. Panel Endorses a Diet Pill," *New York Times*, February 23, 2012, B1, B5.

10. Steve Lohr, "Digital Records May Not Cut Health Costs, Study Cautions," *New York Times*, B1.

11. Katie Thomas, "J & J Fined $1.2 Billion in Drug Case," *New York Times*, April 12, 2012, B1.

12. Roni Caryn Rabin, "The Consumer: How Much Aspirin Is Too Much of a Good Thing?" *New York Times*, March 27, 2012, D2.

13. Jane E. Brody, "Forging Social Connections for Longer Life," *New York Times*, March 27, 2012, D7.

14. Jane E. Brody, "Too Much Medicine, and Too Few Checks," *New York Times*, April 17, 2012, D7.

15. Theresa Brown, "Cases: Feeling Strain When Violent Patients Need Care," *New York Times*, health section, January 31, 2012, D5.

16. Peter J. Papadakos, "Electronic Distraction: An Unmeasured Variable in Modern Medicine," *Anesthesiology News* 37, no. 11 (2011), http://www.anesthesiologynews.com/ViewArticle.aspx?d=Commentary&d_id=449&i=November+2011&i_id=785&a_id=19643&tab=Most Read (accessed October 30, 2012).

17. Matt Richtel, "As Doctors Use More Devices, Potential for Distraction Grows," *New York Times*, December 15, 2011, A1.

18. Jordan Rau, "Test for Hospital Budgets: Are the Patients Pleased?" *New York Times*, November 7, 2011, A1.

19. Brooks Barnes, "In Customer Service Consulting, Disney's Small World Is Growing," *New York Times*, April 22, 2012, A1.

20. Liz Kowalczyk, "Nurses Balk at Bid to Guide Dealings with Patients," *Boston Globe*, metro section, March 21, 2012, A1, A7.

21. Nina Bernstein, "Chefs, Butlers, Marble Baths: Hospitals Vie for the Affluent," *New York Times*, January 22, 2012, 1.

22. Katie Thomas, "Generic Drugs Prove Resistant to Damage Suits," *New York Times*, March 21, 2012, A1.

23. Donald G. McNeil Jr., "A Cheap Drug Is Found to Save Bleeding Victims," *New York Times*, March 21, 2012, A13.

24. Jaimee Rose, "Gabrielle Giffords' Doctors, Husband Share Details on Her Progress," *Arizona Republic*, April 24, 2011, http://www.azcentral.com/news/articles/2011/04/24/20110424-gabrielle-giffords-medical-condition.html (accessed January 29, 2012). To read more, see http://www.azcentral.com/news/articles/2011/04/24/20110424gabrielle-giffords-medical-condition.html#ixzz1zaVDjnsW.

8. Reaching Out to the Media

1. Ross Koppel and Suzanne Gordon, eds., *First, Do Less Harm: Confronting the Inconvenient Problems of Patient Safety* (Ithaca, N.Y.: Cornell University Press, 2012).

2. Liz Kowalczyk, "Patient Alarms Often Unheard, Unheeded," *Boston Globe*, February 13, 2011, http://www.boston.com/lifestyle/health/articles/2011/02/13/patient_alarms_often_unheard_unheeded/ (accessed May 28, 2012).

3. Ross Koppel et al. in Koppel and Gordon, *First, Do Less Harm*; http://www.umaryland.edu/offices/communications/news/?ViewStatus=FullArticle&articleDetail=11776.

4. http://www.newsline.umd.edu/health/nurse-shifts-012811.htm (accessed July 2, 2012).

5. http://rnao.ca/news/media-releases/2012/06/28/provincial-task-force-action-plan-will-ensure-same-day-access-patient (accessed July 2, 2012).

9. In Your Own Voice

1. The Milwaukee Journal Sentinel Online http://www.jsonline.com/news/30627794.html (accessed October 10, 2012).

2. "Can Stop-and-Frisk Be Mended?" *New York Times*, editorial, June 19, 2012, http://www.nytimes.com/2012/06/19/opinion/can-stop-and-frisk-be-mended.html (accessed June 21, 2012).

3. Elizabeth Gross Cohn, *New York Times*, letter to the editor, June 22, 2012, http://www.nytimes.com/2012/06/22/opinion/stop-and-frisk-through-the-prisms-of-race-and-health.html?_r=1&partner=rssnyt&emc=rss (accessed June 22, 2012).

4. Atul Gawande, "Personal Best: Should Everyone Have a Coach?" *New Yorker*, October 3, 2011, 53.

5. Virginia Tyack, Letter to the *New Yorker*, October 24, 2011, http://www.newyorker.com/magazine/letters/2011/10/24/111024mama_mail2 (accessed June 5, 2012).

6. Kelly Clow, Letter to the Editor, *Keene Sentinel*, July 19, 2011, http://www.sentinelsource.com/opinion/letters_to_the_editor/nurses-are-overworked/article_09959d48-e59f-5697-9609-bc93f1ebd66e.html#user-comment-area (accessed October 10, 2012).

7. Wikipedia, "Blog," http://en.wikipedia.org/wiki/Blog (accessed October 10, 2012).

8. Ibid. (accessed October 10, 2012).

9. Wikipedia, "The Huffington Post," http://en.wikipedia.org/wiki/The_Huffington_Post (accessed October 16, 2012).

10. Wikipedia, "Blog," http://en.wikipedia.org/wiki/Blog (accessed October 10, 2012).

11. http://www.impactednurse.com/, (accessed June 2, 2012).

12. Ian Miller, "The Re-Identification of Our Patients," http://www.impactednurse.com/?p=4953 (accessed October 25, 2012).

13. http://notratched.net/ (accessed July 2, 2012).

14. Kathleen McPhaul, Jane Lipscomb, and Matt London, "The Public, Should Care That Healthcare Workers Face Dangerous Working Conditions," *Baltimore Sun*, September 22, 2010.

15. Theresa Brown, *Critical Care: A New Nurse Faces Death, Life, and Everything in Between*, New York, HarperStudio 2010.

16. Theresa Brown, "Physician, Heel Thyself," *New York Times*, Sunday opinion section, May 7, 2011, http://www.nytimes.com/2011/05/08/opinion/08Brown.html?_r=1 (accessed June 18, 2012).

17. Theresa Brown, "When the Nurse Is a Bully," *Well* (blog), *New York Times*, February 11, 2010, http://well.blogs.nytimes.com/2010/02/11/when-the-nurse-is-a-bully/ (accessed June 18, 2012).

18. Kevin Pho, "It's Nurse vs Doctor on the New York Times Op-Ed Page." *Atlantic* (blog), May 8, 2011, http://www.theatlantic.com/health/archive/2011/05/its-nurse-vs-doctor-on-the-new-york-times-op-ed-page/238549/ (accessed June 18, 2012).

19. Lucian L. Leape et al., "A Culture of Respect, Part 1: The Nature and Causes of Disrespectful Behavior by Physicians," *Academic Medicine* 87, no. 7 (2012), http://journals.lww.com/academicmedicine/Abstract/publishahead/Perspective___A_Culture_of_Respect,_Part_1__.99622.aspx (accessed June 8, 2012); "A Culture of Respect, Part 2: Creating a Culture of Respect," *Academic Medicine* 87, no. 7 (2012), http://journals.lww.com/academicmedicine/Abstract/publishahead/Perspective___A_Culture_of_Respect,_Part_2__.99622.aspx (accessed June 8, 2012).

20. Robert Fraser, *The Nurse's Social Media Advantage: How Making Connections and Sharing Ideas Can Enhance Your Nursing Practice*, Indianapolis, Sigma Theta Tau International 2011.

21. Megen Duffy, "iNurse: Facebook, Twitter, and LinkedIn, Oh My!" *American Journal of Nursing*, V111 4, April 2011, 59.

22. Seema Marawha, CICC, Toronto General Hospital. Wash Your Hands—it just makes sense. http://www.youtube.com/watch?v=M8AKTACyiB0, (accessed June 30, 2012).

23. Megen Duffy, "iNurse: Patient Privacy and Company Policy in Online Life," *American Journal of Nursing*, V111–9, September 2011 68.

24. Ibid., 67.

25. Patti Neighmond, "Need a Nurse? You May Have to Wait," National Public Radio, May 25, 2012, http://www.npr.org/blogs/health/2012/05/25/153634317/need-a-nurse-you-may-have-to-wait (accessed October 22, 2012).

26. Help a Reporter Out, www.helpareporter.com.

27. National Labor Relations Board, Office of the General Counsel, Division of Operations Management, *Report of the Acting General Counsel on Social Media Cases*, May 30, 2012, http://links.govdelivery.com/track?type=click&enid=ZWFzPTEmbWFpbGluZ2lkPTIwMTIwNTMwLjc5MTMxNzEmbWVzc2FnZWlkPU1EQi1QUkQtQlVMTIwMTIwNTMwLjc5MTMxNzEmZGF0YWJhc2VpZD0xMDAxJnNlcmlhbD0xNzAxMDI0MiZlbWFpbGlkPWRhbGllbC5xLmIubWl5YW5lkZXJjb24udWNzYS5lZHUmdXNlcmlkPWRhbGllbC5xLmIubWl5YW5lkZXJjb24udWNzYS5lZHUmZmw9JmV4dHJhPU1bHRpdmFyaWF0ZUlkPSYmJg==&&&101&&&http://mynlrb.nlrb.gov/link/document.aspx/09031d4580a375cd.

10. Getting It Right

1. Hospital for Special Surgery advertisement, *New York Times*, September 6, 2011, A9.
2. Hospital for Special Surgery advertisement, *New York Times*, December 13, 2011, A13.
3. Todd Sloane, "Raising the Bar Even Higher," *Partners*, November/December 2011, 8–11, http://www.hss.edu/newsroom_raising-the-bar-press-ganey.asp (accessed March 31, 2012).
4. Ibid.
5. Press Ganey, "2011 Pulse Report, Perspectives on American Health Care," 2011, 3, http://www.pressganey.com/researchResources/medicalPractices/pulseReports.aspx (accessed March 31, 2012).
6. The Swiss Nurses Association displays an image of Powernurse on its homepage, http://www.sbk-asi.ch/webseiten/deutsch/0default/frameset.htm and on its Facebook page, http://www.facebook.com/sbk.asi (both accessed November 1, 2012).
7. Pierre-André Wagner, "Remaking the Power Nurse," in *When Chicken Soup Isn't Enough: Stories of Nurses Standing Up for Themselves, Their Patients, and Their Profession*, ed. Suzanne Gordon, 159–161 (Ithaca, N.Y.: Cornell University Press, 2010).
8. "Vital Signs," Alison Whittaker, http://www.nursealison.com/Alison_Whittaker_VITAL_SIGNS/Welcome.html (accessed November 4, 2012).

11. Appearing on Television and Radio

1. Courtney H. Lyder et al., "Quality of Care for Hospitalized Medicare Patients at Risk for Pressure Ulcers," *Archives of Internal Medicine* 161 (2001): 1549–1554; Joseph V. Agostini, Dorothy I. Baker, and Sidney T. Bogardus, "Prevention of Pressure Ulcers in Older Patients," in *Making Health Care Safer: A Critical Analysis of Patient Safety Practices*, Evidence Report/Technology Assessment 43, Agency for Health Care Research and Quality, http://www.ahrq.gov/clinic/ptsafety/chap27.htm (accessed May 28, 2005).

12. Opportunities and Challenges Ahead

1. Institute of Medicine, *The Future of Nursing: Leading Change, Advancing Health* (Washington, D.C.: National Academies Press, 2011), http://books.nap.edu/openbook.php?record_id=12956.

2. HealthLeaders Media, Release, "Two Proven Strategies to Shrink Nurse Labor Costs," program announcement, e-mail to author, received June 2, 2012.

3. Dominick L. Frosch et al., "Patients Fear of Being Called 'Difficult' Impedes Shared Decision-Making," *Health Affairs* 31, no 3 (2012): 1030–1037.

4. For permission to reproduce the "Just a Nurse" script, please submit your request in writing to Suzanne Gordon.

Appendix

1. Bernice Buresh, Suzanne Gordon, and Nica Bell, "Who Counts in News Coverage of Health Care?" *Nursing Outlook* 39, no. 5 (1991): 204–208.

INDEX

Note: Italic page numbers refer to figures.

advanced practice registered nurses (APRNs), 59, 78, 84–85, 148, 237, 265, 266
Advancing Men in Nursing, 47, 49
Affordable Care Act, 162–63, 167–68, 173
agency of nurses, 67–73, 76–77, 78, 110, 126, 129. *See also* voice of agency
Aiken, Linda, 2, 221–22
Allnurses.com, 60
American Academy of Nursing, 55
American Association of Colleges of Nursing, 47, 55, 85
American Association of Critical-Care Nurses (AACN), 27, 47, 50, 55
American Association of Heart Failure Nurses, 33–34
American Hospital Association, 55
American Journal of Nursing (AJN), 217
American Medical Association (AMA), 65
American Nurses Association (ANA), 2, 35–36, 55, 99–100, 166, 262
American Nurses Credentialing Center (ANCC), 20, 23, 24, 25, 52
American Organization of Nurse Executives (AONE), 45, 47, 55
American Student Nurses Association, 55
anchoring effects, 4–5
Anderson, Peggy, 213
anecdotes: all-purpose anecdotes, 146–47; audiences for, 147–50; checklist for, 150–51; construction of, 130–31, 134; facts and statistics in, 140–41; and holistic narratives, 7–8, 80, 131–33; and jargon, 138–40, 256; makeovers of, 138, 144–45; and nursing practice, 31, 129, 130, 143–44; painting a picture, 134–38;

painting the whole picture, 143–44; painting yourself into picture, 142–43; and television and radio appearances, 243–45, 256, 257–58
Anesthesiology News, 166–67
Angell, Marcia, 64
Annals of Internal Medicine, 164
API Healthcare, 42, 52, 53
Association of Registered Nurses of Newfoundland and Labrador (ARNNL), 104, 123

Baker, Ashlynn, 39
Banner Good Samaritan Medical Center, Phoenix, 25–26
Barnes, Bonnie, 40, 44–46, 48–50, 52, 54, 74
Barnes, J. Mark, 40, 44–46, 48–50, 52, 54, 74
Barnes, J. Patrick, 40, 45, 48
Barnes, Tena, 40
Becker, Kathy, 37
Belenky, Mary, 84
Benner, Patricia, 6, 44, 70, 77, 84, 228
Berenson, Alex, 17
Bernstein, Nina, 169
Beth Israel Hospital, Boston, 194
Beth Israel Hospital, New York, 79
blogs, 157, 158, 180, 196, 202–5
Bloomberg, Lawrence, 236
body language, 31, 106–10, 120, 130, 250
books, writing of, 196, 209, 213
Boston Globe, 22, 37–40, 70, 74, 168–69
breaking news, 160, 161–62, 165, 173
Brigham and Women's Hospital, Boston, 39–40
Brody, Jane E., 166
Brown, Theresa, 81–82, 122, 166, 212–16
Brusseau, Jerilyn, 48

Buerhaus, Peter, 55–56, 60
bullying, 214–16, 220
bumper stickers, 254–56, 257
Bureau of Labor Statistics, 97
Buresh, Bernice, 63, 72, 254–56
Burke, Kathleen, 175–78

California Nurses Association, 192
Canadian Association of Critical-Care Nurses, 47
Caplan, Arthur L., 209
caring aspect of nursing practice: care narrative, 5–8, 36, 58, 70–73, 84, 265–67; and DAISY Award, 42–44, 48, 49, 72; and documentaries, 52–53; and expertise, 6–9, 44, 48, *51*, 53, 71–72, 73, 132, 143, 226, 228, *239*, 253, 267; and Johnson & Johnson, 56, 57–58; and juvenalia problems, 33; and Nurses Week supplements, 37–38, 74; and professional self-presentation, 36, 87, 93–94; and public communication skills, 115, 116; and virtue script, 6, 58, 70–72, 84, 265; and visibility of nursing, 21
cause-related marketing, 61–62, 63
Cedars-Sinai Medical Center, Los Angeles, 169
Centers for Medicare and Medicaid Services (CMS), 77, 81–82, 169, 176, 178
Cheney, Carol, 25
Cheshire Medical Center, Keene, New Hampshire, 200–201
Children's Hospital, Pittsburgh, 164
Cinnabon, 5, 41, 45, 46–49, 53, 65, 80
civil rights movement, 101, 106, 157
Clarke, Sean P., 43
Cleveland Clinic, 247–48
Clifford, Joyce, 194
Clow, Kelly, 200–201
Cohn, Elizabeth Gross, 198–99
communication: definition of, 30–31; and feedback loop, 74–75; internal and external, 174–78, 238; tiers of, 31. *See also* public communication; public communication skills
Culbert, Tracy, 162

Daisy Dilemma, 32. *See also* professional self-presentation
DAISY Foundation: Extraordinary Nurse Award, 5, 40, 41–52, 58, 65, 72–75, 80; mission of, 40–41; and promotion of nursing, 175; sponsors of, 5, 41, 43, 45, 46–48, 49, 53–54, 65
Dalton, Cindy, 243–45, 257
Dana Farber Cancer Institute, 22
Davies, Celia, 110
Davis, Cortney, 213
Delp, Steve, *139*
Discovernursing.com, 55

Doctors Without Borders (Médicins Sans Frontières), 81
Donnelly, Judith, 135
Doonesbury, 51
Dotter, Earl, 226
Douglas, Kathy, 42–43, 51–52, 53
Drummond, Don, 189–90
Duffy, Megen, 217, 220, 221
Durnyeva, Iryna, *232*

editorial pages, 172–73. *See also* op-ed pages
electronic medication administration record (eMAR), 177
Emergency Nurses Association, 47
Emory Health Care, 23
Enloe, Cynthia, 49
enterprise reporting, 160, 170–71
expertise of nurses: and agency of nurses, 71–73, 77; and anecdotes, 131–32, 135–38; awareness of, 7, 13, 48–49, 240; and caring aspect of nursing, 6–9, 44, 48, *51*, 53, 71–72, 73, 132, 143, 226, 228, *239*, 253, 267; and clinical judgment, 4, 6, 18, 20, 22, 23–26, 31, 32–35, 39, 42, 43, 44, 46, 53, 71–74, 78, 84–85, 87, 95, 113, 115–16, 135–36, 143, 147–50, 189, 203–4, 218, 234, 247; and DAISY award, 42–43, 44; and erroneous-assumption questions, 258; and internalized knowledge, 136–38; and Johnson & Johnson, 56–57; and journalists, 14, 157; and letters to the editor, 199, 201–2; and marketing of health care institutions, 226–29, 232–35; and news media, 16, 160, 172; and Nurses Week supplements, 38–39; and op-ed pages, 212; and professional self-presentation, 32, 85–86, 87, 91, 92, 94, 100, 101, 103, 228–33; and public communication skills, 112–16, 119–20, 124, 127–28; and salaries, 14, 80; and skill of involvement, 44, 228; and television and radio appearances, 249, 253; and visibility of nursing, 180, 225–29, 234

Facebook, 159, 179, 196, 218–23
Fagin, Claire, 126, 216
Fairman, Julie, 27
Fanning, Patricia, 210
feminism, 68, 70, 84, 106, 157, 238
Fenton, Joshua, 81–82
Fernald, Phoebe, 119–20
Food and Drug Administration (FDA), 163, 171
Forward, Debbie, 109
framing effects, 4, 5, 74, 83, 172
Fraser, Robert, 217, 218, 219–21
Freedberg, Kate, 37
Frosch, Dominick, 46, 89–90, 267

Gallansky, Adam, 105
Gawande, Atul, 199–200, 213
Geiger-Brown, Jeanne, 3
GetWellNetwork, 53, 54
Giffords, Gabrielle, 161–62, 171–72, 248
Goffman, Erving, 5, 49, 83, 95
Golfinos, John, 28
Goodman, Ellen, 247
Google Alerts, 159, 219
Google Reader, 160
Gordon, Suzanne, 6, 67, 68, 80, 178, 225–27,
    243–45, 268, 269
Grady, Elizabeth M., 92, 142
Grant, Susan M., 22, 23
Green, Christina, 161
Griffith, Ellen B., 169
Grinspun, Doris, 189
Groopman, Jerome, 213

Harris, Katherine, 132–33
Harvard School of Public Health, 221
Hasso, Samantha, 25
HCPro, 168
Health Affairs, 60, 61, 89, 163–64
health care administration, 20–21, 122, 123, 213,
    264–67
health care business, 160, 163–67
health care institutions: cultural practices
    within, 100–102; and DAISY Award, 41–42,
    44, 45, 46–50, 51, 54; history of, 69; and
    images of nursing, 33, 77–78, 225; and
    lifting equipment, 59, *165*; and long-term care,
    17–18; and Magnet Recognition, 20, 21, 23–27,
    225, 234; marketing practices of, 18–28, 30,
    71–72, 74, 78–79, 194, 226–29, 232–35;
    media conferences of, 161–62, 247–48;
    minimizing violence in, 98; and Nurses Week,
    35; and patient satisfaction surveys, 77–78,
    81–82, 168–69; and public communication
    skills, 125–28, 193; and public relations
    professionals, 174, 193–94, 225–26, 248;
    restructuring of, 273; and social media policies,
    221, 222–23
health care policy: and editorials, 173; and news
    media, 160, 162–63, 191; and nursing practice,
    5, 15, 51, 146; and nursing research, 14–15;
    and public communication skills, 15, 128, 178,
    181, 191, 203, 205, 210, 217, 222, 224, 245; and
    television and radio appearances, 246, 257; and
    visibility of nursing, 14, 71
health care resources, 2, 3, 6, 71, 75
Health Insurance Portability and Accountability
    Act (HIPAA), 121, 122, 220, 221
HealthLeaders Media, 266
Help a Reporter Out (HARO), 222

Hemenway, Nancy, 169
Herbert, Sidney, 155
Heron, Echo, 213
Higham, Andrea, 56
Hospital Consumer Assessment of Healthcare
    Providers and Systems Survey, 81
Hospital for Special Surgery (HSS), New York
    City, 233–35
Hospital of the University of Pennsylvania
    (HUP), 104, 225–31
Howard, Jewell, *229*
human interest and features, 160, 163, 171–72,
    248

ImpactedNurse.com, 203–4
Institute for Safe Medication Practice, 176, 178,
    215
Institute for Staffing Excellence and Innovation,
    42, 53
Institute of Medicine (IOM), 5, 38, 65, 140, 266
International Council of Nurses (ICN) Code for
    Nurses, 121
Internet, 156, 157, 196, 219. *See also* social media;
    websites
interprofessional education and practice, 6, 14, 264
interviews: and anecdotes, 243–45, 256; and
    appearance, 250–52; and bridging technique,
    257–63; etiquette of, 253–54; ground rules for,
    252–53; preparation for, 246–48, 254–56, 257;
    setting of, 249–50; tips for, 260

jargon, 138–40, 256
Jarvis, David, 17
Johns Hopkins Hospital, Baltimore, 210
Johnson, Ruth, 138
Johnson & Johnson: Campaign for Nursing's
    Future, 54–58, 61–64, 65, 73–75, 80; and care
    narrative, 5, 6, 8, 73; and health care business,
    164; and promotion of nursing, 175
Josey, Karen, 25
journalists and journalism: advertising distin-
    guished from, 158; assembling written materi-
    als for, 182–83; and coverage of nursing, 29,
    194; and enterprise reporting, 170–71; and
    focusing the story, 182; function of, 158–59;
    and Help a Reporter Out, 222; and letters to
    the editor, 201; news releases for, 183–90,
    191, 192, 195; and news values, 157, 170, 180;
    and nursing research, 210; and public
    communication skills, 174–75, 179, 180;
    and sources of health care information, 157,
    271, 272–73. *See also* news media
Journal of Marketing, 62
*Journal of the American Medical Association
    (JAMA),* 164

Jurkowitz, Mark, 201
"Just a Nurse" (Gordon), 227, 268, 269

Kadri, Maureen, *78*
Kahneman, Daniel, 4, 83
Karpeh, Martin S., Jr., 79
Kassiere, Jerome, 64–65
Katz, Brian, 169
Kesey, Ken, 96
Kessler, David A., 47–48
Kimberly-Clark, 45, 53, 54, 63
King, Samantha, 61–62
Kleenex, 5, 41, 43, 45, 74
Kleinman, Arthur, 94
knowledge work, 53, 136–38, 225. *See also* expertise of nurses
Koppel, Ross, 100, 178, 209
Kowalczyk, Liz, 168–69

Labrador Nurses Union, 104
Lake, Nancy, 70
Lakoff, George, 4
Leape, Lucian, 6, 216
Lefton, Cindy, 50, 51
Lehman, Betsey, 22
Lemole, G. Michael, Jr., 162
Leonard, Michael, 6
letters to the editor, 173, 196, 197–202, 205, 216–17
Levine, Diana, 170
Lewin, Ann, 168–69
Lewis, Siobhainn, 123
licensed practical nurses (LPNs), 109–10
Lindaman, Crystal, 92
LinkedIn, 218
Lipscomb, Jane, 210–12
Listservs, 176, 179
Living in Emergency (documentary), 18
London, Matthew, 210–12
Lydon, Christopher, 254
Lynaugh, Joan, 27, 88, 94, 156

Ma, Ralph, 28
Maimonides Medical Center, Brooklyn, New York, 232–33
Marcus, Isabel, 48–49, 68
Martin, Roger, 236
Martineau, Harriet, 155–56
Massachusetts General Hospital (MGH), Boston, 21–22, 37–38, 71–72
Massachusetts Medical Society, 64
Massachusetts Nurses Association (MNA), 192
Mayo Clinic, Rochester, Minnesota, 112
McCarthy, Karen, 181
McInaney, Maureen, 194

McPhaul, Kathleen, 210–12
media kits, 182–83
medical associations, 191
medical journals, 210
Medicare, 17, 77, 81, 168, 169
medicine, 64, 69, 175, 193, 209–10, 272
Memorial Hermann Hospital, Institute for Rehabilitation and Research, Houston, 162
Mendeley.com, 218
men in nursing, 9, 14, 49, 69, 70, 118
Miller, Ian, 203–4
Monteiro, Lois, 156
Morley, Barry, 126–28
Morley, Ben, 127
Morley, Grace, 126–27
Mount Sinai Medical Center, New York, 169
Moyers, Bill, 258–59
Ms. Foundation for Communication and Education, 273
multiauthor blogs (MABs), 202
Myers, Barbara, *187*

National Council of State Boards of Nursing, 46
National Institute for Occupational Safety and Health, 98
National Labor Relations Act, 126, 222, 223
National Labor Relations Board (NLRB), 222–23
National League for Nursing (NLN), 47, 55
National Patient Safety Foundation, 176
National Public Radio, 160
Neighmond, Patti, 221
Nelson, Sioban, 6, 43, 68, 69, 235–38
Newbert, Gordon "Ed," 37–38
New England Journal of Medicine (NEJM), 64, 164
Newfoundland and Labrador Nurses Union (NLNU), 109–10, 123
news media: and breaking news, 160, 161–62, 165, 173; and enterprise reporting, 160, 170–71; and health care business, 160, 163–67; and health care coverage, 3, 14, 16, 17–18, 157–63, 271–72; and health care policy news, 160, 162–63, 191; and human interest and features, 160, 163, 171–72; and Nightingale, 155; and nursing research, 16, 166; and nursing shortages, 16, 255; and nursing stereotypes, 74; and op-ed pages, 207; and public communication skills, 174, 175, 179; and reader/viewer feedback, 197; and research news, 160, 164–67; and trend stories, 160, 163, 167–70; and visibility of nursing, 14, 16, 29, 158, 174, 175, 272–74. *See also* journalists and journalism
newspapers: and images of nursing, 271; and multiauthor blogs, 202; and Nightingale, 155; and Nurses Week supplements, 36–40, 74, 75;

public's trust in, 156; websites of, 159, 161, 183. *See also* op-ed pages

news releases, 182, 183–92, 195

Newton-Wellesley Hospital, Massachusetts, 74

New Yorker, 27, 104, 199–200

New York Presbyterian/Weill Cornell hospital, 169

New York Times: and breaking news, 161–62; comprehensive coverage of, 159, 160; and editorial pages, 173; and enterprise reporting, 170–71; and health care business, 163–64; and images of nursing, 17–18, 29, 81–82, 162, 233–34; and images of physicians, 79, 233–34; and letters to the editor, 200; and op-ed page, 198–99, 212, 213; and research news, 165–66; and trend stories, 167–70

New York Times Magazine, 3, 233–34

New York University Langone Medical Center, 26–28, 168

New Zealand Nurses Organization, 34

Nightingale, Florence, 35, 44, 76–77, 102, 155–56

Nixon, Richard, 262

nonverbal communication: body language, 31, 106–10, 120, 130, 250; and professional self-presentation, 84; and public communication, 30–31

Not Nurse Ratched, 204–5

NPR (National Public Radio), 221–22

nurse executives, 54, 62, 194, 209, 265

nurse managers, 108, 122, 123, 148–49, 265

nurse midwives, 138, 148

nurse/physician relationship: and agency of nurses, 69–71, 78; and anecdotes, 137, 142–43, 147; collaboration in, 229–30; and expertise of nurses, 4; and letters to the editor, 199; and nurses' professional self-presentation, 87–92, 100, 101, 229–31; and nursing stereotypes, 15–16, 71, 107, 108–9; and op-eds, 214–16; and patient safety, 6, 215, 264; and public communication skills, 115, 116; and television and radio appearances, 247–48

nurse practitioners (NPs), 148, 207–8, 265

nurse recruitment, 50, 55, 73, 174, 225–26, 234

Nurses Day/Week: and care narrative, 5, 36, 72; history of, 227; newspaper supplements, 36–40, 74, 75; and nursing stereotypes, 34, 35–36, 38, 44, 53; and public communication, 22; sponsorship of, 48, 80

Nurses (documentary), 51–53

Nurses of America (NOA) project, 271, 273

Nursing Economics, 42, 51

nursing education: and anecdotes, 149–50; and caring aspect of nursing practice, 6; continuing education, 14; and DAISY Foundation, 41; and Johnson & Johnson, 55; and juvenalia

problem, 33; and professional self-presentation, 85; and public communication skills, 5, 235–38; and public relations professionals, 174; visibility of, 26

"The Nursing Gang" video, 57–58

Nursing Notes, 55

nursing organizations: and blogs, 203; and DAISY award, 47; and Johnson & Johnson, 55; and journalists, 29; and juvenalia problem, 33–34; and media strategies, 175, 272–73; and news releases, 191; and patient confidentiality, 123; and professional image, 30, 35–36, 84, 174, 271; and public communication skills, 9, 180, 238–40; and public relations professionals, 174–75, 179–80, 238, 271, 273

nursing practice: conflict in discussion of, 123–28; and health care business news, 163; and health care policy, 5, 15, 51, 146; holistic narrative of, 7–8, 80, 131–33; nurses' framing of, 5, 28, 74; and professional self-presentation, 39–40; public attitudes toward, 1, 2, 4, 5, 8, 9, 15–16; and public communication skills, 30, 111–13, 180; and silence of nurses, 25, 113, 115. *See also* caring aspect of nursing practice

nursing profession: accurate coverage of, 29–30; assertive nurses, 6, 264; and blogs, 203–4; devaluation of, 148–49; gendered images of, 33, 45, 49, 66; holistic narrative of, 7–8; and Johnson & Johnson, 56; and juvenalia problem, 33–35, 58; motivations for entering, 59–60; and naming practices, 24–27, 58, 86, 87–102, 103, 104, 108, 109, 233, 252–53; public attitudes toward, 2–4, 29, 32, 34, 65, 85, 271; and public relations professionals, 194; religious and secular influences on, 68–75; and trustworthiness, 1, 2–4, 5, 8, 64, 65, 87, 93–94, 100, 267

nursing research: and anecdotes, 141; and blogs, 203; and DAISY Foundation, 41; highlighting importance of, 15; and news media, 16, 166; and op-ed pages, 209–12; and social media, 218; visibility of, 26, 227

nursing shortages: advertisement on nursing profession, *158*, 225–26; and health care resource allocation, 2; and Johnson & Johnson, 55–56, 58, 61–64, 65; and necessary nursing care, 15, 222; and news media, 16, 255; and public relations, 271; and working conditions, 58–61, 184, 255, 260

Nursing Spectrum, 55

nursing stereotypes: and angelic images, 16, 29, 34, *34*, 35, 57, *68*, 71, 74, 232, 234; and health care resources, 6; and Johnson & Johnson, 58; "just a nurse" stereotypes, 111–12, 123, 124, 129, 187, 214, 217, 268; and nurse/physician

nursing stereotypes (*cont.*)
relationship, 15–16, 71, 107, 108–9; and patient safety, 264; persistence of, 15–16, 66; replacement of, 14, 16; and television and radio appearances, 248; and virtue script, 9, 32–33, 53, 69, 70, 74, 232, 237–38, 274

obesity epidemic, 46–48, 163
On Nursing Excellence (ONE), 51, 52, 53
op-ed pages, 160, 172–73, 196, 205–17
Opinionator blog, 213

Palmer, Helen, 192
Papadakos, Peter J., 166–67
Parker-Pope, Tara, 213
Parkland Memorial Hospital, Dallas, 258
Parsee, Mary, 146
Parsons, Talcott, 46
patient care: and agency of nurses, 76; anecdotes concerning, 133, 135; and digital devices, 167; evidence-based care, 6; and Johnson & Johnson, 57; and patient acuity, 59; and professional image, 4; and public communication skills, 113–16, 125–26, 180, 267; societal beliefs about, 2; and visibility of nursing, 25
patients: bill of rights for, 100; confidentiality of, 113, 121–23, 134, 204, 213, 220, 241, 244; and health care coverage, 272; nurses' advocacy for, 7, 8–9, 64, 65, 76, 92, 106, 125, 240; and nurses' professional self-presentation, 86, 87, 93–96, 103–4; role in clinical decision making, 46, 89–90, 115, 267; satisfaction surveys, 77–78, 81–82, 168–69
patient safety: advertisement for infection prevention, *267*; advertisement for medication administration, *178*; advertisement for operating room safety, *142*; and health care costs, 264; and letters to the editor, 200–201; and nurse/physician relationship, 6, 215, 264; and physician work hours, 2–3; and professional self-presentation, 90, 91; and public communication skills, 175–76, 267; and social media, 175–78; and teamwork, 28, 90–91, 106; and working conditions, 211
"Patient's Perspective" videos, 57
patriarchal culture, 49, 69, 70, 88–89
The PBS NewsHour, 160
Penrose, Joyce, 207–8
Pew Charitable Trusts, 271
Pew Research Center, 156, 201
pharmaceutical industry, 54, 55, 63, 64–65, 158, 163, 164
Phipps, Marion, 67
Pho, Kevin, 216

physicians: book publishing of, 213; and media coverage of health and health care, 3, 14, 16, 17–18, 161–62, 167, 172, 182, 193–94, 272; and op-ed pages, 212; and patient confidentiality, 123; professional image of, 3, 4, 18, 71, 78–79, 84, 86, 88, 94, 95; and public communication, 209; relationship to patients, 94; and television and radio appearances, 247–48; and work hours, 2–3. *See also* nurse/physician relationship
"Portrait of Thanks Project," 55
Poteet, Kristy, 172
Power Nurse, 238–40
Press Ganey Associates, 235
Prideaux, Mary, 123
privacy rights, 99–100
problem narratives, 16
professional self-presentation: and advanced practice nurses, 84–85; and appearance, 31, 34, 86, 102–10, *103*, 228–31, 250–52; and DAISY Award, 41–42, 46, 50; and enclothed cognition, 105; and expertise of nurses, 32, 85–86, 87, 91, 92, 94, 100, 101, 103, 228–33; and first name use, 86, 87–91, 92, 93–95, 96; and introductions, 86–102, *86, 88*, 107–8, 109, 110; and juvenalia problems, 33–35, *34*, 71; and naming practices, 58, 86, 87–102, 232, 233; and nurse as title, 92–102; and nurses as "girls," 105–6; and nursing stereotypes, 15–16; and personal safety, 96–99; and television and radio appearances, 247, 250–52
pseudoevents, 164
public, definition of, 30
public attitudes: and news media, 156; toward nursing practice, 1, 2, 4, 5, 8, 9, 15–16; toward nursing profession, 2–4, 29, 32, 34, 65, 85, 271
public communication, 7–8, 30–31, 157, 174, 271
public communication skills: accepting thanks, 119–20, *120*; assembling written materials, 182–83; changes in, 5; and conversational openings, 116–19, *117*; defining audience, 147–50, 178–80; development of, 9, 266, 273; and enthusiasm, 120–21; and expertise of nurses, 112–16, 119–20, 124, 127–28; fears/inhibitions concerning, 123–25; and focusing the story, 181–82; and health care policy, 15, 128, 178, 181, 191, 203, 205, 210, 217, 222, 224, 245; and introductions, 180; and news media, 174, 175, 179; and news opportunities, 181; and news releases, 182, 183–92, 195; and Nightingale, 155–56; and nursing practice, 30, 111–13, 180; and patient care, 113–16, 125–26, 180, 267; and patient confidentiality, 113, 121–23; and patient safety, 175–76, 267; and working conditions, 125–28. *See also* anecdotes

public/private space, 49, 69, 110, 112, 219–20
public relations, 112, 158, 174, 271
public relations professionals: duties of, 174–78; and health care institutions, 174, 193–94, 225–26, 248; and nursing organizations, 174–75, 179–80, 238, 271, 273; and television and radio appearances, 175, 246
Pulse, 235–38, *237*

Rabkin, Mitchell, 194
radio, 190–91, 192. *See also* television and radio appearances
Rampersaud, Rook, 232, 233
Raphael, Sally Jesse, 247, 248
Rau, Jordan, 168
Reason, James, 3
Registered Nurses Association of Ontario (RNAO), 188–90
registered nurses (RNs): and conflict in public communication, 126; credentials of, 187, 198; four *R*s for, 15, 79–80, 88, 147; and nursing shortages, 61; personal safety of, 97; and professional self-presentation, 104, 109–10, 230, 231; and staffing, 13; and workplace injuries, 59
Reverby, Susan M., 70
Rhee, Peter, 161
Rich, Victoria L., 104, 225, 226, 228–31
Richtel, Matt, 167
Roberts, Laura Morgan, 84
Roberts, Leslie, 244–45
Robert Wood Johnson Foundation, 221, 266
Roll, John M., 161
Rose, Jaimee, 172
Rosner, David, 169–70
RSS (Really Simple Syndication), 159–60
Rubin, Amir Dan, 24
Rubinstein, Arthur, 229–30
Ruddick, Sara, 70
Russell, William Howard, 155

St. Mary's (Magnet) Hospital, Madison, Wisconsin, 71
Sanghavi, Darshak, 3
SBAR (Situation, Background, Assessment, Recommendation), 91
Schork, Debbie, 170–71
Schreiber, Elliot, 64
Schwartz, Pearl, 168
Science in the Public Interest, 47
Seidman-Carlson, Rhonda, 188
Select Specialty Hospital, Kansas City, Kansas, 17–18
Selzer, Richard, 213
Sen, Amartya, 75–76

Shannon, Claude Elwood, 74
Sharp, Kathleen, 63
Sigma Theta Tau International, 47, 55
silence of nurses: ending of, 13, 20–21; and external communication plan, 175; and nursing practice, 25, 113, 115; and public communication skills, 123–28, 274; as threat to profession, 75; and virtue script, 70–72
Simpson, Kate, 126–28
Smith, Cathy, *114*
Smith, Tom, 233
social media: health care institutions' policies on, 221, 222–23; and journalists, 158–59; and letters to the editor, 202; as news source, 157; and patient safety, 175–78; and public communication skills, 156, 196, 197, 216, 217–24, 241; recommendations on using, 218–19; setting boundaries, 219–24
Somerville, Jackie, 39
Stanford Hospital and Clinics, 24–25
Stanford Nurses, 25
Stanford University Medical Center, 167
Stecher, Jo, 134, 135, 137–38
Steele, Claude, 129–30
stereotype threat, 129–30
storytelling, 129–30. *See also* anecdotes
Strunk, William, Jr., 187
Surridge, Judie, 189
Swartz-Lloyd, Tony, 193, 194
Sweeney, Susan, 142–43
Swiss Nurses Association (ASI), 238–40

Tannen, Deborah, 105, 106
television, 79, 159, 190–91
television and radio appearances: and anecdotes, 243–45, 256, 257–58; basic rules for, 246; and call-in shows, 247, 262–63; feeling in control, 246–48; and interviews, 249–50, 253–54, 257–63; and naming practices, 101–2, 253; preparation for, 254; and professional self-presentation, 247, 250–52; and public relations professionals, 175, 246; setting ground rules, 252–53; types of questions, 257–62
trend stories, 160, 163, 167–70
Trinkoff, Alison M., 3, 184–85
trustworthiness: and Nurses Week, 36; and nursing profession, 1, 2–4, 5, 8, 64, 65, 87, 93–94, 100, 267; and virtue script, 74
Tumblr, 196, 203
Twitter, 196, 202, 217, 218, 221
Tyack, Virginia, 199–200

Ulrich, Laurel Thatcher, 70
unions, 34, 104, 109–10, 126, 149, 222–23
University Medical Center, Tucson, 161–62

University of California San Francisco Medical Center, 176, 194, 240–42
University of Iowa Hospitals and Clinics, 168
University of Maryland School of Nursing, 47
University of Pittsburgh Medical Center (UPMC), 212–13
University of Rochester Medical Center, 166–67
University of Toronto, Faculty of Nursing, 235–38
U.S. News & World Report, 20, 24, 26, 234
U.S. Supreme Court, 162–63, 170–71

Vanderbilt University, 55
Vanderbilt University Medical Center, 23–24
verbal communication, 30, 84
Verghese, Abraham, 167
virtue script: and care narrative, 6, 58, 70–72, 84, 265; expertise contrasted with, 6, 9, 30, 32, 43; and feedback loop, 74–75; history of, 68–69; and nurse recruitment, 73; and nursing stereotypes, 9, 32–33, 53, 69, 70, 74, 232, 237–38, 274; and silence of nurses, 70–72
visibility of nursing: and expertise, 180, 225–29, 234; and letters to the editor, 198; and marketing practices, 18–28, 30, 226–29, 232–35; and news media, 14, 16, 29, 158, 174, 175, 272–74; and news releases, 187–88; and professional image, 72; and silence of nurses, 13
"Vital Signs" (Whittaker), 240–42

voice of agency, 8, 66, 67–68, 75–82. *See also* agency of nurses

Wagner, Pierre-Andre, 238, 240
Wall Street Journal, 173
Weaver, Warren, 74
websites: blogs on, 203; and media coverage of nursing, 175; of newspapers, 159, 161, 183; and news releases, 191; op-ed pieces on, 205; and public communication skills, 179, 196, 241
Weeden, Curt, 62–63, 64
Well blog, 212, 213
White, E. B., 187
Whittaker, Alison, 240–42
Wolper, Carla, 48
Woods, Michael, 6
working conditions: and juvenalia problems, 35; and medical errors, 59, 176–78, 180; and news releases, 184–85; and nursing shortages, 58–61, 184, 255, 260; and obesity risks, 47; public awareness of, 2, 3, 13, 53; and public communication skills, 125–28; and recognition programs, 50–51; and social media, 221–22; and staffing issues, 266; and workplace violence, 210–12

Yahoo, 159
Young, Christina, 32, 218, 219
YouTube videos, 183, 196, 219

Zion, Libby, 2